Schizophrenia

Medical Psychiatry

Series Editor

William A. Frosch, M.D.
Weill Medical College of Cornell University
New York, New York

1. Handbook of Depression and Anxiety: A Biological Approach, *edited by Johan A. den Boer and J. M. Ad Sitsen*
2. Anticonvulsants in Mood Disorders, *edited by Russell T. Joffe and Joseph R. Calabrese*
3. Serotonin in Antipsychotic Treatment: Mechanisms and Clinical Practice, *edited by John M. Kane, H.-J. Möller, and Frans Awouters*
4. Handbook of Functional Gastrointestinal Disorders, *edited by Kevin W. Olden*
5. Clinical Management of Anxiety, *edited by Johan A. den Boer*
6. Obsessive-Compulsive Disorders: Diagnosis • Etiology • Treatment, *edited by Eric Hollander and Dan J. Stein*
7. Bipolar Disorder: Biological Models and Their Clinical Application, *edited by L. Trevor Young and Russell T. Joffe*
8. Dual Diagnosis and Treatment: Substance Abuse and Comorbid Medical and Psychiatric Disorders, *edited by Henry R. Kranzler and Bruce J. Rounsaville*
9. Geriatric Psychopharmacology, *edited by J. Craig Nelson*
10. Panic Disorder and Its Treatment, *edited by Jerrold F. Rosenbaum and Mark H. Pollack*
11. Comorbidity in Affective Disorders, *edited by Mauricio Tohen*
12. Practical Management of the Side Effects of Psychotropic Drugs, *edited by Richard Balon*
13. Psychiatric Treatment of the Medically Ill, *edited by Robert G. Robinson and William R. Yates*
14. Medical Management of the Violent Patient: Clinical Assessment and Therapy, *edited by Kenneth Tardiff*
15. Bipolar Disorders: Basic Mechanisms and Therapeutic Implications, *edited by Jair C. Soares and Samuel Gershon*
16. Schizophrenia: A New Guide for Clinicians, *edited by John G. Csernansky*

ADDITIONAL VOLUMES IN PREPARATION

Schizophrenia

A New Guide for Clinicians

edited by

John G. Csernansky

*Washington University School of Medicine
and Metropolitan St. Louis Psychiatric Center
St. Louis, Missouri*

MARCEL DEKKER, INC. NEW YORK • BASEL

ISBN: 0-8247-0642-0

This book is printed on acid-free paper.

Headquarters
Marcel Dekker, Inc.
270 Madison Avenue, New York, NY 10016
tel: 212-696-9000; fax: 212-685-4540

Eastern Hemisphere Distribution
Marcel Dekker AG
Hutgasse 4, Postfach 812, CH-4001 Basel, Switzerland
tel: 41-61-261-8482; fax: 41-61-261-8896

World Wide Web
http://www.dekker.com

The publisher offers discounts on this book when ordered in bulk quantities. For more information, write to Special Sales/Professional Marketing at the headquarters address above.

Current printing (last digit):
10 9 8 7 6 5 4 3 2 1

PRINTED IN THE UNITED STATES OF AMERICA

Series Introduction

American psychiatry was preoccupied with schizophrenia in the decades following the second World War. Nathan Kline's published précis of Eugen Bleuler's great work, followed closely by Joseph Zinkin's full translation of it as *Dementia Praecox, or the Group of Schizophrenias,* stimulated interest, and most patients admitted to psychiatric hospitals (in the era before the spread of general hospital units) were so diagnosed. Kraepelin was a relatively forgotten man. The introduction of lithium and of effective antidepressants, and the findings of the joint British-American study of diagnosis, redirected attention to the affective disorders. Bleuler and his "schizophrenias" moved to the back burners of research and clinical interest. This shift of focus was reinforced by the growing awareness of the inadequacies of our research methods in investigating such a complex problem as schizophrenic illness.

New ways of looking at the brain (as distinct from the mind), such as the ever-expanding variety of imaging techniques (e.g., SPECT, PET, MRI, and CAT), increasing knowledge of the complexities of neurotransmission, and the development of criteria sets for DSM-III with accompanying structured interviews, drew the attention of investigators back to the problems of understanding the etiologies and pathologies of schizophrenia, this all too often crippling illness. Researchers and clinicians became more aware of the importance of negative as well as positive symptoms, of affective lability and the role of family-expressed emotion, and of the subtleties of cognitive dysfunction that the disease imposed. These new data, in a setting of interested attention, have resulted in the development of new and more effective and less toxic medications, and of focused psychotherapies, including family work, cognitive and behavioral techniques, and sociotherapies. Perhaps most importantly, in the best of settings, it has ended the war between biological and psychological approaches to treatment and resulted in a collaborative rapprochement that works in the patient's best interests.

Csernansky and his colleagues present us with this new world. While the illness(es) is (are) more complex than we realized decades ago, recent findings and advances also hold out more promise, both for our ability to intervene more effectively than ever before and for the future, as we build on our recently acquired knowledge. The authors are distinguished and experienced; their book tells us where we are, what to do, and where we need to go in the future.

William A. Frosch

Preface

Schizophrenia remains one of the most common psychiatric disorders, affecting approximately 1% of the world's population. It occurs with a similar frequency in all races and cultures, and while men and women are equally likely to be affected by schizophrenia, its age of onset is earlier and its severity is greater in men. If left untreated, schizophrenia is almost always a lifelong, disabling disease.

Despite the seriousness of this disease, over the past decade we have witnessed major advances in our understanding of schizophrenia and our ability to mitigate its disabling effects. Systematic diagnosis based on well-defined symptom categories has become a worldwide standard. An increased number of symptom categories are now recognized as being central to schizophrenia, including psychotic symptoms, symptoms of thought disorganization, negative symptoms, and mood instability. In addition, subtle deficits in fundamental elements of cognition, such as attention and memory, have been identified in patients with schizophrenia. These deficits, which may predate the onset of more obvious clinical symptoms, appear to be the major block to patients' attempts to return to school or work.

The recognition of new symptom categories and cognitive deficits in schizophrenia patients offers important new avenues for treatment.

The efficacy of antipsychotic drugs developed in the 1950s was largely limited to psychotic symptoms and symptoms of thought disorganization. A new generation of drugs for schizophrenia, called atypical antipsychotics, has recently been shown to have at least equivalent efficacy for psychotic symptoms and thought disorganization as well as increased efficacy for negative symptoms, mood instability, and cognitive deficits. Improved treatment of negative symptoms and cognitive deficits in schizophrenia patients offers the promise that more patients with this disease will return to school or work and resume their lives as satisfied and productive members of society. Improved treatment of mood instability offers the possibility of reducing the rate of suicide in patients with schizophrenia, which is second only to that in patients with major forms of depression. Finally, second-generation antipsychotic drugs have fewer neurological side effects, such as pseudoparkinsonism, which should improve compliance with treatment.

This book is intended as a guide for clinicians who care for patients with schizophrenia and other major psychotic disorders. While recent research has improved our understanding of schizophrenia, it has also provided us with many new tools and increased the complexity of decision-making for clinicians. Psychiatric residents in training as well as more experienced psychiatrists should find this book of value because of its emphasis on recent diagnostic and therapeutic advances. In addition, clinicians from mental health disciplines should find this book useful because of its emphasis on the integration of drug treatment with other modalities of assessment, treatment, and case management. The information in this book is based on evidence from systematic clinical research studies, although findings from these research studies are presented in such a way as to be easily understood by clinicians without extensive backgrounds in research methodology.

The book is divided into three major sections: Assessment and Diagnosis, Treatment, and Special Management Issues. In the Assessment and Diagnosis section, some chapters reflect a more cross-sectional analysis of symptom clusters, while others emphasize a longitudinal or life-cycle perspective. The integration of cross-sectional and longitudinal information is needed to develop a thorough understanding of schizophrenia as a multimodal, lifelong disease. In the Treatment section, chapters are offered on both drug treatments and rehabilitative approaches. The chapters in the Special Management Issues section discuss forensic issues, primary prevention, family education, and service delivery. This last section reflects the realization that the treatment of patients with schizophrenia must be carried out within a community context, and that there are multiple stakeholders in the outcome of treatment and resources management.

Clinicians working with schizophrenia patients today are fortunate in having new and improved tools available for diagnosis, treatment, and case management. The diagnosis and treatment of patients with schizophrenia have become more strongly based on an understanding of the neurobiology of this disease and the realization that patients with schizophrenia have human needs that go far beyond the straightforward goals of "biological" treatments. There are still too many patients who do not benefit from the best treatments available for schizophrenia. The ultimate purpose of this book is to educate clinicians about these treatments so that more patients can share in their benefits.

John G. Csernansky

Contents

Series Introduction *William A. Frosch* iii
Preface v
Contributors xi

ASSESSMENT AND DIAGNOSIS

1. Interviewing the Patient with Schizophrenia 1
   C. Peter Rosenbaum

2. Symptom Clusters in Schizophrenia 29
   William O. Faustman and Shelley Fleming Ficek

3. Differential Diagnosis of Schizophrenia 53
   Del D. Miller and Susan K. Schultz

4. Cognitive Assessment in Schizophrenia Patients 69
   Anne L. Hoff

5. Laboratory Tests to Aid in the Diagnosis of Schizophrenia 89
Jose Mathews and John G. Csernansky

TREATMENT

6. Treatment of Acute Psychotic Episodes 107
Michael D. Jibson and Rajiv Tandon

7. Maintenance Treatment for Schizophrenia Patients 141
John G. Csernansky

8. Management of Treatment-Refractory Patients 163
Robert R. Conley

9. Psychosocial and Cognitive Rehabilitation 183
Gitry Heydebrand

10. Antipsychotic-Drug Side Effects: Assessment, Treatment, and Prevention 213
Gary Remington, Shitij Kapur, and Robert Zipursky

SPECIAL MANAGEMENT ISSUES

11. Violence and Forensic Issues in Schizophrenia 247
John Rabun and Susan K. Boyer

12. Impact of Substance Abuse and Dependence on Patients with Schizophrenia 267
Collins E. Lewis

13. Family Education: A Guide for Developing a Program 285
Mary Will

14. Schizophrenia from the Life-Cycle Perspective 301
John Lauriello, William P. Horan, and Juan Bustillo

Index **323**

Contributors

Susan K. Boyer, M.D. Instructor of Psychiatry, Washington University School of Medicine, and Supervising Psychiatrist, St. Louis Psychiatric Rehabilitation Center, St. Louis, Missouri

Juan Bustillo, M.D. Assistant Professor, Department of Psychiatry, University of New Mexico, Albuquerque, New Mexico

Robert R. Conley, M.D. Associate Professor of Psychiatry and Pharmacy Science, University of Maryland School of Medicine, and Director, Treatment Research, Maryland Psychiatric Research Center, Baltimore, Maryland

John G. Csernansky Gregory B. Couch Professor of Psychiatry, Washington University School of Medicine, and Medical Director, Metropolitan St. Louis Psychiatric Center, St. Louis, Missouri

William O. Faustman, Ph.D., C.Psychol. Veterans Affairs Palo Alto Health Care System, Palo Alto, and Department of Psychiatry and Behavioral Sciences, Stanford University School of Medicine, Stanford, California

Shelley Fleming Ficek, Ph.D. Veterans Affairs Palo Alto Health Care System, Palo Alto, and Department of Psychiatry and Behavioral Sciences, Stanford University School of Medicine, Stanford, California

Gitry Heydebrand, Ph.D. Instructor, Department of Psychiatry, Washington University School of Medicine, St. Louis, Missouri

Anne L. Hoff, Ph.D. Associate Professor, Department of Psychiatry, University of California Davis School of Medicine, Sacramento, and UC Davis Napa Psychiatric Research Center, Napa, California

William P. Horan, Ph.D.* Department of Psychiatry, University of New Mexico, Albuquerque, New Mexico

Michael D. Jibson, Ph.D., M.D. Clinical Associate Professor, Department of Psychiatry, University of Michigan Health System, Ann Arbor, Michigan

Shitij Kapur, M.D., Ph.D., F.R.C.P.(C) Section Head, Schizophrenia Research, Schizophrenia and Continuing Care Program, Centre for Addiction and Mental Health, Department of Psychiatry, University of Toronto, Toronto, Ontario, Canada

John Lauriello, M.D. Associate Professor and Vice Chairman, Department of Psychiatry, University of New Mexico, Albuquerque, New Mexico

Collins E. Lewis, M.D. Associate Professor of Psychiatry, Emeritus, Department of Psychiatry, Washington University School of Medicine, St. Louis, Missouri

Jose Mathews, M.D. Staff Psychiatrist, Metropolitan St. Louis Psychiatric Center, St. Louis, Missouri

Del D. Miller, Pharm.D., M.D. Associate Professor, Department of Psychiatry and Mental Health Clinical Research Center, The University of Iowa, Iowa City, Iowa

---

**Current affiliation*: Western Psychiatric Institute and Clinic, University of Pittsburgh School of Medicine, Pittsburgh, Pennsylvania

John Rabun, M.D. Supervising Psychiatrist, Forensic Evaluation Unit, St. Louis Psychiatric Rehabilitation Center, St. Louis, Missouri

Gary Remington, M.D., Ph.D., F.R.C.P.(C) Director, Medication Assessment Program for Schizophrenia, Schizophrenia and Continuing Care Program, Centre for Addiction and Mental Health, Department of Psychiatry, University of Toronto, Toronto, Ontario, Canada

C. Peter Rosenbaum, M.D. Professor Emeritus, Department of Psychiatry and Behavioral Sciences, Stanford University School of Medicine, Stanford, California

Susan K. Schultz, M.D. Associate Professor, Department of Psychiatry and Mental Health Clinical Research Center, The University of Iowa, Iowa City, Iowa

Rajiv Tandon, M.D. Professor and Director, Schizophrenia Program, Department of Psychiatry, University of Michigan Health System, Ann Arbor, Michigan

Mary Will, M.S.W., L.C.S.W. Director of Social Services, Metropolitan St. Louis Psychiatric Center, St. Louis, Missouri

Robert Zipursky, M.D., F.R.C.P.(C) Head and Tapscott Chair, Schizophrenia and Continuing Care Program, Centre for Addiction and Mental Health, Department of Psychiatry, University of Toronto, Toronto, Ontario, Canada

1

Interviewing the Patient with Schizophrenia

C. Peter Rosenbaum
Stanford University School of Medicine
Stanford, California

INTRODUCTION

The Purpose of this Chapter

This chapter is intended to help you enter into conversations with patients who have schizophrenia (referred to more briefly, if less accurately, in the remainder of this chapter as schizophrenic patients), conversations that will allow the two of you to begin to get to know each other and that might hold the promise of developing the therapeutic alliance on which successful treatment so heavily depends. Treatment includes individual psychotherapy (Chapter 9); structured living, learning, and working situations, such as day hospitals and psychosocial and cognitive rehabilitation (Chapter 9); use of medications (Chapter 7); and working with patients and their families (Chapter 13).

For therapists new to working with schizophrenic patients, the prospect of entering into an intimate conversation with the patient can be anxiety-provoking. Medical students starting their first psychiatry rotations are almost uniformly scared of patients, of craziness and unpredictability, of contact with the unreal and the bizarre. Some (or more than some) psychiatrists remain uncomfortable working with such patients on a psychological level, preferring to serve only as psychopharmacologists or confining their practices to nonpsychotic patients. Sometimes fears of verbal or physical attack are realistic, and later I describe some ways in which safety for both patient and interviewer can be secured.

Schizophrenic patients can sometimes home in on the interviewer's own unconscious or at least private conflicts and worries and thus stir up a great deal of anxiety. For beginning interviewers, having a trusted consultant or supervisor with whom one can discuss sessions is a virtual necessity. Some mental health professionals are reluctant to work with schizophrenic patients because they have fears about their own emotional stability or they have had to deal with psychotic members of their own families, and the prospect of such work with patients hits too close to home. For such persons in particular, but for people in training in general, being in one's own personal therapy often makes approaching difficult situations easier and broadens the personal and professional growth that should be the product of working with patients.

It is through such challenges that we mature and develop as therapists. For those trained in psychodynamic psychiatry, working with schizophrenic patients can contribute much to professional growth. These days, the difficulty of finding the time to do it makes it a rarity, but once undertaken, it can add a dimension to one's therapeutic abilities that cannot be found in any other way.

The chapter starts with five vignettes of interviews with schizophrenic patients. In all cases, names and other identifying information about patients and therapists have been changed for reasons of confidentiality. The vignettes are given in order of difficulty of entering into and sustaining a conversation, from Ernestine, who was pleasant and helpful, to Gordon, who became furious and bolted from the room. We come back to some of these patients later in the chapter.

After the vignettes, there is a discussion of the ambivalence and reservations that many patients have at a first interview. The next section contains ideas about sidestepping some of these ambivalences and getting off to a productive start. This is followed by theoretical material about the dynamics of interviewing patients with schizophrenia. A number of matters of practical technique are then addressed. After providing follow-up information on the patients previously presented, the chapter closes with a list of tips for interviewers.

The Five Vignettes

Ernestine

Ernestine was in her 50s. She had been diagnosed with schizophrenia 30 years earlier, had been hospitalized in the early years of her illness, and for the last 20 years had lived in her own apartment and saw her psychiatrist twice a week to talk about things and get medications renewed. Her treatment had been paid for by the state mental health department. The department was considering ending the payments and had asked an outside consultant to evaluate the situation. Ernestine's psychiatrist had, with her consent, already given the consultant his psychiatric records prior to the consultation interview.

The consultant found Ernestine to be a classic sweet old woman. Her hair was white; her manner was demure; she was polite and soft-spoken. She said, "I go to see my doctor twice a week and he helps me a lot. I get very confused by what the voices keep telling me. I get very mad at them for bothering me all the time, but I know by now that I can't make them go away. But when I go to my doctor's office, I tell him about what they said, and what went on in my life during the week, and he helps me figure out what is true and what is not, and what I can tell people about and what I should keep to myself. I feel so much better each time I talk with him. I hope they don't make me stop seeing him." The consultant recommended that the state continue to pay for her treatment, which was keeping her functioning and out of the hospital. The state agreed and her treatment continued.

Ernestine had already been told by her psychiatrist that the consultant was a "nice guy" and that she should be open and honest with him. The consultant felt that his rapport with Ernestine was good from the beginning of the interview.

Comment. Ernestine left her psychotherapy sessions much less deluded and confused by what the voices had been telling her and much clearer on what was real and what was unreal. It was as if she had left in the psychiatrist's office a portion of the toxins of psychosis that had built up between sessions. It was a kind of *psychological dialysis* that she needed regularly if she was to remain relatively sane and able to conduct her life without the supervision of others. Seeing the patient twice a week for half an hour rather than once a week for an hour may enhance the dialysis-like effect that patients like Ernestine benefit from.

Many patients who have been sick for a long time develop ways of trying to cope with their voices and delusions—ways of trying to ignore them or blunt their impact on their lives. If your interview gets to the point where you and the patient can comfortably discuss voices or delusions, it can frequently be useful to ask, "Have you developed any tricks over the years to keep the voices [or delusions] from bothering you as much as they did in the beginning?" Knowing these tricks and supporting the patient in using them at stressful moments can be a useful part of treatment.

Irma

Irma was in her teens when she was admitted for her first schizophrenic episode, before many current medications effective against catatonia had been discovered. She was in a severe catatonic stupor, standing motionless and mute for hours at a time, seemingly oblivious to her surroundings. A psychiatric resident who was responsible for her care would go over to her each day at around 2 P.M. and spend 10 to 15 minutes standing or sitting by her, sometimes silently, sometimes talking to her in a soft voice, commenting on how terrified she seemed, or how preoccupied she looked, or guessing how she might be feeling.

One day the resident was called for an emergency and had to miss his meeting with Irma. Weeks later, when she had come out of her catatonia and was much more communicative, he asked her how she had felt about the missed session, wondering to himself whether she had even noticed. "I felt terrible," she said. "I wondered what had happened to you. You were my bread and butter."

Comment. Clearly the resident's visits with Irma had laid the groundwork for a therapeutic alliance. *One must never treat the patient as if he or she were not in the room or unable to perceive what is going on.* It is one more slap in the face to someone whose self-esteem is already extraordinarily low.

Craig

Craig was a 27-year-old graduate student in engineering who dropped out of school because he thought the other students and professors were reading his mind and stealing his ideas for their own gain, and that they were ridiculing him in the process. He thought that a radio transmitter in his brain transmitted all his thoughts to the Federal Bureau of Investigation. He wandered around the country, winding up on the doorstep of a physician cousin in Arizona, whom he asked to take him in for a while. The cousin did so, and asked Craig to see a psychiatrist, Dr. Coulter. Craig agreed.

At the first visit, Craig said, "I know you will think this is crazy, all the rest of them have," and then described the transmitter. Dr. Coulter agreed that it was hard to believe. Craig had requested skull x-rays, but Dr. Coulter pointed out that if the x-rays did not show any transmitter Craig would probably conclude that either the transmitter was not made of substances that could be detected by x-ray or that the x-ray was of the wrong part of his brain to find it, and that they would then be right back where they had started. Craig agreed; both were baffled.

Then Dr. Coulter said, "You know, having all your thoughts transmitted to the FBI must be driving you crazy. You don't have any privacy at all. Lord, if all my thoughts were open for other people to know about, I don't know what I would do. How do you live with it?" Craig quickly picked up on this theme of how much he was troubled by the lack of privacy and entered willingly into a discussion of how to proceed.

Comment. The late Norman Reider, M.D., of the Mt. Zion Hospital Psychiatric Clinic in San Francisco, used to say, "No collusion with delusion." This is a rule worth observing. With Craig, Dr. Coulter did not endorse the notion that there really was a transmitter, but he still tried to be sensitive to the bind Craig felt he was in because his thoughts were known. Had Craig asked point-blank "Do you think I have a transmitter in my head?," Dr. Coulter probably would have replied, "No, I don't think you do, but I know that you are convinced that there is one there, and that because of it you have no privacy, which is very troubling, and that is what I think we should work on."

Finding an area of agreement with the patient, identifying something that is bothersome or tormenting to him, can help start a therapeutic alliance and allow both parties to sidestep embarrassing debates, for example, about what is real and what is not or whether or not the patient is mentally ill.

Steven

One Friday afternoon at the Mt. Zion Psychiatric Clinic, the receptionist said that there were two gentlemen in the waiting room who wanted to see me. A concerned-looking middle-aged man told me that his name was Fredrick Weitzer and that the young man sitting next to him was his son, Steven. Steven, in his 20s, looked very psychotic, and I took him into my office first.

He gave me a very suspicious look and asked rather gruffly, "Are you Dr. Rosenbaum?" I said I was. He asked, "Are you Dr. C. Peter

Rosenbaum, of Chicago, Illinois?" "Yes." "Do you know Dr. J. R. Tanzer in Chicago?" I said very gravely, "Yes, I do. If I remember right, he has an office in the Pittsfield Building, which is on Washington near Wabash. Is that the person you mean?" Steven said yes, and he relaxed and a good deal of the paranoia drained out of his face and manner.

During our brief session, Steven told me how he had been in therapy with Dr. Tanzer (a friend of mine) since he was 17, that he had paranoid schizophrenia, that he had been hospitalized several times for it, and that Stelazine seemed to help him considerably. His father had left the family when Steven was 4; he was brought up by his mother, a maiden aunt, and a sister and had been reared under his mother's maiden name of Sheridan. Steven had decided to escape "the matriarchy" by flying out to San Francisco and taking his father's last name in hopes of becoming more of a man.

After I had seen the father as well, it looked as if Steven would be welcome at his house over the weekend. We set an appointment for Steven on Monday for an hour and, at his request, I made out an appointment card, writing as legibly as possible and making sure that I spelled all three of his names correctly, *Steven Sheridan Weitzer.* I also provided the phone number at which they could reach the psychiatrist on call if needed during the weekend. Both father and son seem relieved that we had established contact. We resume the story of Steven's treatment later in the chapter; remember the appointment card.

Comment. It is usually a mistake to counter paranoia with sweetness or affability. My manner with Steven was initially reserved, even a little grave, almost a mirror of his paranoid suspiciousness. Suspicious patients are inclined to view affability as an attempt to trick them into trust, whereas a very businesslike attitude on the part of the therapist may reassure the patient that even if the world is full of malevolent souls, the interviewer isn't trying to pull a fast one.

Gordon

In a mock psychiatry-board interview, a candidate was introduced to Gordon, who didn't want to give his last name. Gordon looked to be in his 40s, had a gray scraggly beard and a slightly unkempt appearance, and was dressed very casually. He had volunteered to be interviewed for a small cash reward. The candidate explained that he was being tested on his interview skills, that the interview would last half an hour, and that he would be asking Gordon lots of questions to get to know him. A faculty "examiner" was present to observe the interview, listen to the postinterview case presentation, and offer a critique of the candidate's performance.

Gordon said, "My psychiatrist told me that I don't have to talk about anything I don't want to talk about. That's right, isn't it?" The candidate said that that was correct. He then asked Gordon why he was in treatment. "Personal problems," said Gordon. When the candidate inquired about the problems, Gordon was evasive and said he didn't want to talk about them. Asked if he ever heard voices, Gordon mumbled and looked a bit agitated. The candidate asked if he heard troubling things from the voices. "I don't want to talk about that," Gordon responded.

It soon became obvious that the candidate had memorized a list of diagnostic criteria for schizophrenia, and, come hell or high water, he was going to go down his list and arrive at a diagnosis. Gordon was getting increasingly agitated under the onslaught. The faculty examiner was slow on the uptake. Just as he sensed imminent disaster and was about to intervene, Gordon shouted at the candidate, "I damn well told you I didn't want to talk about these things, and you can take your stinking interview and shove it!" and bolted from the room. The examiner, along with the staff member who had accompanied the patients to the interviews, found Gordon, who was calming down. Both felt that Gordon would be all right after a cooling-off period. The examiner then returned to the interview room to discuss what had happened.

Comment. Everyone has needs for privacy; boundaries must be respected. The interrogation of the patient, who had given numerous warning signs that the candidate was treading into unwelcome territory, rapidly alienated him. The candidate would have been much more effective if he had dropped his dogged pursuit of diagnostic criteria and instead said to the patient at the outset, "OK, I don't want to ask you about things that are private for you. Tell me if I start doing that. In the meantime, I'd like to get to know you a little. Can you tell me a little bit about yourself that you feel it's OK to talk about?" Even for what was to be a single, half-hour interview, the interviewer's failure to try to establish some kind of rapport, to show some signs of empathy for the patient's obvious distrust and suspiciousness, resulted in a predictable, disastrous outcome.

This does not mean that being forceful with a patient is always a mistake. Experienced therapists sometimes use an assertive approach profitably, but for those new to such work, being respectful and responsive are usually the best attitudes to start with.

COMMON AMBIVALENCES PATIENTS HAVE ABOUT THE FIRST MEETING

There are several possible reasons for schizophrenic patients to be ambivalent about initial interviews, including neophobia, paranoid or delusional projections, unhappy experiences in nonmedical settings, and unhappy experiences in medical settings.

Neophobia and the Fear of Strangers

In his pioneering research at Worcester State Hospital in the 1930s and thereafter, David Shakow (1) concluded that one characteristic of schizophrenic patients was a fear of novelty, of the unknown, a trait he termed *neophobia*. The interviewer is at first a stranger to the patient, and no matter how much each party hopes that something good may come of their meeting, the interviewer is one more stranger to cope with. Just as 8-month-old infants show "stranger anxiety," so do schizophrenic patients feel apprehensive when meeting someone new. For this reason, it is often useful to let the patient look you over: approach him from the front, not the side or the rear (none of us likes to be snuck up upon). Anecdotes abound among experienced clinicians about paranoid patients fearing anal assaults, e.g., a transmitter being placed in the rectum or electric shocks entering the body through the anus.

Paranoid patients may also wear sunglasses indoors, to keep people from reading their minds ("the eyes are the windows to the soul"). Professor Nathaniel Apter once told our medical school class: "There are three main reasons why people wear dark glasses indoors: 1) they are paranoid people who don't want others looking into them; 2) they are narcissistic Hollywood actors; or 3) they have just had their eyes refracted."

Paranoid and Delusional Projections

Patients bring with them their own notions about the interviewer's intentions and abilities, and often these are negative. Steven from Chicago took some convincing that I was really who I represented myself as being. Gordon, who fled from the overzealous interviewer, was skeptical about the respect for privacy that he would get from the candidate who interviewed him, and, unfortunately, his fears were a self-fulfilling prophecy. The interviewer should be prepared to be tested and misperceived.

Nonmedical Experiences

Schizophrenic patients often frighten other people, and the patients have had more than enough experience to know that they are an often despised minority. When patients undergo their first psychotic break, they often have a sense of something going terribly wrong, of being in the grip of a nightmare over which they have no control. Patients live on the streets, or get thrown into jail for crimes instigated by their voices or delusions. Many have to live in board-and-care homes, which can be unsupportive of the patients' social needs. Meeting someone new may remind the patient of other failed beginnings.

Medical Experiences

Many patients have had to endure being put on involuntary holds and being hospitalized against their will, spending hours in corridors, being asked—sometimes forced—to take medications. They may overhear themselves being disparagingly referred to by staff. To be referred to as a "schiz" must, for many patients, be akin to a racial slur.

For these many reasons, patients for the most part come to the initial encounter with the interviewer with considerable apprehension, and the interviewer should be willing to hear about these early on if they seem to stand in the way of getting to know the patient.

GETTING OFF TO A GOOD START

Given the ambivalences that both patient and interviewer may feel, there are a number of things interviewers can do to lessen apprehension, increase the openness to the experience, and establish rapport as part of a first interview.

Psychosis as a Dream

Many authors have likened the psychotic state to a dream—Jung was especially eloquent on this topic (2). But these dreams are usually closer to nightmares than otherwise. If we listen to someone relate a dream, we try to conjure up images that coincide with the dreamer's report. We willingly suspend our powers of disbelief, not focusing on the irrational, the bizarre, the mutually contradictory themes that are so typical of dreams.

When interviewing a patient with schizophrenia, if the interviewer can assume the stance of entering into someone else's interesting and sometimes frightening dream world, the process should be more tolerable.

The Strategy of the Strange Cousin from Kankakee

It is sometimes a useful strategy for an interviewer to imagine that she has been told that she will be meeting a cousin from Kankakee, Illinois, on his first visit to Bridgeport, Connecticut, and that family lore has it that the cousin is a bit on the strange side. Being a decent and polite person, she meets the cousin and seeks to make him comfortable for his visit. The cousin may start talking about voices, mystical experiences, religious beliefs, or firmly held notions that seem quite strange, but the cousin/interviewer knows that it is not her part to challenge these things, but to listen attentively and do what she can to make her cousin feel at home.

In the same manner, one can interview a new patient, being receptive and responsive to what the patient is saying. If the patient asks whether the interviewer believes that what he is saying is true, the interviewer can politely say, "No, that's not what I believe, but what I'm interested in is how things look to you."

Even though there should not be collusion with delusion, the ways in which delusions are received and reflected back to the patient should be flexible. Sometimes the interviewer can label them openly as delusions (or, often more acceptable to patients, "unrealistic thoughts" or "tricks your mind plays on you"), once rapport has been achieved, as Ernestine's therapist was able to do. Sometimes he accepts them with a symbolic grain of salt, as with Craig, the student who believed there was a transmitter in his brain.

Introductions and Explaining the Purpose of the Interview

The interviewer should introduce himself to the patient, mention the purpose of the interview, see how this accords with the patient's perceptions, and give the patient an opportunity for comment (this is true for virtually all psychiatric interviewing, not only with schizophrenic patients). For instance, Dr. Coulter told Craig something of this sort: "Craig, I'm Dr. Coulter. I'm a psychiatrist. Your cousin John told me that you are concerned about a radio transmitter that's been planted in your brain and transmits all your thoughts, and you'd like to see if it can be removed. Do I have it right?"

The consultant who saw Ernestine said: "I'm Dr. Green. I'm a psychiatrist. The state of California is wondering about your psychotherapy bills in your treatment with Dr. Brown, and they have asked me to learn more about it. When we are done, I will have to write a report to the state, and I will be sure that both you and Dr. Brown get a copy of it. Is that OK with you?"

In the following case, of Mr. Williams, there is an example of an introduction, and later an example of picking up on a subtle cue (in this instance, an unusual proverb interpretation) that led to a revelation about the patient's psychosis.

A psychiatrist, Dr. Cook, was asked to see Mr. Williams, who was incarcerated at a state hospital for the criminally insane after he had been found not guilty by reason of insanity for shooting a delicatessen owner, who, fortunately, had survived the attack. Mr. Williams and his attorney maintained that he was no longer dangerous and therefore eligible for release back into the community. The staff felt that even though he was no longer overtly psychotic (he had been diagnosed with paranoid schizophrenia), he still had a dangerous and unstable feel to him, in spite of his protestations, and they wanted an independent evaluation.

Dr. Cook told him, "Mr. Williams, I am Dr. Cook. I'm a psychiatrist. The staff here [several of whom were in the room to observe the interview] has asked me to talk with you and see if you are no longer dangerous and ready for release. Whatever we talk about might wind up in the staff report, and that report will be going to a judge in the court that sent you here. Is that OK with you?" Mr. Williams said it was.

As they started the interview, Dr. Cook noticed that Mr. Williams had an excoriated-looking area on the inside of his right wrist. Even though the patient said nothing psychotic, Dr. Cook had the very strong feeling that psychosis (and the violent feelings that were part of the psychosis) was barely beneath the surface, under tight but brittle control. Still, Mr. Williams avoided saying anything psychotic-sounding during the interview. Finally, Dr. Cook asked him to interpret proverbs and offered: "No use crying over spilt milk."

Mr. Williams hesitated, and then said, "If you spill your milk, you don't get no good dinner?"

"No good dinner?" Dr. Cook repeated. "I guess getting a good dinner is pretty important to you?"

"I really need a good dinner," Mr. Williams replied, and stuck his wrist in his mouth and started sucking and chewing on the excoriated areas. When Dr. Cook asked if he was getting a good dinner now, Mr. Williams nodded. This led into a discussion about the importance of food, how he had wanted (but could not afford) some of the food in the delicatessen, and how he had "known" that it was the delicatessen owner's responsibility to give him some food and that the owner had to be punished for evading this responsibility. He had gone to his room, gotten a gun, and shot the owner. A delusional system about food was apparent.* With the psychosis once more very much in evidence, it was easy to persuade Mr. Williams's attorney and the court that continued treatment in the hospital was necessary.

The Beginnings of the Therapeutic Alliance

The seeds of a potential therapeutic alliance are often sown during the first interviews. Irma, the catatonic girl, came to rely on the brief daily visits of her resident. Craig with the imagined transmitter found a psychiatrist who was willing to take his beliefs and fears seriously. Steven from Chicago was desperate for help, and eagerly accepted an appointment for what later became several years of psychotherapy with a succession of residents who worked with him.

Diagnosis

First interviews often require a diagnosis to be part of an interview report or a case presentation. The fourth edition of the *Diagnostic and Statistical Manual of Mental Disorders* (DSM-IV) (3) lists the characteristic symptoms of schizophrenia as: 1) delusions, 2) hallucinations, 3) disorganized speech (e.g., frequent derailment or incoherence), 4) grossly disorganized or catatonic behavior, and 5) negative symptoms (i.e., affective flattening, alogia, or avolition). It requires generally that two of more of these be present for a significant portion of time during 1 month.

Arriving at a diagnosis need not be an intrusive process. By simply listening to and observing a patient during the first interview, disorganization of speech, disorganized or catatonic behavior, and affective flattening will often become obvious. As the interview proceeds, the patient may spontaneously refer to "the voices," and interest by the interviewer—"Can you tell me more about the voices?"—may be sufficient to establish their presence. If there is no such spontaneous mention, the interviewer can ask, "Have you had any unusual or strange experiences, such as hearing voices that no one else seems to hear?" This may be sufficient to get into a discussion of voices, and

*Oral concerns are very common in schizophrenic patients, and a proverb containing the word "milk" will often elicit such concerns. Similarly, "People who live in glass houses shouldn't throw stones" may pull for themes of destruction and being under surveillance, and "A stitch in time saves nine" may pull for themes of hostility and aggression—needles and all that.

then the interviewer can follow up by asking about other kinds of hallucinatory phenomena—"Have you seen things that other people haven't seen, or felt things when there was nothing there?" Likewise, for delusions the interviewer can say, "Sometimes people worry more than they should that other people are spying on them, or planning to get them into trouble. They get paranoid. Has anything of that sort ever happened to you?" Similarly, questions about thought insertion—"Do you ever get the feeling that other people or the radio or TV are putting thoughts into your head?"—or thought broadcasting—"Do you ever get the feeling that your thoughts are being transmitted to other people or come out on the radio or TV?"—are easily enough asked.

Once the patient can talk about such matters, the interviewer can ask, "When was the first time in your life that you remember hearing voices?" "When was the last time you heard the voices?" "Are you hearing the voices now?" At this point, the interviewer asks, "How does it make you feel to hear the voices [think people are spying on you]?" This is a point at which the patient may express some anguish at the mental torture the voices or the delusions cause him (as did Craig), and the interviewer can strengthen an alliance with the patient by empathizing with the patient's distress. From this point, the interviewer can inquire about areas of potential danger.

Potential Dangers: Suicide, Assault, and Homicide

The time-honored dictum *Primum non nocere* (first, do no harm) can be recast as *Primum non noceat* (first, let no harm be done*). Thus, we have to know about the patient's potential for suicide, assault, and homicide. For schizophrenic patients, these impulses often enter consciousness as hallucinations and delusions. The interviewer can initiate such an inquiry with a statement such as "We are always concerned about people's safety—yours and other people's—so I am going to ask you a few questions about experiences you may have had that involve safety." The interviewer can then ask whether the voices or the delusions that they have already been talking about ever give the patient commands to obey or suggestions to follow, especially ones that might involve hurting themselves or someone else. If the patient has had such thoughts, it is important to know when he last had them, how close he came to acting on them, whether he is having such thoughts now, and whether he wants any help with controlling his

*Translation by Romolo Rossi, M.D.

impulses. If there is a current risk of dangerous behaviors, the patient needs to be helped with these before any other matters are addressed. Many patients, having been helped to control or overcome destructive impulses before they acted on them, have later thanked those who aided them.

SOME THEORETICAL CONSIDERATIONS

The Schizophrenic Patient's World Is at Least Partially Understandable

Prior to the work of Freud and Eugene Bleuler, the Swiss psychiatrist who first coined the term *schizophrenia*, the utterances of schizophrenic patients were regarded by most physicians as incomprehensible babble not worth paying attention to. Our examples have shown the falsity of this belief: some sense could be made of each of our patients' words and actions. If one is to interview patients intelligently and profitably, it is a necessary assumption that some sense is to be made of virtually every patient's words and actions, no matter how bizarre they may seem at first, just as the seeming irrationality of dreams can be turned to psychotherapeutic gain.

Psychiatrists Don't Read Minds

The terms "shrink" and "head candler" are suggestive of the public's fear/belief that psychiatrists can read minds and perform mental magic. Many psychiatrists have developed a cocktail-party strategy of responding, when asked what they do for a living, with some variant on "I'm a psychiatrist, but I leave my work at the office," hoping this will avoid an embarrassed hitch in the conversation.

Schizophrenic patients are all the more fearful about such matters, and therefore the interviewer should be careful to avoid pronouncements that might seem like mind reading. For instance, if a patient seems to be getting more agitated, furrows appear on the forehead, and his speech becomes even more disorganized, if the interviewer merely says "You're nervous," the patient may believe that his mind is being read. If the interviewer, in the interest of helping the patient's reality testing, says, "I notice your hand is trembling more than it was, and your forehead looks tense and your words are harder to follow; are you feeling nervous about something?," the patient is again anchored to the here-and-now, mutually observable, phenomena that led to the interviewer's question.

Schizophrenic Patients Have Trouble Moderating Social Closeness and Distance

The degree to which nonpsychotic people interact socially with others, entirely unconsciously, is impressive. Healthy 8-year-olds know almost instinctively whose lap they can jump into without asking permission, whose hand is to be shaken, who is to be addressed as "Mrs.," and who can harmlessly be called "Doo-Doo Head." They often know without prompting which family matters are private and not to be discussed with grandma, no matter how much she pries.

It is as if we can shift our several social gears almost automatically. Schizophrenic patients, on the other hand, often seem to have only two gears—or sometimes to be stuck in one gear. In my first full, one-hour session with Steven from Chicago, things were going well for about the first 10 minutes. He was looking at me with the kind of adoring gaze seen normally only in children who have not yet learned that it is not polite to stare or between lovers. All of a sudden, with his hand scratching in his lap, his face clouded; he looked very fearful and said, "I'm afraid of you!" Surmising on some level that the degree of intimacy we had been having was suddenly taking on some sexual overtones, I said, "Steven, if you're afraid we are going to get sexually involved, that's not what's going to happen. We're here for your psychotherapy and to help you get settled in San Francisco." He relaxed and we resumed on a friendly note. But later in that session, a fearful irruption from his unconscious again upset him, and we had to deal with it before anything else. Steven was in many ways stuck in first gear, in which his ego boundaries were poor and he felt at the mercy of his impulses, some of which he projected onto me. He didn't know how to shift up to third, where he could feel a little more distance.

In contrast, Gordon, the man who bolted from his interview, had many years' practice at being vague and guarded, concealing personal information from strangers. Even if the candidate had been empathetic and in tune with Gordon's presentation of himself, it is doubtful that Gordon would have revealed much of a personal nature. It was as if he were perpetually stuck in third gear and unable to shift down to a more intimate first gear.

Schizophrenic Patients Form Transferences, Often Very Powerful Ones

By *transference,* Freud meant the unconscious attribution of a quality or characteristic to another person that is not warranted by reality. These attributions—kinds of projections, if you will—are the result of the person's psychodynamics. He who has been raised by a tyrannical father may fear teachers and bosses, no matter how benign they may be. She who has been raised by an overpraising, never-critical set of parents may always want to be the center of attention and become excessively histrionic with people who refuse to act as obedient audiences. The analysis of such transferences is a central part of the techniques of psychoanalysis.

Freud did not work with psychotic patients because he felt they did not develop transferences, and therefore analysis of transference was not possible. We now know that schizophrenic patients do indeed form transferences, often very powerful ones. With the neurotic patient, transference has an "as-if" quality. The analyst may interpret to the patient, "You are reacting to me as if I am your father."

With schizophrenic patients, transferences often feel very real and lack the distance of the "as-if" formulation. Steven was truly afraid I wanted to have sex with him during our first hour. Craig was truly prepared to believe that I would laugh at him and be dismissive when he talked about the transmitter in his head.

A rule of psychoanalysis of neurotics is that the positive transference is as much to be analyzed as the negative—paying the analyst a compliment is just as worthy of scrutiny as disparaging the analyst's intelligence. In working with schizophrenic patients, certain kinds of transference or feelings about the interviewer deserve immediate attention; others should simply be acknowledged without further comment. With schizophrenic patients, it is perhaps better to use the terms *conjunctive* and *disjunctive* feelings. Conjunctive feelings, which help the patient enter into and maintain a working alliance, should simply be accepted, uncommented on, with good grace by the interviewer, such as Craig's willingness to be hospitalized for skull x-rays and to try Stelazine (described more fully later in the chapter). Disjunctive feelings, those that threaten to rupture the often fragile alliance, should be dealt with directly, in hopes of averting an impasse, as was the case with Steven and his fears about a sexual encounter.

The dilemma of wanting contact and yet being afraid of it was very poignantly expressed by Vivian, a 19-year-old woman with hebephrenic (now officially called *disorganized*) schizophrenia during a therapy hour in about the eighth month of treatment. She and her therapist had been having a lively interchange. Toward the end of the hour, she became remote and silent. The therapist commented on this shift and asked if she had noticed it. She had, and she said that it had to do with "friendship." The therapist asked her to explain further. "Too much friendship is like when a bear is cold and he sees the hunter's fire, and he comes over to get warm, and instead he gets scorched."

TECHNIQUE

The Physical Setting and Limits

Primum, ne noceat (first, let no harm be done)—we must ensure safety from harm for all parties involved before any interview can proceed. The patient who is out of control must be subdued and brought back under control as humanely as possible, often by putting him in restraints and in seclusion, and/or by giving medications. Being in restraints and in a seclusion room is not necessarily a barrier to starting an interview, assuming that contact with the interviewer will not inflame the patient further. In fact, sitting with the patient in restraints, explaining what is being done and why, and simply being present may be extremely important for a patient who fears that through her imagined omnipotence she has destroyed or at least alienated the very treatment staff she needs most.

Some patients who are in good control still feel too confined in an office, get paranoid about being trapped, and may respond very well to talking in a day room, or near the nurses' station, or during a walk on the grounds. Other patients are willing to sit in an office but may want the door left ajar and to have the seat closest to the door, and these sensitivities should be respected. Usually, as rapport develops, such patients will agree to having the door closed if privacy becomes an issue. Thus it may be useful to start the session by saying, "Let me suggest that you sit here [indicating the patient's chair] and I will sit over there. Are you comfortable with that?"

Timing and Length of Sessions

Somewhere in the beginning of the session, tell the patient about how long the interview will last, and that if it begins to feel too long to be sure to let you know. Although traditional admission or outpatient interviews often last about an hour, sometimes patients can only tolerate briefer periods, and two half-hour sessions a day may be far more productive than a single one-hour session.

In any event, be as precise about sessions with the patient as circumstances allow, e.g.: "For this week, while you are on the unit, I'll spend at least 15 minutes with you every day. We'll meet at 10 A.M. each day except Wednesday, when I have staff meeting, and I'll find a time Wednesday afternoon when we can meet and will tell you about it tomorrow." Then make every effort to be on time or get word to the patient if you are going to be late. As was the case with Irma, the catatonic girl, the interviewer may come to be the patient's "bread and butter," and being even a few minutes late may feel like a devastating betrayal to the patient, similar to the plight of the trusting, disappointed child: "But you promised me you would be here!"

Building Rapport

Sullivan advises starting by telling the patient the purpose of the interview and what you know about him or her. Try to frame this information in the way that is least likely to upset the patient's already precarious self-esteem. Many patients don't believe they are mentally ill, so starting off by saying "We're here to talk about your mental illness" is almost guaranteed to have awful results. Other patients know they are mentally ill but have been treated so shabbily because of it that, again, the phrase is odious to them and should be avoided. Likewise, many patients find the term *schizophrenia* obnoxious and recoil from it.

If initial rapport is to form, it is much better to find some problem about which the patient is concerned and with which he or she might want help. The admission sheet that says "Patient has become increasingly erratic and talking about voices and delusions and had to be taken by ambulance from her board-and-care home" can be translated to that patient as "It sounds like the people at your board-and-care home and you are not understanding each other very well these days and it made you very upset" rather than "Your talking about voices and crazy thoughts has freaked out the people who run your board-and-care."

In the following case, a patient named James was initially very suspicious about what Dr. Adams had in mind for him. It was only after they were able to agree on a common goal that the therapeutic alliance began to form.

James

In the spring of 1968, James, a disheveled man, was picked up by highway patrolmen. He had been walking on a California freeway, carrying a sign endorsing the candidacy of Robert Kennedy. The police found out that he was an engineer who had missed work for a week. He was brought to a nearby psychiatric clinic, where he was seen by Dr. Adams.

James told Dr. Adams straight off that if Dr. Adams diagnosed him as schizophrenic and tried to put him in a psychiatric ward, he would leave the office right away. He said this had happened to him two years previously, and that it had been a gross misuse of medical authority. Dr. Adams told him that he wasn't so much interested in diagnosis as he was curious about what had been going on in James's life. Somewhat reluctantly, James described a growing preoccupation with Kennedy and how the whole fate of the country lay in getting him elected, and that was why he had quit his job to work full time for Kennedy's candidacy. He was monomaniacal in his zeal. He had not slept much and admitted that it was difficult to keep himself organized.

As the interview went on, Dr. Adams told James that he too wanted to see Kennedy elected, and that he would like to help James to be more effective in his campaign efforts. He also told James that he thought he wasn't thinking or planning very clearly, partly because of lack of sleep; James agreed. The doctor said that if he were the average motorist driving on that freeway and saw James walking along it in his disheveled condition, he'd probably think, "Kennedy really has some strange-looking people working for him; I wonder if I want to vote for him after all." James took this in and asked what Dr. Adams could do about it. The doctor explained that a medicine called Trilafon (perphenazine) sometimes helped people to sleep better and think more clearly. James, knowing that Trilafon was an antipsychotic, wondered if the suggestion meant that Dr. Adams thought that he was schizophrenic. Dr. Adams replied that James was much too complicated a person to try to diagnose solely on the basis of a single interview, and that he as a physician was more concerned about getting him in shape to help the Kennedy campaign. (Privately Dr. Adams was thinking about mania, a schizophreniform psychosis with grandiosity and schizophrenia as possible diagnoses.) James accepted this formulation and took a Trilafon tablet that Dr. Adams had on hand, and they set up daily meetings for the rest of the week. By avoiding odious diagnoses and finding some area of mutual concern, they were able to establish a working alliance. I discuss James again later.

The Problem of Anxiety

For most of us, a little anxiety is a good thing for getting coping juices flowing. It is a spur to thought and action. But which of us has not had the miserable experience of completely blanking on an exam question for which we had been well prepared, simply because we were too anxious? Sullivan said he would "again and again suggest that severe anxiety probably contributes no information. The effect of severe anxiety reminds one in some ways of a blow on the head, in that it simply wipes out what is immediately proximal to its occurrence. If you have a severe blow on the head, you are quite apt later to have an incurable, absolute amnesia covering the few moments before your head was struck. Anxiety has a similar effect" (4).

Most of us have what the psychoanalysts call a "strong ego," meaning that we can cope with a significant amount of anxiety without serious deterioration in functioning—that we can "muddle through," as the English did during the dark days of World War II. Schizophrenic patients generally can tolerate much less anxiety before their rational abilities begin to suffer. It is important for the interviewer to try to help patients keep their anxiety levels low, so that their reality testing and abilities to cope with the interview are not compromised.

Nonpsychotic people usually recognize anxiety by feelings of impending doom, rapid heartbeat, sweat on the palms and brows, frequent urination, and other indications. Many schizophrenic patients, however, may not be aware of these simple cues. Instead, there may be a sudden rise in the level of psychotic thinking (louder voices, more intrusive delusions, looser associations), as was true for Steven from Chicago when he was afraid we would have sex or for Vivian when she got concerned about "too much friendship."

Sometimes schizophrenic anxiety is contagious (even if the psychosis is not): if the interviewer finds himself suddenly becoming anxious for no discernible reason, he should consider the possibility that he is picking up the patient's anxiety and wonder if something going on in the interview itself is making the patient anxious.

When the interviewer detects what may be anxiety, it is wise to address the issue promptly. Again, give the patient the basis for your conclusion, e.g.: "I notice you've been squirming in your chair a lot the last few minutes, and you seem more preoccupied than usual with thoughts of electric shocks going through your body. Have you noticed this? What do you think is going on? Does it have anything to do with our session or me or what we've been talking about?"

Benzodiazepines and related medications, given in addition to antipsychotic medications, may help the anxious patient.

Moderating Catharsis; Listening for Unlabeled Metaphors

Movies and TV programs about psychotherapy to the contrary, the uninhibited expression of strong emotion—catharsis—is not always a good thing. The ego has to be big enough and strong enough to contain the flood of feeling, or it becomes overwhelmed and reality testing and judgment suffer, as murders of passion so amply demonstrate. The egos of schizophrenic patients are weaker than those of neurotics, and the interviewer must be sensitive to signs that the patient is being overwhelmed by feeling.

If patients seem to be getting too anxious, too angry, or too sad, or too anything, it is wise to move away from the charged topic to something more neutral, perhaps employing what Sullivan referred to as an abrupt transition, e.g., "Those activities of the Antichrist outside Mexico City are important, but first, tell me, what was it like growing up in Tulsa?"

If a session is simply too hot for a patient to handle, the therapist may say, "It feels to me like there is an awful lot getting stirred up here right now. Maybe more than we can handle at one time. What do you say to our taking a time out for a little while and coming back together this afternoon at around 2?" If the session has been on an inpatient service, add, "I'm going to mention to the nurses that this has been a rough session, so they can be with you if you'd like."

Schizophrenic patients have difficulties with the use of metaphor* and often unwittingly use private symbols as unlabeled metaphors for their perceptions of the relationship with the interviewer. If a patient starts talking about volcanic eruptions in the Philippines, it makes sense for the interviewer to inquire, "Are you afraid something is close to exploding in here?"

Don't Just Do Something; Sit There!

Medical education fosters two kinds of furors that can adversely affect establishing rapport: *furor diagnosticus* (the frenzy to reach a DSM-IV diagnosis) and *furor therapeuticus* (the frenzy to treat, aggravated by pressures from managed-payment insurance companies). A particularly awful example of the former attitude is the interviewer in the case of Gordon, the man who bolted. Both furors imply that the interviewer should be *doing* something: make a diagnosis; start a treatment. Both

---

*Proverbs are common metaphors. Some schizophrenic patients respond with standard answers, but those who are acutely ill and/or have a prominent thought disorder often give abnormal responses. Contrary to the common assertion that schizophrenic patients interpret proverbs concretely, in my experience these abnormal responses much more frequently tend to be highly idiosyncratic and personalized, or overly generalized, e.g., Mr. Williams's interpretation of "spilt milk" as meaning "you don't get a good dinner." It is patients with moderately to severely compromised brain function who are likely to be concrete, responding, for example, "Well, if some milk spills on the floor, wipe it up and don't make a big fuss about it."

stand in the way of letting a dialog unfold between the interviewer and the peculiar cousin from Kankakee. The interviewer should try to minimize both furors during the initial interview, even though some conclusions about diagnosis are often requisite after a first interview, as described previously.

One can approach an interview with one of two sets of expectations, just as one might approach a morning's fishing expedition: 1) "If I don't bring home three trout by noon, the whole morning will have been wasted" or 2) "I hope to catch some trout, but even if I don't, wading in the stream, watching the dragonflies darting back and forth, hearing the hum of the bees, seeing the fields and their flowers, all these are wonderful and make the whole thing worthwhile." The interviewer who can adopt the latter stance has a better chance of communing with the patient and perhaps coming out of the interview with many more fish than he had anticipated.

Lewis Hill, in discussing psychotherapy of schizophrenia, cautioned as follows: "I would urgently advise any [therapist] beginning his training to subject himself to a rule. The rule is that he will not cure or analyze anyone during the first several months of his training. The purpose of this rule is to remove the temptation to *do* something rather than to *be* something in therapy. The temptation is strong to invade a patient's extremely precarious balance with the intention of doing him good without the skill to avoid doing him harm" (italics added) (5).

Picking Up on Subtle Cues

Sometimes patients will use a word with an intonation, emphasis, or gesture that is a bit different from their usual stream of speech when some particularly psychotic, but until now hidden, theme is being touched on. By keeping an ear cocked for these little grace notes of expression, and responding to them, the interviewer can sometimes get to some very important issues very quickly, issues that might otherwise have escaped notice.

Mr. Williams, who responded to the "spilt milk" proverb by talking about "a good dinner" and sucking on his wrist, was letting the psychosis he was trying so hard to keep hidden make an appearance. A simple inquiry about the importance of a good dinner allowed the psychosis to come spilling out.

Another patient, Tom, seemed very normal and nonpsychotic during the first part of an initial interview with Dr. Burton. For the first 15 minutes, it felt like a conversation struck up at a bar—about the weather, how the local sports teams were doing, current politics, etc.

Somehow the topic of travel came up, and Dr. Burton asked if he liked to travel (he did) and whether he had been to any interesting places. "I was in Mexico last December," Tom said, "and there were some funny things going on"—the latter said with a bit more edge to his voice than previously. "What kind of funny things?" Dr. Burton asked. Tom looked at Dr. Burton closely and said, "Is this conversation confidential?" The psychiatrist told him it was. "The Antichrist has a coven just outside Mexico City," Tom said, and they were off to the races. A very elaborate delusional system, replete with transmitters that sent confidential information from Mexico to the Vatican and Jerusalem, came to the fore, and Tom was getting more and more exercised about the perfidies that he had uncovered during his trip. His face darkened, and Dr. Burton, fearing that Tom was working up too great a head of steam, changed topics back to more neutral territory, telling him that this was all very important but shouldn't be talked about too much at one time.

The Interviewer as Auxiliary Ego

Schizophrenic patients can often "borrow" the interviewer's reality orientation and ego strength to use in their own struggles toward better adjustment. For example, after several months of treatment, I asked Steven from Chicago about the appointment card I'd given him at our first, 15-minute interview on that Friday afternoon. "That card was a lifesaver," he said. "All during the weekend, I wasn't sure whether I was in Chicago or San Francisco, whether I was dreaming or not, and I would keep taking out the card and reading it and seeing your name, and my name, and the Mt. Zion Clinic name on it, and I knew where I was."

On another occasion, Steven was worried about going out with friends to dinner. One of his fears was that his voices would get loud, as they often did in a group of people, and accuse him of disgusting practices, and that he would become so upset that he would run from the restaurant to the embarrassment of all concerned. We anticipated several aspects of the dinner and I told him that I hoped he could ignore his voices during what promised to be a pleasant time. At the next visit he reported, "My voices started to get loud after dinner, but then I heard *your* voice telling me not to listen to *my* voices, and it was just like a radio. I could turn the volume control on my voices almost all the way down—not quite completely off—and I was able to stay for the whole evening."

FOLLOW-UP ON THREE OF THE PATIENTS

In each of the three cases followed up below, the initial interview, in addition to letting the interviewer know a good deal about the patient (enough for an informal diagnosis and the beginnings of a treatment plan), served as the entry to a psychotherapeutic experience.

Craig with the Transmitter

Craig came into the hospital for a few days, and had a neurological examination and skull x-rays. He was dubious about taking the Stelazine (trifluperazine) that had been suggested, but agreed to give it a 3-day try when it was pointed out that taking it or not taking it was entirely under Craig's control and he could refuse it any time he wanted to.

The neurological examination and the skull films failed to show the transmitter, surprising no one. After 3 days of Stelazine, he wasn't nearly as worried and preoccupied about the transmitter as he had been, and that was a relief to him. In a final outpatient visit a few days later, Craig accepted a prescription for a 2-week supply of the medication and said he felt it was time to leave his cousin's house and head for Seattle, where he knew some people. He took down the name of a psychiatrist in Seattle who could renew his prescription. How Craig did after that session is not known. But for a few days, at least, he had been willing to engage, he had been willing to try the medicine, and he had derived some benefit from it.

James Who Campaigned for Robert Kennedy

In the days and weeks following his first visit, James slept better and his thinking gradually cleared. At first he saw Dr. Adams every day. The psychiatrist helped him get medical leave from his employer (who valued James and had kept his position open), and many weeks later was able to certify that he thought James was ready to go back to work. The psychosis slowly disappeared over those weeks. After his return to work, James confined his political activities to handing out leaflets and campaign buttons at organized rallies.

Steven from Chicago

During the year that I worked with him, Steven achieved a level of independence and autonomy that was new for him. As I was leaving the clinic, an incoming resident was glad to start working with him, and each year, Steven, who had become well liked at the clinic, would start work with a new resident. Several of us had encouraged him to get a job, but he had stoutly resisted all our efforts.

Four years after our last session, I had parked near the clinic, with my wife and our 2-year-old son in the car, and the boy stepped off the curb when we weren't looking. Out of nowhere a young man in a long coat suddenly appeared, scooped my son out of the street, and planted him on the sidewalk. "Dr. Rosenbaum," said Steven, "how are you? Is that your son?" I thanked Steven for his rescue and we chatted for a few minutes. He proudly told me that he was now down to a half hour of psychotherapy a week (he was just on his way to his appointment), that he was now living in his own apartment, and that he had finally gotten a job! He was, he said, a sales representative for the Hearst Corporation. It turned out that he was delivering copies of the *San Francisco Examiner,* but he couldn't have been more proud than if he had been made CEO of the organization. He still needed hospitalizations once or twice a year, always in conjunction with his mother's visits from Chicago. He had not found a way to discourage her from coming out. Otherwise, though, he was pleased with the way his life was going, and he was enjoying more autonomy than ever before.

SUMMARY: TIPS FOR INTERVIEWERS

Let me summarize this chapter by recasting several of its major points in the form of tips or suggestions on how to proceed.

1. The patient's world is meaningful to himself, and the interviewer can begin to make sense of it by hearing it as a dream (or nightmare).
2. If the interviewer receives the patient as if he were an eccentric cousin from Kankakee, he can befriend the person without necessarily endorsing his psychosis.
3. Establishing rapport whenever possible is more important than immediately trying to come to a firm diagnosis, and diagnostic information is more likely to emerge when the beginnings of a working alliance have already formed.
4. Patients with schizophrenia are often afraid of strangers, including interviewers. Care with introductions and explaining the purpose of the interview can diminish the patient's distrust.
5. Inexperienced interviewers are often afraid of schizophrenic patients. Having a trusted consultant with whom one can discuss the interview, and being in one's own personal psycho-

therapy, can both reduce the interviewer's anxiety and lead to unique kinds of personal and professional growth.

6. Rapport is more likely to develop when patient and interviewer can agree on some problem or distress that the patient is experiencing than by looking first for diagnostic information or arguing about the truth or falsity of the patient's experiences. Still, there should not be "collusion with delusion."
7. Interviewers who can establish rapport can help patients by letting the patient "borrow" parts of the interviewer's ego and by letting the patient discharge in the interviewer's office some of the toxins of the psychosis, in a kind of psychological dialysis.
8. Schizophrenic patients have trouble with maintaining comfortable social closeness and/or distance—they may be "stuck in third gear." Respecting their ego boundaries and needs for privacy may enhance the development of rapport. Exaggerated sweetness or affability by the interviewer may put some patients off, especially those with paranoia. It is better to start off in a business-like manner and let mutual warmth develop naturally if and when it can.
9. Even modest amounts of anxiety can have crippling effects on patients' ability to cope. The presence of such anxiety may be revealed by unlabeled metaphors or a rise in the level of psychosis in the patient's speech. When the interviewer suspects rising levels of anxiety, he or she should try to work with the patient to identify and deal with them.
10. Diagnoses have to be made and assessments of the potential for violence have to be part of an initial interview. Going after such information gently, after a modicum of rapport has been established, is much more likely to yield useful information than abrupt interrogations.
11. Beware of *furor diagnosticus* and *furor therapeuticus*. If the situation permits, commune with the patient while fishing for information. When in doubt, don't just do something; sit there!
12. Schizophrenic patients can develop powerful transferences. Some transferences are friends of the therapeutic alliance; others are its enemy. Accept the friends without much comment, but try to talk about the enemies before they strain the relationship too badly. Moderate catharsis when too-strong emotion threatens to overwhelm the patient.

ACKNOWLEDGMENTS

I thank Joseph Belanoff, M.D., Ari Harrison, M.D., and Irvin Yalom, M.D., for their comments.

REFERENCES

1. Shakow D. Some observations on the psychology (and some fewer, on the biology) of schizophrenia. J Nerv Ment Dis 1971; 153:300–330.
2. Jung CC. The psychology of dementia praecox. In: Collected Works of C. G. Jung. Vol III. Princeton, NJ: Princeton: Princeton University Press, 1960:297–298.
3. American Psychiatric Association. Diagnostic and Statistical Manual of Mental Disorders. 4th ed. Washington, DC: American Psychiatric Association, 1994:285–286.
4. Sullivan HS. The Interpersonal Theory of Psychiatry. New York: Norton, 1953:151–152.
5. Hill LB. Psychotherapeutic Intervention in Schizophrenia. Chicago: University of Chicago Press, 1955:191.

2

Symptom Clusters in Schizophrenia

William O. Faustman and Shelley Fleming Ficek
Veterans Affairs Palo Alto Health Care System
Palo Alto
and Stanford University School of Medicine
Stanford, California

INTRODUCTION

Schizophrenia has been recognized for over 100 years as a form of severe mental illness, typically, although not always, showing an onset in late adolescence or early adulthood. Extensive biological research searching for a unique diagnostic marker has failed to yield a means of diagnosing the illness from a medical test. Accordingly, clinicians remain wholly dependent on the observation of clinical symptom clusters to diagnose the disorder. Since schizophrenia may represent a complex syndrome with diverse etiological bases and disorder outcomes, the identification of specific symptom clusters is vital in the understanding of the nature of the disorder.

The goal of this chapter is to provide an overview of symptom presentation and assessment in schizophrenia. It begins with a historical review chronicling the evolution of diagnostic criteria from the early descriptions of Kraepelin to the fourth edition of the *Diagnostic and Statistical Manual of Mental Disorders* (DSM-IV). Detailed descriptions of currently recognized symptom clusters (e.g., positive, negative, and disorganized symptoms) are presented. Given the increasing emphasis on the documentation of outcomes in clinical practice, the review includes information on commonly used rating scales for the measurement of symptom clusters in schizophrenia.

HISTORICAL OVERVIEW

The history of a psychiatric disorder can be traced through the evolution of the diagnostic criteria that define it. The first descriptive classification system in psychiatry is usually credited to Emil Kraepelin, who considered course and outcome as critical factors in the diagnostic process. Kraepelin viewed mental illness as the result of brain dysfunction with clusters of co-occurring symptoms, or syndromes, reflecting a common etiology. Indeed, Kraepelin's notion of syndromes sparked international controversy when he combined previously independent categories of illness under a common disorder rubric, providing the first description of "manic-depressive insanity" and "dementia praecox." With respect to the early descriptions of schizophrenia, Kraepelin focused on common symptoms (i.e., disturbances of attention and comprehension, hallucinations, affective flattening, and disturbances in the flow of thought) and a chronic, declining course leading to "psychic invalidity" (1).

Eugen Bleuler retained the basic concepts of Kraepelin's descriptive system. However, he elaborated the notion of a somatic etiology to include a pathogenic cascade from molecular biological dysfunction to the manifest clinical symptoms. Bleuler also extended Kraepelin's descriptive work by proposing operational criteria for psychiatric diagnoses. Much of this work focused on delineating the basic and accessory symptoms of psychiatric disorders. Basic symptoms, also referred to as primary symptoms, are those that directly reflect the illness process and therefore must be present for diagnosis of the disorder. With respect to schizophrenia, basic symptoms included hallucinations, disturbances of association, and melancholia. Accessory, or secondary, symptoms are those that may or may not be observed in any given patient. In schizophrenia, accessory symptoms include thought disorder, affect disturbance, cognitive deficits, and avolition (2).

In the late 1930s Kurt Schneider established a pragmatic system for the assessment of schizophrenic symptoms. He defined "first-rank" symptoms as those that maximized diagnostic specificity, including audible thoughts; voices arguing, discussing, or commenting; influenced thought (i.e., thought withdrawal, thought broadcasting); and delusional perception (1). Perplexity, depressive or euphoric mood changes, and emotional impoverishment were viewed as second-rank symptoms (1). Schneider's reliance on clinically relevant and readily recognized symptoms was a strength of his system and a factor in his influence on the development of diagnostic criteria. Interestingly, some recent work (3) suggests that Schneiderian first-rank symptoms may not be useful in differentiating schizophrenia from other psychotic disorders.

In an attempt to create a nationally recognized standard, the American Psychiatric Association adopted a descriptive classification system based largely on the work of Kraepelin. However, the criteria derived by clinical consensus were not universally accepted, and several competing systems grew out of the paradigmatic struggle between the psychoanalysts and biologically oriented psychiatrists. This struggle continued until 1952, when the first DSM was drafted.

In 1968, DSM-II was published and included revisions for an internationally accepted standard as part of the International Classification of Disease (ICD-8) criteria published by the World Health Organization (summarized in Ref. 4). Schizophrenia was defined as a group of psychoses involving a "fundamental disturbance of personality, a characteristic distortion of thinking, often a sense of being controlled by alien forces, delusions which may be bizarre, disturbed perception, abnormal affect out of keeping with the real situation, and autism" (1, p. 35). Further, this revision provided one of the first formal classifications of subtypes, including simple type, hebephrenic type, catatonic type, paranoid type, schizoaffective type, and acute schizophrenic episode.

A significant advancement in psychiatric diagnosis came in 1972, when a group of psychiatrists from Washington University in St. Louis published a paper entitled "Diagnostic Criteria for Use in Psychiatric Research" (5). The paper focused on the beliefs that psychiatry had moved too far away from its roots in medicine and that psychiatric diagnosis should be based on scientific evidence instead of clinical consensus. Proposed diagnostic criteria were presented for 15 mental disorders and were later expanded into the Research Diagnostic Criteria (RDC). The RDC included a broader set of categories focusing primarily on the schizophrenic and affective disorders developed with an associated structured interview called the Schedule for Affective Disorders and Schizophrenia.

The development of the RDC was quickly followed by DSM-III, the first classification system based on scientific evidence rather than clinical consensus. DSM-III also began the use of a multiaxial diagnostic system. An updated version (DSM-III-R) was published in 1987, and in 1994 DSM-IV was published in conjunction with the World Health Organization revision of ICD-10 to make the classification as universal as possible.

DESCRIPTION OF SYMPTOM CLUSTERS

Observations by the early diagnostic clinicians and more recent scientific analysis of symptom presentation suggest that multiple replicable groupings of symptoms can be found in schizophrenia. These include: 1) positive symptoms such as hallucinations and delusions, 2) thought-disorder features demonstrated by impairments in thought process, 3) negative symptoms typified by the absence of behaviors (e.g., emotional affect) common in unaffected individuals, and 4) other symptoms found in schizophrenia but also common in other major psychiatric disorders (e.g., depressed mood). Some uncertainty exists as to which symptoms are primary features of the illness and which symptoms are actually secondary, occurring as a result of the expression of the primary symptoms. The following sections provide a detailed description of these symptom dimensions and their assessment.

Positive Symptoms

Schizophrenia is a heterogeneous disorder with symptoms that often vary over the course of the illness. One of the characteristic clinical features is the marked distortion of reality, often referred to as positive symptoms. These symptoms are typically associated with the acute phase of the disorder, and include hallucinations, delusions, and other experiences that would be considered grossly abnormal. Positive symptoms are typically the targets of treatment with antipsychotic medication.

Delusions—false beliefs that are not subject to reason or contradictory evidence—represent one of the most common positive symptoms associated with schizophrenia. In fact, one source estimated that approximately 90% of patients describe delusional beliefs at some point in the illness (6). Such beliefs may take on different themes (e.g., paranoia or grandiosity) and may or may not be bizarre in nature. Bizarre delusions are thought of as beliefs that are totally out of the realm of physical possibility. For example, an individual may believe that his or her thoughts are being controlled by outside forces as a result of an electronic device that has been placed in the brain. It should be noted that DSM-IV (7) accords the presence of a bizarre delusion primary diagnostic significance in that no other characteristic symptom need be present for diagnosis of schizophrenia. Specific auditory hallucinations (described below) also hold this level of diagnostic significance.

Hallucinations (i.e., perceptions that are disconnected from an appropriate source) are another characteristic symptom of acute schizophrenia. Auditory hallucinations are the most common, occurring in nearly 50% of all patients (6). Several categories of auditory hallucinations were included among Schneider's first-rank signs, including voices speaking thoughts aloud, voices arguing, and voices commenting on the patient. DSM-IV (7) emphasizes the diagnostic importance of some forms of auditory hallucinations (e,g,. a voice that provides a running commentary on the patient's thoughts or behavior). It has been estimated that approximately half of patients reporting auditory hallucinations will describe a voice as directing or commanding behavior. These specific hallucinations may be of clinical importance as predictors of violent or suicidal behavior (8).

Measurement of Positive Symptoms

The Scale for the Assessment of Positive Symptoms (SAPS) (9) is dedicated to the detailed assessment of different types of hallucinations, delusions, and thought disorganization (see below). The scale's broad array of symptoms are listed in Table 1. Each of the positive-symptom domains is broken down into ratings of specific symptoms thought to constitute each domain, and a global severity item is included at the end of the symptom ratings for each domain. Scoring is based on a six-point scale ranging from 0 (not present) to 5 (severe). The scale is often used in conjunction with the Scale for the Assessment of Negative Symptoms (see below).

Thought Disorder

Thought disorder refers to a discontinuity or disorganization of thought resulting in fragmented or illogical speech and grossly disorganized behavior. It is often included under the rubric of positive symptoms although recent research suggests that it represents an independent dimension of symptomatology in schizophrenia (10). In fact, thought disorder has historically been described as a defining feature of schizophrenia, although it may best be conceptualized as a prominent clinical feature most often observed in the acute phase of an illness. Thought disorder, however, is not unique to schizophrenia; manic patients may show elements of it. Indeed, some work has demonstrated that thought-disorder ratings in a group of nonpsychotic manic patients were equal

Table 1 Items in the Scale for the Assessment of Positive Symptoms (SAPS) (the full version of the scale should be consulted for detailed definitions)

Hallucinations
1. Auditory hallucinations
2. Voices commenting
3. Voices conversing
4. Somatic or tactile hallucinations
5. Olfactory hallucinations
6. Visual hallucinations
7. Global rating of severity of hallucinations

Delusions
1. Persecutory delusions
2. Delusions of jealousy
3. Delusions of sin or guilt
4. Grandiose delusions
5. Religious delusions
6. Somatic delusions
7. Ideas and delusions of reference
8. Delusions of being controlled
9. Delusions of mind reading
10. Thought broadcasting
11. Thought insertion
12. Thought withdrawal
13. Global rating of the severity of delusions

Bizarre behavior
1. Clothing and appearance
2. Social and sexual behavior
3. Aggressive and agitated behavior
4. Repetitive or stereotyped behavior
5. Global rating of severity of bizarre behavior

Positive formal thought disorder
1. Derailment (loose associations)
2. Tangentiality
3. Incoherence (word salad)
4. Illogicality
5. Circumstantiality
6. Pressure of speech
7. Distractible speech
8. Clanging
9. Global rating of positive formal thought disorder

Inappropriate affect (single item rating of degree of inappropriate affect)

Source: Copyright © Nancy C. Andreasen.

to ratings from a group of psychotic manic patients during the acute phase of the illness (11). This finding challenges the diagnostic specificity of thought disorder by showing that it may be simply a component of acute psychosis.

Symptoms of thought disorder are typically grouped into two broad categories: disorder of form and disorder of content. However, it should be noted that the familiar distinction of "formal thought disorder" refers specifically to symptoms representing an intrinsic thinking disturbance (i.e., disorder of form). These symptoms include loosening of associations, derailment, neologisms, echolalia, poverty of speech content, and pressure of speech. In contrast, symptoms that reflect disorder of content include delusions regarding the independence and control of one's own thought processes. Examples include thought withdrawal and thought insertion. Appendix C of DSM-IV (7) includes an excellent Glossary of Technical Terms to help clinicians with the finer distinctions between symptoms. Overall, elements of thought disorder vary in frequency, with 2% of schizophrenia patients exhibiting neologisms, 40% demonstrating poverty of speech content, and 56% demonstrating derailment (6). Other work (12) notes that approximately 50% of patients in a large research trial showed conceptual disorganization.

Research suggests that thought disorder is not a unitary construct, but rather is best understood in terms of its multidimensional nature (13). In fact, thought disorder may consist of somewhere between two and six independent dimensions. One of the primary obstacles in this research is the tremendous difficulty encountered in measuring thought disorder (see below). Consequently, our current understanding of the construct is guided as much by theory and clinical experience as it is by empirical research. Features of thought disorder include disorganization, negative thought disorder or alogia, positive thought disorder or mania, attention disturbance, and semantic anomalies (13).

Measurement of Thought Disorder

There is a relative paucity of assessment techniques providing thorough and reliable measurement of thought disorder. One difficulty in this work relates to the process of measuring thought disorder itself, since structured social interactions that take place in interviews may actually reduce the expression of thought disorder in schizophrenic patients. One approach, referred to as the Thought Disorder Index, evaluates the verbal productions of schizophrenic patients in an unstructured interaction (14). Another approach, the Assessment of Thought, Language, and Communication (15), provides for a clinical rating of a range of elements of thought disorder. In addition, broad-scope rating scales (see below) often used in schizophrenia research provide for some global summary measures (e.g., severity of conceptual disorganization) of thought disorder.

Negative Symptoms

Broadly defined, negative symptoms may be taken as those that are absent or diminished in schizophrenic individuals but are typically present in unaffected persons. It should be noted that there is some disparity regarding exactly what should be grouped under the heading of negative symptoms. However, definitions of negative symptoms have nearly universally included affective flattening (16), typically observed through specific features such as unchanging facial expression, affective nonresponsivity, and decreased movements. Negative symptoms have also been taken to include deficits in mental activity (i.e., alogia) as observed by lack of speech and increased latency of response. Features of amotivation and apathy have been included in some definitions.

As noted previously, both Kraeplin and Bleuler noted disorder features such as disturbances in volition, drive, and affect (2). However, probably due to several factors, there has been a significant increase in interest in negative symptoms over the past 20 years. Typical antipsychotic medications may well be useful for reducing positive symptoms in many patients, but many patients continue to have persistent negative symptoms. An increasing interest in negative symptoms may be related to the introduction of atypical antipsychotics (e.g., clozapine) that may have relatively greater efficacy in treating such symptoms.

The observation that typical antipsychotic agents are relatively ineffective in treating negative symptoms, as well as other research data, has led to speculation that negative symptoms may have a biological basis that could be at least somewhat independent from the biological underpinnings of positive psychotic symptoms. Alhough there are some discrepant findings, some studies have linked negative symptoms to cognitive impairments frequently observed in schizophrenia. Schizophrenic patients tend to show differences in brain morphology (e.g., ventricular enlargement and gray-matter deficits) when compared with unaffected individuals, and some (17), although not all (18), work has suggested that such abnormalities may relate to negative symptoms. Auditory evoked potentials such as the P300 may reflect the electrophysiological basis of novel information processing, and numerous studies have noted abnormalities in P300 amplitude and latency in schizophrenia. Several works have noted relationships between abnormalities in the P300 and the severity of negative symptoms (19). Some work (20) has suggested unique neurochemical correlates of negative symptoms.

Negative symptoms are present at illness onset and subsequently may be stable following longitudinal measurement (21). Thus, negative symptoms are likely one of the core disabling features of schizophrenia and among the most difficult to treat. Attempts at social rehabilitation are often focused on overcoming negative symptom features such as avolition.

Deficit Symptoms and Primary vs. Secondary Negative Symptoms

The construct of negative symptoms has been refined and expanded in recent years. Notions of deficit and primary and secondary negative symptoms have been advanced. While some definitions and clinical measures of negative symptoms reflect clinical symptomatology (e.g., blunted affect) that fluctuate over time with both treatment and disorder remission/exacerbation, deficit symptoms (or a deficit syndrome) have been defined as intrapsychic, interpersonal, and instrumental functioning deficits that fluctuate less over time (22). Deficit-syndrome symptoms are characterized by what have been called primary negative symptoms, or symptoms judged to be primary manifestations of the avolitional aspects of schizophrenia (23). Secondary negative symptoms have been advanced as being actually more closely related to other causes such as medication side effects (e.g., masked facies and bradykinesia, both pseudoparkinsonian features), depression, or suspiciousness.

Deficit symptoms can be reliably assessed, although it has been questioned as to how one can make an accurate distinction between primary and secondary negative symptoms in a given patient. The categorization of patients into deficit and nondeficit groups has been shown to have a high degree of stability over an approximate 4-year follow-up period (24). Deficit symptoms relate to disorder characteristics such as neuropsychological functioning (25) and MRI-derived structural brain measures (26). Interestingly, some work (27) suggests that nondeficit schizophrenic patients could benefit from intensive social-skills training, but patients with significant deficit symptoms had difficulties in acquisition of social skills.

Measurement of Negative/Deficit Symptoms

There has been some speculation that the measurement of negative symptoms can be more difficult than that of positive symptoms, perhaps because the assessment of the absence of an expected behavior is somewhat more difficult than measuring the presence of psychotic symptoms that are rarely present in the general population. However, research suggests that with some degree of education and training one can achieve adequate reliability levels for negative-symptom assessment.

One of the first and primary rating scales for evaluating such symptoms is the Scale for the Assessment of Negative Symptoms (SANS) (28). The item coverage of the SANS is provided in Table 2. It

Table 2 Items in the Scale for the Assessment of Negative Symptoms (SANS) (the full version of the scale contains needed descriptors)

Affective flattening or blunting
1. Unchanging facial expression
2. Decreased spontaneous movements
3. Paucity of expressive gestures
4. Poor eye contact
5. Affective nonresponsivity
6. Lack of vocal inflections
7. Global rating of affective flattening

Alogia
1. Poverty of speech
2. Poverty of content of speech
3. Blocking
4. Increased latency of response
5. Global rating of alogia

Avolition–apathy
1. Grooming and hygiene
2. Impersistence at work or school
3. Physical anergia
4. Global rating of avolition-apathy

Anhedonia–asociality
1. Recreational interests and activities
2. Sexual interest and activity
3. Ability to feel intimacy and closeness
4. Relationships with friends and peers
5. Global rating of anhedonia–asociality

Attention
1. Social inattentiveness
2. Inattentiveness during mental status testing
3. Global rating of attention

Source: Copyright © Nancy C. Andreasen.

should be noted that the full scale provides detailed descriptions for each item that are too lengthy to reprint here, but are vital for the proper use of the instrument. The instrument breaks down negative symptoms into five domains: affective blunting, alogia, avolition/apathy, anhedonia/asociality, and disturbance of attention. Scoring is similar to that described above for the SAPS, with items being scored on a six-point scale ranging from 0 (not present; patient shows no features of the item) to 5 (severe). The SANS has been shown to be reliable and has been extensively validated.

Several techniques have been offered for the documentation of the deficit syndrome. The Quality of Life Scale (22) is a 21-item scale that offers a measure of interpersonal relationships, instrumental role functioning, intrapsychic foundations (e.g., sense of purpose, motivation), and the presence of commonplace objects and activities. The scale is scored on a 0-to-6 scale. Items included in the scale are detailed in Table 3.

More recent work (29) has offered a further technique for the categorization of schizophrenic patients into deficit and nondeficit groups. A clinical interview and review of other information (e.g., reports of family and treating clinicians) are conducted to assess the characteristics of a patient across long periods of clinical stability. The schedule provides suggested questions and procedures to collect data in order to determine whether patients formally meet the diagnostic criteria listed in Table 4.

The documentation of negative symptoms may also be performed using more broad-scoped instruments that assess a wide range of symptoms. The Brief Psychiatric Rating Scale (BPRS) (30,31) provides a range of items (e.g., blunted affect, emotional withdrawal, psychomotor retardation) that reflect current symptom severity of aspects of negative symptoms. These BPRS items correlate fairly well with negative-symptom measures derived from the SANS (32), thus yielding a rapid assessment of current negative symptoms. The Positive and Negative Syndrome Scale (PANSS) contains a modified and behaviorally anchored version of the BPRS negative-symptom items noted above plus additional items reflecting negative symptoms as well as other symptoms commonly found in schizophrenia (33).

Symptoms Found in Schizophrenia and Shared with Other Disorders

Research in symptom expression in schizophrenia has emphasized dimensions of thought disorder, negative symptoms, and positive

Table 3 Items in the Quality of Life Scale to Assess Deficit Symptoms in Schizophrenia

1. Intimate relationships with household members
2. Intimate relationships (i.e., with people other than family/household members)
3. Active acquaintances
4. Level of social activity
5. Involved social network
6. Social initiatives
7. Social withdrawal (i.e., active avoidance)
8. Sociosexual relations
9. Occupational role functioning
10. Level of accomplishment (i.e., level of success in fulfilling the role chosen)
11. Degree of underemployment (i.e., utilization of potentiality and opportunities)
12. Satisfaction with occupational role functioning
13. Sense of purpose
14. Degree of motivation
15. Level of curiosity
16. Anhedonia (i.e., capacity to experience pleasure)
17. Time utilization (i.e., amount of time passed in aimless inactivity).
18. Commonplace objects (e.g., whether patient has common objects such as a watch)
19. Commonplace activities (e.g., whether patients engage in specific common activities)
20. Capacity for empathy
21. Capacity for engagement and emotional interaction with interviewer

Source: Courtesy of W. T. Carpenter.

symptoms. However, other dimensions of psychopathology may be present in schizophrenia. Two such dimensions that have received some attention are depressive and obsessive-compulsive symptoms.

Depression

Schizophrenic patients may present with significant symptoms of depression. One work (34) noted that 20% of older (age 45–79) schizophrenic women had Hamilton Depression Scale scores greater than 17, a level suggestive of depression. Schizophrenic patients at the time of first hospitalization may have a high prevalence of depression (35). Another study (36) of patients early in the course of schizophrenia found a similar high frequency of depression. Depression was noted to be associated with age and suicidal tendencies. In sum, depression may

Table 4 Diagnostic Criteria for the Deficit Syndrome of Schizophrenia (criteria are used in conjunction with the Schedule for the Deficit Syndrome)

1. At least two of the following six symptoms must be present:
   a. Restricted affect
   b. Diminished emotional range
   c. Poverty of speech
   d. Curbing of interests
   e. Diminished sense of purpose
   f. Diminished social drive
2. Some combination of 2 or more of the negative symptoms listed above have been present for the preceding 12 months and were always present during periods of clinical stability (including chronic psychotic states). These symptoms may or may not be detectable during transient episodes of acute psychotic disorganization or decompensation.
3. The negative symptoms above are primary, i.e., not secondary to factors other than the disease process. Such factors include:
   a. Anxiety
   b. Drug effect
   c. Suspiciousness (and other psychotic symptoms)
   d. Mental retardation
   e. Depression
4. The patient meets DSM-III-R criteria for schizophrenia.

Source: From Kirkpatrick B, Buchanan RW, McKenney PD, Alphs LD, Carpenter WT Jr. The Schedule for the Deficit Syndrome: an instrument for research in schizophrenia. Psychiatry Res 1989; 30:119–123. Copyright © 1989 Elsevier Science.

be an important symptom dimension (e.g., suggestive of suicide risk) that can be easily overlooked given the usual emphasis on positive and negative symptoms in the clinical care of schizophrenic patients.

Obsessive-Compulsive Disorder

Clinicians may note that patients with schizophrenia periodically show obsessive and/or compulsive symptoms. Such symptoms may take the form of persistent thoughts on a particular topic or persistent repetitive actions that the patient feels compelled to perform. One recent study (37) used a variety of assessment methods to show that approximately 8% of patients met criteria for obsessive-compulsive disorder (OCD) in addition to schizophrenia or schizoaffective disorder. Other work (38) noted a 13% rate of OCD in a diagnostically mixed group of patients with diagnoses of schizophrenia, schizoaffective disorder, and bipolar disorder. In sum, OCD features may not be rare in schizophrenia. The biological and prognostic importance of such symptoms remains to be clarified, although the incidence of OCD symptoms suggests that formal treatment studies for such symptoms are warranted (37).

AN IMPORTANT DIMENSION OF COGNITIVE IMPAIRMENT

There has been a growing recognition that schizophrenic patients frequently display impairments in memory, attention, and executive cognitive functioning (see Chapter 5 for a full review). These impairments are currently rarely considered when one details the traditional symptom clusters of schizophrenia, because such features typically require formal testing to be documented, yet cognitive impairments in schizophrenia may be among the best predictors of outcome and functioning. These impairments are not merely the result of medication side effects, but represent a core component of the illness (39). One recent review (40) has suggested that measures of psychosis are poorly associated with outcome. However, neuropsychological deficits and negative symptoms are related to important outcome dimensions such as community functioning, social problem solving, and skill acquisition (40). These findings suggest that cognitive deficits are probably underassessed in the clinical care of schizophrenic patients, since such problems may better predict outcome than the psychotic symptoms that are frequently the predominant focus of treating clinicians.

BROAD-SCOPE MEASURES OF SYMPTOM SEVERITY IN SCHIZOPHRENIA

As reviewed in Table 5, multiple specific rating scales have been offered for the measurement of symptoms such as positive or negative symptoms. An alternative approach to symptom measurement is the use of broad-scope measures of global symptom severity. One of the most widely employed rating scales in psychiatric research is the 18-item BPRS (31), mentioned earlier. The scale has gained extensive use in psychopharmacology research. The 18 items contained within the BPRS, listed in Table 6, are scored from 1 (not present) to 7 (extremely severe) following a 20–30-minute clinical interview of the patient. Although the scale was developed with the goal of measuring psychopathology found in a range of severe psychiatric disorders, it has been used most extensively in schizophrenia research. Each item in Table 6 has detailed definitions that should be used in the clinical applications of the scale (31). Various combinations of items have been thought to provide an

Table 5 Knowing Which Symptoms Are Which

Positive symptoms

1. Defined as grossly abnormal experiences/behaviors not typically observed in nonpatient groups
2. Typically observed in the acute phase of the disorder and represent a primary target of antipsychotic medications
3. Includes delusional ideation, hallucinations, and other anomalous perceptual experiences
4. Measured by scales such as Scale for the Assessment of Positive Symptoms (SAPS)

Thought disorder

1. Defined as discontinuity of thought resulting in fragmented of illogical speech and grossly disorganized behavior
2. Typically observed in acute phase of disorder with residual thought-disorder symptoms associated with poor prognosis
3. Symptoms include neologisms, derailment, thought blocking, circumstantiality
4. Measured by the Scale for the Assessment of Thought, Language, and Communication (TLC) and other techniques

Negative and deficit symptoms

1. Defined as symptoms that are altered or diminished in patients but typically present in the general population
2. Commonly include features such as affective flattening, avolition, affective nonresponsivity
3. Negative symptoms may be present over the entire course of the illness, and represent one of the most difficult to treat aspects of the disorder
4. Deficit symptoms include enduring deficits in intrapsychic, interpersonal, and instrumental functioning
5. Related to poor social outcome, including skill acquisition
6. Negative symptoms measured by the Schedule for the Assessment of Negative Symptoms and other scales; deficit symptoms measured by the Quality of Life Scale

acceptable rapid assessment of features of negative and positive symptoms (32,41).

A relatively new broad-scope rating instrument for the assessment of schizophrenia is the PANSS (33). As explained above, this scale contains a modified and behaviorally anchored version of the 18 core BPRS items plus 12 additional items (33). This instrument seeks to provide expanded coverage of negative symptoms as well as other positive and general psychiatric symptoms commonly found in schizophrenia (33). As reviewed below, the instrument has been included in factor-analytic work seeking unique symptom clusters in schizophrenia.

Table 6 Symptom Coverage Provided by the Brief Psychiatric Rating Scale (items are scored on a seven-point scale ranging from not present to extremely severe)

1. Somatic concern
2. Anxiety
3. Emotional withdrawal
4. Conceptual disorganization
5. Guilt feelings
6. Tension
7. Mannerisms and posturing
8. Grandiosity
9. Depressed mood
10. Hostility
11. Suspiciousness
12. Hallucinatory behavior
13. Motor retardation
14. Uncooperativeness
15. Unusual thought content
16. Blunted affect
17. Excitement
18. Disorientation

Source: Adapted from Ref. 30.

Use of the PANSS has been growing in clinical treatment trials in schizophrenia. A structured clinical interview has been offered to assist in the assessment of symptoms for completing the scale. The PANSS and supporting materials are available from Multi-Health Systems, 908 Niagara Falls Blvd., North Tonawanda, NY 14120.

Defining Symptom Clusters in Schizophrenia

A major goal of research in symptom expression in schizophrenia is the identification of replicable clusters of symptoms that tend to be associated with one another and are, at least to some degree, independent of other groups of symptoms. To achieve this goal, researchers employ statistical techniques called factor analysis—often using a specific technique called principal-components analysis, which generates groupings of symptoms that are independent of one another. Such studies can be either exploratory (entering large numbers of items derived from many patient observations to determine relationships) or confirmatory (testing whether specific hypothesized models of clusters of symptoms can be fit from the clinical ratings).

The findings of factor-analytic work are obviously dependent on the type of symptom measures entered into the analysis. In reviewing this work it is important to note that research restricted to the evaluation of core schizophrenic/psychotic-disorder symptoms will yield different results than work employing rating scales (e.g., BPRS and PANSS) that include symptoms that are not specific to schizophrenia (e.g., depressed mood).

Numerous works have performed factor analyses of ratings of schizophrenic patients who were evaluated with the SANS and SAPS. These works have generally identified three major symptom factors (42): 1) negative symptoms (e.g., SANS measures such as affective flattening, avolition), 2) positive psychotic symptoms (e.g., delusions, hallucinations), and 3) what has been deemed a disorganization factor (e.g., formal thought disorder). Table 7 provides the factor loading for the global SANS and SAPS items that were entered into analysis and demonstrates the relative factor loadings for the measures.

There has been significant clarification of the nature of some symptoms in schizophrenia. For example, inappropriate affect may well relate more to disorganized symptoms than to negative symptoms (the

Table 7 Varimax Rotated Factor Structure of the Global Items from the Scale for the Assessment of Negative Symptoms and the Scale for the Assessment of Positive Symptoms

	Factor		
Symptom	Negative	Disorganized	Psychotic
Avolition	**0.832**	0.131	0.172
Anhedonia	**0.818**	0.179	0.110
Affective flattening	**0.809**	–0.105	0.036
Inappropriate affect	0.057	**0.796**	–0.114
Thought disorder	–0.050	**0.754**	0.267
Bizarre behavior	**0.426**	**0.598**	0.249
Delusions	0.071	0.175	**0.821**
Hallucinations	0.168	0.012	**0.759**
Variance explained	2.235	1.652	1.440
Percentage	27.938	20.650	18.000

Boldface = highest correlations ($r > 0.4$) on a factor for a given item.
Source: From Ref. 10. Copyright © 1995 American Medical Association.

item is now placed on the SAPS rather than the SANS) and attentional impairment relates to multiple symptom factors, including disorganization, negative symptoms, and, to some degree, psychotic symptoms (43). The SANS construct of alogia is somewhat complicated, with elements (e.g., poverty of speech content) loading on a disorganized factor while other items (e.g., poverty of speech) fall on the negative symptom factor

One interesting recent work (44) has expanded prior factor-analytic work with the SANS and SAPS. This study examined a large sample (N = 630) using a principal-component analysis of global items and noted the negative, positive, and disorganized factors. Interestingly, an individual-item-level (rather than global-item level) factor analysis found two negative-symptom factors (disordered relating and diminished expression), two positive-symptom factors (bizarre delusions and hallucinations), and a single disorganization factor. This finding suggests that information in the SANS and SAPS is lost when only global ratings are used (44).

Factor-Analytic Work with the BPRS and PANSS

As noted above, the BPRS is among the most widely used clinical rating scales in psychiatric research. This scale was developed nearly 40 years ago without being linked to any specific diagnostic group, thus having utility in settings where diagnostically diverse samples require rapid symptom assessment (e.g., in inpatient general psychiatric units). Accordingly, much of the factor-analytic work with this scale has been performed in samples of patients with a broad range of severe mental illness diagnoses. This work has suggested factors that include thinking disturbance, withdrawal/retardation, hostility/suspiciousness, and anxiety/depression (31). Although these factors have gained widespread use in clinical research, it should be stressed that they were not originally derived in samples composed exclusively of schizophrenic patients. This fact has recently been criticized in an article (45) that suggests that these factors derived from diagnostically diverse samples may not fit the data well in a confirmatory factor analysis using exclusively schizophrenic patients. The authors used a further exploratory analysis to note that a three-factor model could be derived showing negative, positive, and disorganization factors.

As noted above, the PANSS represents a broad-scope symptom assessment that includes additional items thought to reflect a broad range of symptoms. The original scoring for the instrument (33) divided symptomatology into dimensions of positive, negative, and general psychopathology. Subsequent factor-analytic work has suggested that the scale is somewhat more factorially complicated than this division. A five-factor solution (negative, positive, excitement, depressive, and cognitive) has been suggested in multiple studies (46–48).

A recent confirmatory factor analysis in a large sample tested the goodness of fit of 20 PANSS-based models of schizophrenic symptoms (49). None of the proposed models, including the original three-factor model (33), was found to adequately fit the data derived from 1233 schizophrenic subjects. Further analyses suggested a five-factor model (positive, negative, dysphoric mood, activation, and autistic preoccupation) that used 25 of the 30 PANSS items (49). The authors expressed concerns about characteristics of the scale, since multiple PANSS items were found to fall on several factors. Further concern was noted regarding the ability of the PANSS to adequately assess the commonly found disorganization factor derived from work with the SANS and SAPS (49). The authors provide suggestions for revision of the instrument.

SUMMARY AND CONCLUSIONS ON THE IMPORTANCE OF SYMPTOM CLUSTERS

Observations about symptom expression in schizophrenia date back over 100 years. Despite significant developments in symptom measurement (e.g., detailed and reliable rating scales) and analysis (e.g., sophisticated factor-analytic techniques), it is remarkable how many similarities there are between the current empirically derived symptom clusters in schizophrenia and the observations of early writers. As noted in Table 8, current work suggests that the unique core syndrome of schizophrenia consists of dimensions of positive, negative, and disorganized symptoms. Further work using instruments (e.g., the PANSS) sampling symptoms shared with other disorders suggests the presence of other clusters that may include dimensions such as dysphoric mood/depression, activation or excitement, and autistic preoccupation (48,49).

Table 8 Main Points in Factor-Analytic Studies

1. Studies making use of rating scales tapping specific schizophrenic features (SAPS and SANS) often note unique groups of symptoms that include positive, negative, and disorganized symptom clusters.
2. Studies using instruments (e.g., the PANSS) that evaluate a broad range of symptoms find clusters that often include positive, negative, dysphoric mood, excitement, and cognitive (i.e., disorganized) features.

Symptom clusters tend to show different levels of severity in different phases of the illness, and the importance of various symptom dimensions may well depend on the context of disorder exacerbation or remission. For example, some work has shown that the severity of psychosis and paranoia relates to overall quality of life when patients are stabilized, but that positive and paranoid symptoms are unrelated to overall quality of life if one considers symptom severity only in acutely exacerbated patients (50). Other work indicates that thought disorder may also relate to the acute phase of the illness and may not be unique to schizophrenia.

Negative and cognitive symptoms may be of importance in that they strongly relate to greater levels of disability in individuals affected with schizophrenia. The presence of negative symptoms early in the illness may have predictive validity for outcome and prognosis five years later (51). Other work suggests that negative symptoms measured by scales such as the PANSS relate to poor social adjustment, poor prognosis, and diminished medication response (52). Negative symptom may be associated with diminished verbal and visual memory as well as poor verbal fluency (53). Patients with enduring negative symptoms may show greater deficits on cognitive measures sensitive to frontal- and parietal-lobe functions (54). Some authors have suggested that positive-symptom severity may not be related to deficits in cognitive functioning (53). Negative symptoms and cognitive impairments have been found to be the strongest correlates of functional status in geriatric, poor-outcome schizophrenic patients (55).

The differentiation of negative and deficit symptoms may also be an important subgrouping dimension in schizophrenia. Negative symptoms may be taken to include features of the illness (e.g., blunted affect reflected in reduced emotional tone) that have some degree of treatment response to medications such as atypical antipsychotics. Some work suggests that negative symptoms are stable over time and are a major target of psychosocial treatment interventions. Deficit symptoms have been more broadly defined to include enduring deficits in social, vocational, and instrumental functioning. These deficits are judged to be at the core of the avolitional aspects of schizophrenia. Deficit symptoms may be of broad prognostic and biological importance, with prior work showing relationships between deficit symptoms and social-skills acquisition, cognitive functioning, and brain morphology.

Symptom clusters may well have unique biological underpinnings and may relate to greater or lesser degrees to disorder outcome. In essence, symptom clusters may be thought of as the unique behavioral expressions of the brain mechanisms that likely underlie this complicated and disabling disorder.

REFERENCES

1. Berner P, Gabriel E, Katschnig H, Kieffer W, Koehler K, Lenz G, Sinhandl C. Diagnostic Criteria for Schizophrenic and Affective Psychoses. World Psychiatric Association, 1983.
2. Arieti S. Interpretation of Schizophrenia. 2nd ed. New York: Basic Books, 1974.
3. Peralta V, Cuesta MJ. Diagnostic significance of Schneider's first-rank symptoms in schizophrenia: comparative study between schizophrenic and nonschizophrenic psychotic disorders. Br J Psychiatry 1999; 174:243–248.
4. Blashfield RK. Models of psychiatric classification. In: Hersen M, Turner SM, eds. Adult Psychopathology and Diagnosis. New York: John Wiley & Sons, 1991:3–22.
5. Feighner JP, Robins E, Guze S, Woodruff RA, Winokur G, Munoz R. Diagnostic criteria for use in psychiatric research. Arch Gen Psychiatry 1972; 26:57–63.
6. Cutting J. The Right Cerebral Hemisphere and Psychiatric Disorders. Oxford: Oxford University Press, 1990.
7. American Psychiatric Association. Diagnostic and Statistical Manual of Mental Disorders. 4th ed. Washington, DC: American Psychiatric Press, 1994.
8. Zisook S, Byrd D, Kuck J, Jeste DV. Command hallucinations in outpatients with schizophrenia. J Clin Psychiatry 1995; 56:462–465.
9. Andreasen NC. The Scale for the Assessment of Positive Symptoms (SAPS). Iowa City: University of Iowa, 1984.
10. Andreasen NC, Arndt S, Alliger R, Miller D, Flaum M. Symptoms of schizophrenia: methods, meanings, and mechanisms. Arch Gen Psychiatry 1995; 52:341–351.
11. Harrow M, Silverstein M, Marengo J. Disordered thinking. Arch Gen Psychiatry 1983; 40:765–771.
12. Breier A, Berg PH. The psychosis of schizophrenia: prevalence, response to atypical antipsychotics, and prediction of outcome. Biol Psychiatry 1999; 46:361–364.
13. Cuestra M, Peralta V. Thought disorder in schizophrenia: testing models through confirmatory factor analysis. Eur Arch Psychiatry Clin Neurosci 1999; 249:55–61.
14. Hurt SW, Holzman PS, Davis JM. Thought disorder: the measurement of its changes. Arch Gen Psychiatry 1983; 40:1281–1285.
15. Andreasen NC. Thought, language, and communication disorders: clinical assessment, definition of terms, and evaluation of their reliability. Arch Gen Psychiatry 1979; 36:1315–1321.

16. Fenton WS, McGlashan TH. Testing systems for assessment of negative symptoms in schizophrenia. Arch Gen Psychiatry 1992; 49:179–184.
17. Flaum M, O'Leary DS, Swayze VW 2nd, Miller DD, Arndt S, Andreasen NC. Symptom dimensions and brain morphology in schizophrenia and related psychotic disorders. J Psychiatr Res 1995; 29:261–276.
18. Gur RE, Turetsky BI, Bilker WB, Gur RC. Reduced gray matter volume in schizophrenia. Arch Gen Psychiatry 1999; 56:905–911.
19. Ford JM. Schizophrenia: the broken P300 and beyond. Psychophysiology 1999; 36:667–682.
20. Csernansky JG, King R, Faustman WO, Moses JA Jr, Poscher M, Faull K. 5-HIAA in cerebrospinal fluid and deficit schizophrenic characteristics. Br J Psychiatry 1990; 156:501–507.
21. Arndt S, Andreasen NC, Flaum M, Miller D, Nopoulos P. A longitudinal study of symptom dimensions in schizophrenia: prediction and patterns of change. Arch Gen Psychiatry 1995; 52:352–360.
22. Heinrichs DW, Hanon TE, Carpenter WT. The Quality of Life Scale: an instrument for rating the schizophrenia deficit syndrome. Schizophr Bull 1984; 10:388–398.
23. Kirkpatrick B, Castle D, Murray RM, Carpenter WT Jr. Risk factors for the deficit syndrome of schizophrenia. Schizophr Bull 2000; 26:233–242.
24. Amador XF, Kirkpatrick B, Buchanan RW, Carpenter WT, Marcinko L, Yale SA. Stability of the diagnosis of deficit syndrome in schizophrenia. Am J Psychiatry 1999; 156:637–639.
25. Buchanan RW, Strauss ME, Kirkpatrick B, Holstein C, Breier A, Carpenter WT Jr. Neuropsychological impairments in deficit vs. nondeficit forms of schizophrenia. Arch Gen Psychiatry 1994; 51:804–811.
26. Turetsky B, Cowell P, Gur RC, Grossman RI, Shtasel DL, Gur RE. Frontal and temporal lobe brain volumes in schizophrenia: relationship to symptoms and clinical subtype. Arch Gen Psychiatry 1995; 52:1061–1070.
27. Kopelowicz A, Liberman RP, Mintz J, Zarate R. Comparison of efficacy of social skills training for deficit and nondeficit negative symptoms in schizophrenia. Am J Psychiatry 1997; 154:424–425.
28. Andreasen NC, Olsen SA. Negative versus positive schizophrenia: definition and validation. Arch Gen Psychiatry 1982; 39:789–794.
29. Kirkpatrick B, Buchanan RW, McKenney PD, Alphs LD, Carpenter WT Jr. The Schedule for the Deficit Syndrome: an instrument for research in schizophrenia. Psychiatry Res 1989; 30:119–123.
30. Overall JE, Gorham DR. The Brief Psychiatric Rating Scale (BPRS): recent developments in ascertainment and scaling. Psychopharmacol Bull 1988; 24:97–99.
31. Faustman WO, Overall JE. Brief Psychiatric Rating Scale. In: Maruish ME, ed. The Use of Psychological Testing for Treatment Planning and Outcomes Assessment. 2nd ed. Mahwah, NJ: Lawrence Erlbaum, 1999:791–830.
32. Thiemann S, Csernansky JG, Berger PA. Rating scales in research: the case of negative symptoms. Psychiatry Res 1987; 20:47–55.

33. Kay SR, Fiszbein A, Opler LA. The Positive and Negative Syndrome Scale (PANSS) for schizophrenia. Schizophr Bull 1987; 13:261–275
34. Zisook S, McAdams LA, Kuck J, Harris MJ, Bailey A, Patterson TL, Judd LL, Jeste DV. Depressive symptoms in schizophrenia. Am J Psychiatry 1999; 156:1736–1743.
35. Bottlender R, Strauss A, Moller HJ. Prevalence and background factors of depression in first admitted schizophrenic patients. Acta Psychiatr Scand 2000; 101:153–160.
36. Wassink TH, Flaumm M, Nopoulos P, Andreasen NC. Prevalence of depressive symptoms early in the course of schizophrenia. Am J Psychiatry 1999; 156:315–316.
37. Eisen JL, Beer DA, Pato MT, Venditto TA, Rasmussen SA. Obsessive-compulsive disorder in patients with schizophrenia or schizoaffective disorder. Am J Psychiatry 1997; 154:271–273.
38. Cosoff SJ, Hafner RJ. The prevalence of comorbid anxiety in schizophrenia, schizoaffective disorder and bipolar disorder. Aust N Z J Psychiatry 1998; 32:67–72.
39. Faustman WO, Hoff AL. Effects of antipsychotic medications on cognitive measures. In: Csernansky J, ed. Handbook of Experimental Pharmacology. Vol 120. Antipsychotics. Berlin: Springer-Verlag, 1996:445–477.
40. Green MF. What are the functional consequences of neurocognitive deficits in schizophrenia? Am J Psychiatry 1996; 153:321–330.
41. Nicholson IR, Chapman JE, Neufeld RWJ. Variability in BPRS definitions of positive and negative symptoms. Schizophr Res 1995; 17:177–185
42. Andreasen NC, Arndt S, Miller D, Flaum M, Nopoulos P. Correlational studies of the Scale for the Assessment of Negative Symptoms and the Scale for the Assessment of Positive Symptoms: an overview and update. Psychopathology 1995; 28:7–17.
43. Miller DD, Arndt S, Andreasen NC. Alogia, attentional impairment, and inappropriate affect: their status in the dimensions of schizophrenia. Compr Psychiatry 1993; 34:221–226.
44. Toomey R, Kremen WS, Simpson JC, Samson JA, Seidman LJ, Lyons MJ, Faraone SV, Tsuang MT. Revisiting the factor structure for positive and negative symptoms: evidence from a large heterogeneous group of psychiatric patients. Am J Psychiatry 1997; 154:371–377.
45. Harvey PD, Davidson M, White L, Keefe RSE, Hirschowitz J, Mohs RC, Davis KL. Empirical evaluation of the factorial structure of clinical symptoms in schizophrenia: effects of typical neuroleptics on the Brief Psychiatric Rating Scale. Biol Psychiatry 1996; 40:755–760.
46. Kay SR, Sevy S. Pyramidal model of schizophrenia. Schizophr Bull 1990; 16:537–545.
47. Bell MD, Lysaker PH, Beam-Goulet JL, Milstein RM, Lindenmayer JP. Five-component model of schizophrenia: assessing the factorial invariance of the Positive and Negative Syndrome Scale. Psychiatry Res 1994; 52:295–303.

48. Mass R, Schoemig T, Hitschfeld K, Wall E, Haasen C. Psychopathological syndromes of schizophrenia: evaluation of the dimensional structure of the Positive and Negative Syndrome Scale. Schizophr Bull 2000; 26:167–177.
49. White L, Harvey PD, Opler L, Lindenmayer JP. Empirical assessment of the factorial structure of clinical symptoms in schizophrenia: a multisite, multimodal evaluation of the factorial structure of the Positive and Negative Syndrome Scale. Psychopathology 1997; 30:263–274.
50. Bow-Thomas CC, Velligan DI, Miler AL, Olsen J. Predicting quality of life from symptomatology in schizophrenia at exacerbation and stabilization. Psychiatry Res 1999; 86:131–142.
51. Weiselgren IM, Lindstom E, Lindstrom LH. Symptoms at index admission as predictor for 1–5 year outcome in schizophrenia. Acta Psychiatr Scand 1996; 94:311–319.
52. Peralta V, Cuesta MJ, de Leon J. Positive and negative symptoms/syndromes in schizophrenia: reliability and validity of different diagnostic systems. Psychol Med 1995; 25:43–50.
53. O'Leary DS, Flaum M, Kesler ML, Flashman LA, Arndt S, Andreasen NC. Cognitive correlates of the negative, disorganized, and psychotic dimensions of schizophrenia. J Neuropsychiatry Clin Neurosci 2000; 12:4–15.
54. Putnam KM, Harvey PD. Cognitive impairment and enduring negative symptoms. Schizophr Bull 2000; 26:867–878.
55. Harvey PD, Jacobsen H, Mancini D, Parrella M, White L, Haroutunian V, Davis KL. Clinical, cognitive and functional characteristics of long-stay patients with schizophrenia: a comparison of VA and state hospital patients. Schizophr Res 2000; 43:3–9.

3

Differential Diagnosis of Schizophrenia

Del D. Miller and Susan K. Schultz
The University of Iowa
Iowa City, Iowa

INTRODUCTION

Schizophrenia is one of the first diagnoses that should come to mind when a clinician encounters a patient experiencing delusions, hallucinations, disorganized speech, grossly disorganized or catatonic behavior, or negative symptoms (i.e., affective flattening, alogia, or avolition). However, the clinician must keep in mind that there is no one pathognomonic feature of schizophrenia. The above symptoms can, and often do, occur in other psychiatric, neurological, and medical conditions, as well as with certain medications and substance abuse (1). It cannot be emphasized enough that no single feature (e.g., cross-sectional symptomatology, course, family history, response to treatment, or laboratory findings) will alone determine a diagnosis of schizophrenia. In general, the reliability of differentiating schizophrenia from the other disorders is strengthened by the presence of several of these characteristic features occurring in a manner consistent with the persistent courses and social/occupational impairment as outlined in the fourth edition of the *Diagnostic and Statistical Manual of Mental Disorders* (DSM-IV) (2).

In the absence of a clear pre-existing psychotic disorder, every patient with an acute episode of psychosis should have a thorough medical workup, including medical and psychiatric histories, medication history, physical and mental status examination, and laboratory evaluation, including urinalysis and toxicology screens (3,4). A detailed history should be elicited from the patient and from family members and other informants regarding any previous episodes of psychotic symptoms or other psychiatric symptoms. The time course and treatment response to any previous treatments should be documented as well. Further information such as family history of psychiatric illness, use of alcohol and illicit drugs, social and occupational functioning, and the presence of any recent stressors may yield important clues to the source of the episode at hand.

When applying diagnostic criteria for schizophrenia, it is important to carefully determine the mode, time of onset, and course of each presenting symptom. One should also establish the presence or absence of symptoms required for the diagnosis of schizophrenia using reliable, narrow definitions of such symptoms. It is equally important to review the presence or absence of symptoms of bipolar affective disorder and major depressive disorder because they may account for the psychotic symptoms and the age of first onset coincides with the typical onset of schizophrenia. Similarly, abuse of such substances as crystal methamphetamine (crank) not infrequently results in psychosis and is used primarily by young adults in the age range of a typical onset of schizophrenia. Crystal methamphetamine has been observed to precipitate symptoms that may be somewhat protracted and make more challenging the diagnosis of substance-induced psychosis versus schizophrenia (5). Often these syndromes may be diagnosed and treated empirically regardless of clarity of the underlying source (6), although the ideal is to apply the DSM-IV criteria rigorously and determine diagnoses with the best possible specificity.

In summary, since psychosis can be a symptom of various psychiatric and medical/neurological illnesses and can be related to medications, alcohol, and illegal drugs (Table 1), the evaluation of a patient with an acute episode of psychosis should begin with the formulation of a broad differential diagnosis. This chapter focuses on differentiating schizophrenia from other psychiatric and medical/neurological illnesses and substance-induced psychotic disorders.

Table 1 Disorders To Be Considered in the Differential Diagnosis of Schizophrenia

Psychiatric illnesses
Schizophreniform disorder
Psychotic mood disorders (major depressive disorder, bipolar affective disorder)
Schizoaffective disorder
Delusional disorder
Brief reactive psychosis
Psychotic disorder not otherwise specified
Paranoid, schizotypal, schizoid, and borderline personality disorders
Factitious disorder with psychological symptoms
Malingering
Panic disorder
Obsessive-compulsive disorder
Psychotic disorders due to general medical conditions
Temporal-lobe epilepsy
Tumor, stroke, brain trauma
CNS infections (neurosyphilis, AIDS, herpes encephalitis)
Alzheimer's dementia
Huntington's disease
Wilson's disease
Endocrine/metabolic disorders (e.g., porphyria)
Vitamin deficiency (e.g., vitamin B_{12})
Autoimmune (e.g., systemic lupus erythematosus)
Substance-induced psychotic disorders
Stimulants (amphetamine, cocaine, methampehetamine)
Hallucinogens (lysergic acid diethylamide)
Phencyclidine
Anticholinergics (e.g., belladonna alkaloids)
Glucocorticoids
L-dopa
Histamine H_2 blocking drugs
Alcohol-withdrawal delirium
Barbiturate-withdrawal delirium
Toxic (e.g., heavy metals, carbon monoxide)

Source: Refs. 2, 5, 12, 21, 23, 25, 31, 32.

PSYCHIATRIC ILLNESSES THAT MUST BE EXCLUDED PRIOR TO DIAGNOSING SCHIZOPHRENIA

Many psychiatric disorders share symptoms with schizophrenia or have symptoms that may be confused with those of schizophrenia. The course and outcome of psychotic and other symptoms are the major factors that differentiate schizophrenia from other psychiatric disorders. When based on isolated symptoms alone (e.g., hallucinations, delusions, disorganized speech, and disorganized behavior), the diagnosis of schizophrenia has often been incorrect (7). For example, in a study examining the diagnoses of 116 consecutively admitted patients experiencing hallucinations, Goodwin and associates (8) found that only 32 (28%) had a diagnosis of schizophrenia and the remainder had other psychiatric diagnoses. Likewise, in a study involving 45 patients with a diagnosis of schizophrenia and 32 patients with a diagnosis of mania, Andreasen (9) found similar rates of "thought-language-communication disorder," including poverty of content of speech, tangentiality, derailment, incoherence, illogicality, loss of goal, and preseveration in both the affective and schizophrenic groups. A more recent study, by Docherty and associates (10), confirmed that both patients with schizophrenia and those with mania had greater frequencies of communication disturbances in speech than nonpsychiatric controls. They also found that the two patient groups differed from each other in the specific nature of the communication disturbances in their speech. Although these communication differences yield hope for the future that more sensitive diagnostic methods will help us better separate "first-episode" psychosis into discrete etiologies, at the present time the clinician is often faced with acute psychotic symptoms that are not pathognomonic for any disorder at face value.

Finally, Abrams and Taylor (11) examined 111 patients who met Feighner criteria, research diagnostic criteria (RDC), and DSM-III criteria for bipolar affective disorder, manic type. The majority (62%) of these subjects had at least one of the following symptoms: auditory hallucinations, persecutory delusions, formal thought disorder, catatonic symptoms, and other positive symptoms. The importance of establishing not only the presence of symptoms, but also their pattern and course, has been recognized in current diagnostic strategies. Along these lines, DSM-IV requires that a patient have at least 1 month of symptoms (or less if successfully treated) that meet the "criterion A" symptoms (i.e., active-phase symptoms) with at least 6 months of continuous signs of the disturbance including prodomal or residual symptoms. DSM-IV further requires the exclusion of schizoaffective, mood and substance-induced psychotic disorders, and psychotic disorders due to general medical conditions.

Schizophreniform Disorder

Given that schizophreniform disorder has the same characteristic symptom criteria as schizophrenia, it is at times not easy to differentiate between the two. With regard to schizophreniform disorder, the DSM-IV requires the duration of symptoms (including prodomal, active, and residual phases) to be at least 1 month but less than 6 months. Thus, schizophreniform disorder is likely to be the diagnosis in patients who have an abrupt, rather than an insidious, onset and who have a good premorbid adjustment. The diagnosis of schizophreniform disorder has historically been applied to individuals who have some of the symptoms of schizophrenia but who differ from patients with schizophrenia in ways such as displaying prominent emotional turmoil, intellectual confusion, or perplexity and who have a presumed greater role for psychosocial stresses (12). Be that as it may, in current diagnostic criteria, the most important distinctions between the two disorders are mode of onset and duration of episode.

Schizoaffective Disorder

Differentiating schizoaffective disorder from schizophrenia and from mood disorder with psychotic features is often very difficult. Schizoaffective disorder differs from schizophrenia in that both affective symptoms and the features of schizophrenia are equally prominent and occur together (12,13). In DSM-IV, schizoaffective disorder is distinguished from schizophrenia by the presence of significant mood symptoms that must be present for "a substantial portion of the total duration of the disturbance" (2). In contrast, mood symptoms in schizophrenia may have a duration that is brief relative to the total duration of the disturbance, occur only during the prodromal or residual phases, or do not meet full criteria for a mood episode. Since the DSM-IV does not specifically define "brief," these distinctions are often very difficult to make. Patients with schizoaffective disorder may also have a relatively abrupt onset of illness and fail to meet the 6-month-duration criterion for schizophrenia.

Affective Disorders

Mood disorders (i.e., major depressive disorder or bipolar affective disorder) with psychotic features should be diagnosed when there are psychotic symptoms that occur only during periods of mood disturbance. In the United States–United Kingdom Diagnostic Project, Cooper and colleagues (14) reported that, in the New York sample, mood disorders—particularly mania with psychotic features—were frequently diagnosed as schizophrenia. An abrupt onset of symptoms and a predominance of affective symptoms usually distinguish bipolar mood disorder with psychotic features from schizophrenia (7). However, some patients diagnosed with bipolar disorder may continually display low-level psychotic symptoms. Patients with mania may have a wide variety of psychotic symptoms, such as hallucinations, paranoid delusions, and formal thought disorder. Flight of ideas occurring during a manic episode may be confused with a chronic formal thought disorder, but this rarely occurs without other symptoms of mania, such as euphoria, decreased need for sleep, and hyperactivity. Patients with schizophrenia may sleep poorly and have episodes of hyperactivity, but these symptoms are usually secondary to delusions and hallucinations, rather than to euphoria, grandiosity, and hyperactivity of mania.

Patients with major depressive episodes may also experience hallucinations and/or delusions, which are usually mood-congruent (i.e., consistent with depressive themes of guilt, worthlessness, etc.). Sometimes mood-incongruent delusions may occur in the context of a major depressive episode, but more typical symptoms of depression should precede them to distinguish the presence of an affective source. When patients with depression experience hallucinations, they are typically of shorter duration and fragmented, and occur within the context of predominantly affective symptoms. In this group of patients, the clinician may have difficulty establishing whether the affective symptoms preceded psychotic symptoms or vice versa. In such circumstances, more information can be gathered, often from members of a patient's family, before the final diagnosis is determined, and often an extended period of observation and/or empirical treatment is needed to lend further diagnostic clarity.

Depression in Schizophrenia

On the other hand, individuals with schizophrenia may also experience depression (15). These episodes generally occur along with other symptoms of schizophrenia and within the context of an otherwise typical symptom pattern for schizophrenia (16). Wassink and associates (17) found that in a group of carefully diagnosed and well-characterized patients with recent-onset schizophrenia, the majority had at least one depressive symptom and more than one-third met DSM-III-R criteria for a major depressive disorder. To further complicate things, depressive symptoms of social withdrawal, lack of interest, and psychomotor retardation may resemble the negative symptoms of schizophrenia. If available, a careful history will reveal whether these symptoms occur in the context of a typical depressive illness or with other symptoms such as poor appetite, terminal insomnia, and self-reproach. Furthermore, further history may reveal whether the depressed (sad) mood did or did not precede marked withdrawal, lack of interest, and psychomotor retardation.

Delusional Disorder

Delusional disorder (formerly paranoid disorder) has been shown to be relatively uncommon in clinical settings (18); however, it is frequently confused with schizophrenia. Of the subtypes of delusional disorder, the persecutory type is the most common. Delusional disorder, persecutory subtype, is often difficult to distinguish from paranoid schizophrenia (19). However, in delusional disorder, only a single, well-encapsulated, nonbizarre (i.e., plausible in the sense that the imagined events could conceivably occur) delusional system is present. The diagnosis of delusional disorder does not include hallucinations, disorganized behavior, or negative symptoms, as in typical schizophrenia, and the delusions should not be fragmented. In general, the age of onset of delusional disorder is later than for schizophrenia (often over the age of 50 years) and there is usually less impairment in occupational and social functioning.

Brief Reactive Psychosis

Brief reactive psychosis is a disturbance that has a sudden onset of positive psychotic symptoms (i.e., hallucinations, delusions, disorganized speech, or grossly disorganized or catatonic behavior) that last for at least 1 day but less than a month. The individual with a brief reactive psychosis eventually has a full return to the premorbid level of functioning. It should not be confused with schizophrenia, except in cases in which a coherent history cannot be obtained (12). Brief reactive psychosis may be mistaken for schizophrenia when the patient has a pre-existing personality disorder that bears some similarities to the prodrome of schizophrenia. However, since patients with schizophrenia are usually psychotic for many months before coming to treatment, this is usually not a problem in most clinical settings. For new, acute-onset cases of schizophrenia, this differential diagnosis can be difficult until additional time passes and the course of the illness becomes clear.

Another defining feature of brief reactive psychosis is a precipitating stressful event, hence the nomenclature "reactive." This is typically perceived as a catastrophic event that is out of the range of daily experience but may be any experience deemed catastrophic by the affected individual. The return to premorbid function usually occurs within days to weeks following the stressful event and the severity of symptoms diminishes during this time in a continuous manner.

Psychosis Not Otherwise Specified

Psychosis not otherwise specified (NOS) is a diagnostic category that includes psychotic symptomatology about which there is inadequate information to make a specific diagnosis or about which there is contradictory information, or when there are psychotic symptoms that do not meet the criteria for a specific psychotic disorder. When diagnostic rules outlined by DSM-IV are strictly applied, patients who have been previously diagnosed with schizophrenia may in fact fall into this category. Using this category rather than forcing a choice between the more carefully defined categories may be of substantial clinical importance. It signifies that more information needs to be gathered before deciding on a specific diagnosis and making predictions concerning prognosis. In many cases, the diagnosis of psychosis NOS serves as a temporary category for new-onset patients until the course and nature of their symptoms help to clarify the appropriate diagnosis.

Personality Disorders

Personality disorders may be confused with schizophrenia with surprising frequency. Most obviously, the "cluster A" personality disorders have the greatest similarity to psychotic disorders (Table 2). These include the schizoid, schizotypal, and paranoid personality disorders. These disorders may be conceptualized as having features of the schizophrenia "spectrum," but to a substantially lesser degree such that they are not of sufficient magnitude in either severity or degree of social/occupational impairment to constitute schizophrenia.

The cluster B personality disorder of borderline personality is also a potential source of misdiagnosis of schizophrenia. Unlike the cluster A patients, these patients have symptoms that may mimic the psychosis of schizophrenia, yet their illness is probably not in the schizophrenia spectrum.

Both cluster A and B personality disorders can be distinguished from schizophrenia by the absence of delusions, hallucinations, and

Table 2 Features of DSM-IV "Cluster A" Personality Disorders

Personality disorder	Features
Paranoid	Distrust and suspiciousness of others; reads hidden meanings into benign remarks; is unforgiving of insults, injuries, or slights
Schizoid	Does not desire or enjoy close social relationships and has a restricted range of emotional expression in interpersonal settings; indifferent to praise or criticism of others
Schizotypal	Acute discomfort in close relationships; odd beliefs or magical thinking; unusual perceptual experiences; odd thinking and speech; suspiciousness or paranoid ideation; inappropriate or constricted affect; and odd, peculiar, or eccentric behavior

Source: Ref. 2.

grossly disorganized behavior. There is some evidence that schizotypal personality disorder may be genetically related to schizophrenia (20). The patient with schizotypal personality disorder may appear suspicious and superstitious, and may complain of vague ideas of reference and have few social contacts. They may also report vague hallucinatory experiences, but the hallucinations and other symptoms never quite reach the level of those required to meet the symptoms listed in criterion A of schizophrenia. In paranoid personality, one might initially suspect that delusions lie behind the suspiciousness, guardedness, and hostility, but none can be found. This disorder should not be confused with schizophrenia, since no well-formed delusions, hallucinations, changes in affect, thought disorder, or other symptoms of schizophrenia are present.

The cluster B personality group includes borderline personality disorder, which has also been confused with schizophrenia since it may exhibit the prodromal symptoms of schizophrenia, vague and fleeting psychotic symptoms, or display susceptibility to brief reactive psychoses. Strict application of the diagnostic criteria for schizophrenia, using reliable and narrowly defined symptoms in criterion A of the diagnostic criteria for schizophrenia, helps to reduce these misclassifications. Additionally, the prominent affective instability and behavioral disturbances such as impulsivity and addictive and self-harm behaviors help distinguish the cluster B personalities.

Mental Retardation

In patients with mental retardation, the diagnosis of schizophrenia may be difficult to make even if the diagnostic criteria for schizophrenia, using reliable and narrow definitions of features, are strictly applied. Many features of schizophrenia are symptoms that only the patient can report. Patients with severe communication defects may not be able to communicate whether they are experiencing hallucinations or delusions to an examiner. It is also often difficult to differentiate misperceptions of events or fantasy from delusions or hallucinations (21). Unfortunately, many individuals with mental retardation receive antipsychotic medications that are often initiated during childhood for control of agitated behaviors or aggressiveness. Over time, the presence of an antipsychotic medication may translate into a presumed history of psychotic disorder such as schizophrenia. Because these individuals are at increased risk for tardive dyskinesia, consistent reappraisals of diagnosis and medication management in this population may be of substantial clinical importance. To help clarify the diagnosis when the patient can't give you the history you need, it is particularly important to obtain history from family informants and caregivers focusing on the presence of behaviors suggestive of psychotic symptomatology (i.e., attending and/or responding to hallucinatory experiences, suspiciousness, etc.). It is also very useful to observe the patient closely on the unit, and at times it may be appropriate to withdraw antipsychotic medications with close monitoring in a closely supervised setting.

Other psychiatric disorders that must be ruled out include factitious disorder and malingering. Less commonly, the following may be confused with schizophrenia: somatization disorder, agoraphobia, obsessive-compulsive disorder, antisocial personality disorder, atypical anxiety disorder, and atypical depressive disorder.

PSYCHOTIC DISORDERS DUE TO GENERAL MEDICAL CONDITIONS THAT MUST BE EXCLUDED PRIOR TO DIAGNOSING SCHIZOPHRENIA

Psychotic symptoms can be seen in many general medical and neurological conditions (Table 1). General medical conditions in the differential diagnosis include endocrinopathies (thyroid, adrenal, pancreatic); autoimmune disorders (systemic lupus erythematosus); vascular disorders; vitamin B_{12} deficiency; and hepatic, erythropoietic, or metabolic disorders. These can generally be identified with a general chemistry screen, complete blood count, thyroid-function tests, urinalysis, and serological tests for evidence of an infection with syphilis or human immunodeficiency virus.

Neurological conditions to be considered in the differential diagnosis of first-episode psychosis include head trauma, brain tumors, seizures, multiple sclerosis, metachromatic leukodystrophy, Huntington's disease, and Wilson's disease. Although psychosis due to these conditions is relatively rare, it is important to ask about trauma, head injuries, and seizures. In the medical evaluation of first-episode patients, special tests such as computerized tomography (CT) or magnetic resonance imaging (MRI) of the brain and electroencephalogram (EEG) may be indicated (or useful) in selected cases (3,4).

There are many case reports suggesting that psychotic disorders due to general medical conditions are frequently confused with schizophrenia or schizophreniform disorder. However, most reported cases of psychotic disorders due to general medical conditions that are confused with a diagnosis of schizophrenia describe individuals who do not show the usual profile of symptoms or course of illness seen in schizophrenia. For example, in acute psychotic disorders due to a medical condition such as a metabolic disorder, head trauma, brain tumor, or stroke, symptoms often begin much more abruptly and may include visual hallucinations or bizarre behavior resulting from a clouded consciousness. These symptoms are usually qualitatively different from the positive symptoms that are characteristic of schizophrenia (i.e., auditory hallucinations in the context of a clear sensorium). In more chronic disorders, such as Huntington's disease or Alzheimer's disease, symptoms that might be confused with negative symptoms are actually the result of cognitive deterioration. The patient with schizophrenia typically can describe the course of hallucinations and delusions over the duration of the illness. Patients with these types of cognitive disorders are likely to have little or no recall or awareness of their psychotic symptoms. For greater detail, see the work of Hall (22) and Lishman (23), who have discussed the problems of differentiating psychotic disorders due to general medical conditions from schizophrenia in great length.

The psychotic disorders due to general medical conditions most likely to be confused with schizophrenia are temporal-lobe epilepsy and psychoses related to alcohol and drug abuse. In temporal-lobe epilepsy (complex partial seizures), delusions and hallucinations may follow a course resembling that of schizophrenia. Generally these symptoms occur subsequent to the onset of complex partial seizures (e.g., in one case series, an average of 14 years after the onset of seizures)

(24). Specifically asking about a history of other seizure phenomena is useful in making this differential diagnosis.

SUBSTANCE-INDUCED PSYCHOTIC DISORDERS THAT MUST BE EXCLUDED PRIOR TO DIAGNOSING SCHIZOPHRENIA

Adverse reactions to prescribed medications may manifest as psychotic symptoms. Psychotic symptoms have been reported with glucocorticoids, L-dopa, anticholinergics, and histamine-H_2-blockers (25). A thorough medical history, including a medication history, is necessary to rule out potential psychotic disorders due to medication.

Transient hallucinations and delusions have been reported to occur in alcohol abuse and dependence. Victor and Hope (26) found that, in a series of 76 patients with a diagnosis of alcohol dependence, 15 patients had onset of hallucinations while still drinking. In the 51 patients for whom the time of the last drink could be determined, 32 (60%) had onset of hallucinations within 12 to 48 hours of the last drink. In the 75 patients for whom the duration of hallucinations could be determined, 64 (85%) had a duration of hallucinations of 6 days or less. Only eight of 75 (11%) had a duration of hallucinations of 6 weeks. In a family study of persons with a diagnosis of alcohol abuse/dependence, Schuckit and Winokur (27) found no increase in the incidence of schizophrenia in the relatives of the patients with alcohol abuse/dependence with hallucinosis. These patients were also no more likely than other patients with alcohol abuse/dependence to have a history of schizophrenia. Based on these data, it appears that alcoholic hallucinosis differs from schizophrenia in that it occurs after prolonged alcohol abuse, is usually of abrupt onset and short duration, and is not associated with a family history of schizophrenia. Another characteristic feature of alcoholic hallucinosis is the fact that patients are quite aware that their perceptions are not real; i.e., they experience preserved insight that typically is not present in schizophrenia.

Other Drug-Induced Psychoses

Stimulants (e.g., amphetamine, methamphetamine, cocaine), hallucinogens (e.g., lysergic acid diethylamide), and phencyclidine may produce a paranoid psychosis with visual, auditory, and tactile hallucinations. Unlike the insidious onset typical of true schizophrenia, these psychoses tend to have an abrupt onset (e.g., during a several-day course of high intake of amphetamines) and to resolve within a few days after cessation of drug use (5,28,29). It is more difficult to distinguish between individuals with pre-existing psychiatric illness who may be abusing substances, as well as substance abusers who may have prolonged or repeated psychoses (5,30). Based on DSM-IV criteria, the differential diagnosis between substance-induced psychosis and schizophrenia depends on the degree to which the substance use can be implicated in the maintenance of a chronic disorder. In the clinical setting, this ends up turning on whether the psychotic disorder persists for a designated period of time in the absence of ongoing substance use (e.g., over 1 month according to DSM-IV).

In a family study of substance abusers, Tsuang and associates (30) examined whether "prolonged psychosis" following substance abuse was related to risk factors for schizophrenia. They defined prolonged psychosis as at least 6 months of psychotic symptoms without return to the individual's previous level of functioning. They found that the risk for schizophrenia in the families of 45 substance abusers with prolonged psychosis was 6.5%. This was similar to the risk for families of 46 patients with schizophrenia (6.8%). In addition, families of substance abusers with prolonged psychosis had increased risk for mood disorder, suggesting that this group of patients with psychosis was genetically heterogeneous. The psychoses of these patients, however, resembled schizophrenia in terms of course and symptomatology. Studies examining the effect of methamphetamine "epidemics" in Japan in the 1950s and 1970s showed that, in a minority of patients, apparent methamphetamine-induced psychoses do not resolve within the first month. In a review of approximately 12 such studies, Sato et al. (31) found that around 15% of the patients with a methamphetamine-induced psychosis took 5 years or more to recover in the absence of ongoing use. The chronic psychoses of these patients were described as being indistinguishable from paranoid schizophrenia in terms of cross-sectional presentation and course of illness. Because chronic psychoses in the context of substance abuse may begin at an earlier age than in the onset of schizophrenia in the absence of substance abuse, some authorities have suggested that substance abuse precipitates the illness in the genetically predisposed (5,30,32). In general, it is felt that a psychosis in someone who abuses substances that does not remit after prolonged cessation of drug use and that otherwise meets criteria for schizophrenia probably is schizophrenia.

SUMMARY

In some ways, the diagnosis of schizophrenia should be considered a diagnosis of exclusion due to both the nonspecificity of psychotic symptoms and the severity of the consequences associated with the diagnosis. A diagnosis of schizophrenia must be based on the presence of specific symptoms and a specific course of symptoms as defined in DSM-IV. Other psychiatric disorders can generally be differentiated from schizophrenia if symptoms are narrowly defined and the course of illness is carefully taken into account. It is important to obtain a thorough history and medical evaluation (i.e., physical exam, general chemistry screen, complete blood count, urinalysis, and drug screen) to rule out organic causes (i.e., medical and neurological conditions or substance abuse) for the psychotic symptoms. Atypical presentations, such as abrupt onset of symptoms, clouding of sensorium, or onset after age 30 should be carefully investigated. When the history and psychiatric examination of a psychotic patient do not reveal a pattern of symptoms and symptom duration that clearly corresponds to a diagnosis of schizophrenia or another well-defined disorder, it is best to use the category of psychosis NOS until more information can be obtained.

REFERENCES

1. Flaum M, Schultz SK. Core symptoms of schizophrenia. Ann Med 1996; 28(6):525–531.
2. American Psychiatric Association. Diagnostic and Statistical Manual of Mental Disorders. 4th ed. Washington, DC: American Psychiatric Press, 1994:290–315
3. Carpenter WT, Buchanan RW. Schizophrenia. N Engl J Med 1994; 330:681–690.
4. Treatment of schizophrenia 1999. The expert consensus guideline series. J Clin Psychiatry 1999; 60(suppl 11):3–80.
5. Flaum M; Schultz SK. When does amphetamine-induced psychosis become schizophrenia? Am J Psychiatry 1996; 153(6):812–815.
6. Rosenhan DL. On being sane in insane places. Science 1973; 179:250–258.
7. Pope HG, Lipinski JF. Diagnosis in schizophrenia and manic-depressive illness: a reassessment of the specificity of "schizophrenic" symptoms in the light of current research. Arch Gen Psychiatry 1978; 35:811–828.
8. Goodwin DW, Alderson P, Rosenthal R. Clinical significance of hallucinations in psychiatric disorders: a study of 116 hallucinatory patients. Arch Gen Psychiatry 1971; 24:76–80.
9. Andreasen NC. Thought, language, and communication disorders. II. Diagnostic significance. Arch Gen Psychiatry 1979; 36:1325–1330.

10. Docherty NM, De Rosa M, Andreasen NC. Communication disturbances in schizophrenia and mania. Arch Gen Psychiatry 1996; 53(4):358–364.
11. Abrams R, Taylor MA. Importance of schizophrenic symptoms in the diagnosis of mania. Am J Psychiatry 1981; 138:658–661.
12. Tsuang MT, Loyd DW. Other psychotic disorders. In: Michels R, ed. Psychiatry. Philadelphia: JP Lippincott, 1985; 1(70):1–17.
13. Tsuang MT, Demsey M, Rauscher F. A study of "atypical schizophrenia": a comparison with schizophrenia and affective disorder by sex, age of admission, precipitant, outcome, and family history. Arch Gen Psychiatry 1976; 33:1157–1160.
14. Cooper JE, Kendell RE, Gurland BJ, et al. Psychiatric Diagnosis in New York and London: A Comparative Study of Mental Hospital Admissions. Maudsley Monographs. No. 20. London: Oxford University Press, 1972.
15. Siris SG. Depression in schizophrenia: perspective in the era of "atypical" antipsychotic agents. Am J Psychiatry 2000; 157(9):1379–1389.
16. Guze SB, Cloninger R, et al. A follow-up and family study of schizophrenia. Arch Gen Psychiatry 1983; 40:1273–1276.
17. Wassink TH, Flaum M, Nopoulos P, Andreasen NC. Prevalence of depressive symptoms early in the course of schizophrenia. Am J Psychiatry 1999; 156(2):315–316.
18. Winokur G. Delusional disorder (paranoia). Compr Psychiatry 1977; 18:511–521.
19. Kendler KS, Tsuang MT. Nosology of paranoid, schizophrenic, and other paranoid psychoses. Schizophr Bull 1981; 7:594–610.
20. Faraone SV, Kremen WS, Lyons MJ, Pepple JR, Seidman LJ, Tsuang MT. Diagnostic accuracy and linkage analysis: how useful are schizophrenia spectrum phenotypes? Am J Psychiatry 1995; 152(9):1286–1290.
21. Wright EC. The presentation of mental illness in mentally retarded adults. Br J Psychiatry 1982; 141:496–502.
22. Hall CW. Psychiatric Presentations of Medical Illness: Somatopsychic Disorders. New York: SP Medical and Scientific Books, 1980.
23. Lishman WA. Organic Psychiatry: The Psychological Consequences of Cerebral Disorder. Oxford: Blackwell Scientific, 1978.
24. Slater E, Beard AW. The schizophrenia-like psychoses of epilepsy. I. Psychiatric aspects. Br J Psychiatry 1963; 109:95–150.
25. Guggenheim FG, Erman MK. Medication-induced psychiatric symptoms and disorders. In: Michels R, ed. Psychiatry. Philadelphia: JP Lippincott, 1985:2(91):1–8.
26. Victor M, Hope JM. The phenomenon of auditory hallucinations in chronic alcoholism: a critical evaluation of the status of alcoholic hallucinosis. J Nerv Ment Dis 1958; 126:451–481.
27. Schuckit MA, Winokur G. Alcoholic hallucinosis and schizophrenia. Br J Psychiatry1971; 119:549–550.
28. Grinspoon L, Bakalar JD. Drug dependence: nonnarcotic agents. In: Comprehensive Textbook of Psychiatry. 3rd ed. Baltimore: Williams & Wilkins, 1980.

29. Ellison GD, Eison MS. Continuous amphetamine intoxication: an animal model of acute psychotic episode. Psychol Med 1983; 13:751–761.
30. Tsuang MT, Simpson JC, Kronfol Z. Subtypes of drug abuse with psychosis: demographic characteristics, clinical features, and family history. Arch Gen Psychiatry 1982; 39:141–147.
31. Sato M, Numachi Y, Hamamura T. Relapse of paranoid psychotic state in methamphetamine model of schizophrenia. Schizophr Bull 1992; 18:15–122.
32. Bowers MB, Swigar ME. Vulnerability to psychosis associated with hallucinogen use. Psychiatry Res 1983; 9:91–97.

4

Cognitive Assessment in Schizophrenia Patients

Anne L. Hoff
University of California Davis School of Medicine
Sacramento, and
UC Davis Napa Psychiatric Research Center
Napa, California

INTRODUCTION

Schizophrenia has been considered a disorder involving cognitive deficits from its earliest description. Kraepelin described it as a "disorder of attention" and eventually coined the term "dementia praecox" to describe the deteriorating course of illness, which resembled an organic dementia in some patients (1). With the advent of antipsychotic medications in the 1950s, it is now rare to observe the natural course of schizophrenic illness over a lifetime. Indeed, there is evidence to suggest that antipsychotic medications improve outcome. A group of recent studies suggest that longer duration of untreated psychosis is associated with a longer period of recovery, more negative symptoms, and worse social or occupational functioning (2,3).

What are cognitive deficits in schizophrenia and how are they measured? Cognitive deficits involve mental-processing capacities that range from elementary processes such as simple attention and vigilance to more complex processes such as abstract thinking and higher-order problem solving. The field of neuropsychology that originally focused on the effects of brain damage (from missile wounds, tumors, head injuries, strokes, etc.) on cognitive processes has contributed greatly to a better understanding of cognitive disorders in schizophrenia. Psychological tests created to measure functioning of different parts of the brain are now used routinely to assess patients with schizophrenia. Because many of these tests are based on principles of localization of different functions to certain brain regions established by brain-lesion studies, one could argue that they are inappropriately applied to patients who have a disorder that involves most, if not all, regions of the brain. In fact, many recent hypotheses postulate that schizophrenia is a disorder in which neural pathways connecting brain regions such as the frontal and temporal-limbic regions of the brain are aberrant (4).

Multiple neurotransmitter systems have been implicated in the pathophysiology of schizophrenia, including but not limited to the dopamine, serotonin, adrenergic and noradrenergic, cholinergic, and, more recently, glutamate systems (5). If schizophrenia involves any or all of these neurotransmitter systems that extend throughout many brain regions, it is hard to imagine the point of performing neuropsychological tests purported to measure discrete brain regions. Yet, recent studies characterizing multiple areas of cognitive deficits in schizophrenia have told us a great deal about the kinds of everyday problems that these patients face and also about the clinical outcome one can expect. A recent review of the literature evaluating the relationships of cognitive dysfunction to clinical outcome indicates that certain cognitive functions, especially verbal memory, may have a stronger relationship to clinical outcome than either positive or negative symptoms (6). If this is the case, then assessing and treating cognitive disabilities in schizophrenia, along with positive and negative symptoms, may be essential to reduce the morbidity of this disease.

Many researchers now consider neuropsychological dysfunction in schizophrenia to be a core deficit that is part and parcel of the illness and not secondary to the effects of institutionalization or medication or to psychotic symptoms such as hallucinations, delusions, or thought disorder (7). If schizophrenia is a brain disease, it is logical to assess the cognitive correlates of this disease. A neuropsychological assessment can be of great clinical value in its ability to determine areas of cognitive strengths and weaknesses and to set realistic expectations for patient functioning. While in their preliminary stages, programs (both cognitive rehabilitation and pharmacological) that target cognitive disabilities in schizophrenic patients may be a great benefit to patients in improving their quality of life and allowing them to function effectively in society.

BASIC CONCEPTS

Like any symptom associated with an illness, cognitive dysfunction in schizophrenia is on a continuum ranging from very mild impairment to very severe impairment. Generally, there is an association of greater severity of illness with greater cognitive impairment across different populations of schizophrenic patients, and degree of cognitive dysfunction will certainly depend on the population of patients studied. For example, our research group has recently found similarities in severity of cognitive dysfunction between a first-episode cohort and chronically ill Veterans Administration (VA) patients, but large differences between these two groups and a third group of chronically ill, treatment-refractory state hospital patients. The state hospital group was significantly more impaired than either the first-episode or VA cohort (8).

Although large differences in cognitive functioning may occur between different cohorts of schizophrenic patients, there is surprising inconsistency of findings relating symptom severity and cognitive dysfunction within a particular cohort. The strongest relationships have been observed between negative symptoms and cognitive dysfunction, with stronger negative symptomatology associated with worse cognitive performance (9). Some studies have found relationships of disorganized thinking and negative symptoms with cognitive disability, but no relationship of positive symptoms (hallucinations, delusion) with neuropsychological dysfunction (10) Yet, within our own studies of treatment-refractory state hospital patients, we find stronger relationships of positive symptoms—Brief Psychiatric Rating Scale (BPRS) Positive Symptom cluster of hallucinations, delusions, unusual thought content—with cognitive dysfunction than with negative symptoms (11). Again, results are dependent on the particular sample studied and this issue is far from resolved. The fact that many studies find weak relationships between symptoms and cognition also supports the notion that cognitive dysfunction may be an independent feature of the illness.

What then are the most frequently seen domains of cognitive dysfunction in schizophrenic patients? The following section of the chapter discusses cognitive domains of neuropsychological dysfunction in schizophrenia. Table 1 lists these domains and tests that can be used to measure them. As in our previous papers (12,13), we have organized these tests into cognitive domains based on their intercorrelations with one another (demonstrating that they are measuring the same construct) because we discuss two clinical cases using these particular cognitive domains. However, it should be noted that many tests measure more than one element of cognitive processing so some tests will appear in more than one domain. Tests that appear in more than one domain are designated.

Table 1 Neuropsychological Tests That Are Useful in the Assessment of Schizophrenic Patients

Test	What it measures
Language/verbal ability	
Verbal IQ from the WAIS-III[a]	Current verbal intellectual ability
Wide Range Achievement Test-III–Reading subtest[a]	Premorbid intellectual ability
Word Attack from Woodcock-Johnson Reading Mastery Test[a]	Phonetics/learning disability
Controlled Oral Word Association [a,b]	Verbal fluency
Boston Naming Test[a,b]	Confrontation naming
Executive functioning	
Wisconsin Card Sorting Test[a]	Abstraction/concept formation
Booklet Categories Test[a]	Abstraction/concept formation
Stroop Color and Word Test[a]	Cognitive inhibition
Trails B[b]	Conceptual flexibility
Controlled Oral Word Association[b]	Verbal fluency
Boston Naming Test[b]	Confrontation naming
Verbal memory	
California Verbal Learning Test[a]	List learning
Logical Memory (WMS-III)[a]	Paragraph recall
Verbal Paired Associates (WMS-III)[a]	Word-pair recall
Visual Reproduction (WMS-III)[a]	Recall of geometric designs
Benton Visual Retention Test[a]	Recall of geometric designs
Concentration/speed (attention/perceptual-motor speed)	
Trails A[a]	Number sequencing
Trails B[a,b]	Number-letter sequencing
Symbol Digit Modalities Test[a]	Number-symbol matching
Cancellation Test[a]	Complex attention
Finger Tapping Test[a]	Motor speed
Sensory-perceptual function	
Tactile Finger Recognition[a]	Finger agnosia
Finger-Tip Number Writing[a]	Graphesthesia

[a]Tests contribute to summary scales in Figure 1.
[b]Tests are present in more than one cognitive domain.

CLINICAL DESCRIPTION

Language Function/Verbal Ability

There has been longstanding controversy over whether schizophrenic language is like that of aphasia, in which brain pathology has affected language mechanisms. The alternative is that language dysfunction in schizophrenia is an epiphenomenon secondary to disturbances of thought (14). Some studies have found that schizophrenics, unlike aphasics, have no difficulties with simple language measures of syntax, fluency, or naming (15), while other studies have found that on measures of language patients with formal thought disorder (16) produce errors similar to those made by fluent aphasics. Schizophrenic and aphasic language can be phenomenologically similar, but a review of the literature indicates that only a subgroup of patients resemble aphasics in both their reception and production of speech (17). The issue of assessing language is especially important because many schizophrenic patients have histories of verbal learning disabilities (18). From a clinical standpoint, there are a number of measures of verbal and language ability that are useful in assessing linguistic or language-based difficulties.

Our battery generally includes a measure of *current verbal intellectual functioning* [Verbal IQ from the Wechsler Adult Intelligence Scales (19)], *premorbid intellectual functioning* [Wide Range Achievement Test (WRAT)–Reading (20)], nonsense syllable pronunciation [Word Attack from the Woodcock-Johnson Reading Mastery Test (21)], confrontation naming [Boston Naming Test (22)], and verbal fluency [Controlled Oral Word Association Test (23)]. Both the WRAT-Reading and the Word Attack Test assist in the determination of whether there is a comorbid learning disability. In addition, a *deterioration index* can be computed in subtracting Verbal IQ (current) from the WRAT-Reading IQ equivalent (premorbid). Word pronunciation is generally resistant to the effects of organic brain dysfunction and can be used to estimate premorbid intellectual ability (24). Measures of verbal fluency (or the ability to generate a word list) and confrontation naming (producing the names of objects) can also be sensitive to the effects of dysfunction in the frontal cortex (25).

Executive Function

The behavior of schizophrenic patients, in particular those with negative symptoms, has been noted to bear strong resemblance to that of patients with disorders of the frontal cortex (26). Both syndromes are remarkable for apathy, lack of motivation, flat affect, disorders of attention, difficulties in the formulation of plans for goal-directed behavior, deficient concept formation, inability to maintain and change cognitive set, and perseverative tendencies. Goldstein (27) first referred to this deficit in schizophrenic patients as a "loss of abstract attitude."

Weinberger et al. (28) found that schizophrenic patients exhibited a hypofrontality pattern on a PET scan during the Wisconsin Card Sorting Test (29). This test measures abstract thinking and the ability to shift mental sets by asking subjects to match cards with colored geometric shapes on the basis of color, shape, and number. The principle needed to get the correct answer changes without warning after a preset number of correct responses. Patients with frontal-lobe lesions as well as patients with schizophrenia have difficulty in maintaining the correct cognitive set and switching cognitive sets, and often exhibit perseverative responses. Results from the Weinberger study (28) were interpreted as evidence of impairment of the dorsolateral prefrontal cortex in schizophrenics.

How common is frontal-lobe dysfunction in schizophrenia? In a group of stable outpatient schizophrenics, only 35% of patients performed in the impaired range on the Card Sort (30), similar to the 29% of outpatient first-episode patients tested at 2-year follow-up in another study (12). In a group of 56 schizophreniform patients, frontal-lobe functions were significantly impaired, but there was no evidence that they were relatively more impaired than those of language, verbal memory, spatial memory, concentration, or motor function (12). Saykin and colleagues (31) also did not find evidence for selectivity of frontal-lobe function in their group of unmedicated (and probably less severely ill) patients. Thus, it appears that frontal-lobe function, as measured by the Wisconsin Card Sort, is likely to be a more prominent feature among schizophrenic inpatients than among stable outpatients.

There are other cognitive measures of frontal lobe function, such as word or design fluency tests (32), the Categories Test and Trailmaking Test (Trails B) from the Halstead-Reitan Test Battery (33), the Stroop Color and Word Test (34), and tests of olfactory identification (35). Fluency tests require the production of word lists (purported to measure left frontal functions) or the generation of spatial designs (thought to measure right frontal functions). The Categories Test and Booklet Categories Test (36) are similar to the Wisconsin Card Sorting Test in that they require the individual to formulate a problem-solving strategy based on a concept and to be flexible in changing that strategy in response to feedback from the examiner. The Stroop Color and Word Test (34) involves an inhibition component in which the subject must name the color in which the name of a different color is printed. Trails B requires the subject to connect alternating numbers and letters in order by drawing a line between them, which calls on the ability to cognitively switch back and forth between numbers and letters in linear sequence. The University of Pennsylvania Smell Identification Test (UPSIT) (35) asks the subject to identify common smells using a series of scratch-and-sniff cards. Olfactory deficits are thought to reflect dysfunction in the orbital frontal regions of the brain (37). Given the relatively large size of the frontal cortex, it is not surprising that putative measures do not correlate significantly with one another (38).

Attention/Concentration and Memory

The nature of attention and memory function in schizophrenia is complex because: 1) from a practical standpoint, it is difficult to differentiate attentional processes from memory processes in the measurement process and 2) memory is a multidimensional construct that is measured differently depending on one's model of human memory. One of the most influential models of memory (39) postulates three memory stores: the *sensory register*, the *short-term store*, and the *long-term store*. The sensory register—the entry point for all information—retains information in a preconscious, sensory form for an approximate duration of 250 ms, whereupon stimulus traces are replaced with other incoming information. Information in the sensory register then proceeds to short-term store, where it is processed by conscious memory routines (e.g., rehearsal). It can be maintained there as long as constant attention is devoted to it, but will disappear after about 15 to 30 seconds without constant attention. This stage has recently been referred to as *working memory*, which is characterized as an online, continually updated storage bank of information in which there is conscious manipulation of information. Finally, there is long-term storage, which is a repository of unlimited information that receives and holds information from short-term or sensory storage.

With regard to attentional functions, Shakow (40), using a simple reaction-time paradigm, and Kornetsky and Mirsky (41), using the Continuous Performance Test, highlighted the notion that schizophrenic patients have a central deficit in sustained attention. Since then, paradigms using backward masking, the span of apprehension test, and other techniques (for a review, see Ref. 42) have demonstrated that schizophrenics perform more poorly than controls on elementary information-processing tasks that are likely to involve the sensory register or short-term store. These deficits may be related to a reduction in processing capacity, abnormal allocation of attention, or poor regulation of arousal. At any rate, such deficits in elementary information processing occur in remitted schizophrenic patients (14) and first-degree relatives of schizophrenic patients (43).

Saccuzzo and Braff (44) found that information-processing deficits also occur in schizoaffective and bipolar patients, suggesting that processing deficits are more reflective of psychotic illness and may be a fundamental trait of schizophrenic spectrum disorders. Some investigators have found that patients with negative symptoms have poorer information processing than positive-symptom patients do (45). In summary, the elementary impairments that schizophrenic patients have on simple tasks of information processing speak to a more generalized trait disturbance. From a neuroanatomical standpoint, attentional functioning is mediated by the inferior frontal cortex along with its connections to subcortical areas such as the reticular activating system and basal ganglia, also important in level of arousal.

Some commonly administered clinical neuropsychological measures of attention and concentration are Digit Span and Arithmetic from the Wechsler Adult Intelligence Scales–III (46), although the latter test involves an additional calculation component. Digit Span requires the individual to repeat strings of numbers of increasing length, both forward and backward. Other measures of attention are Trails A (33) and the Cancellation Test. Trails A requires the individual to connect numbered circles in order by drawing a line between them as quickly as possible. The Cancellation Test (47) requires the subject to cancel a target item in a group of non–target items as quickly as possible. There are three target items at the top of three pages: a diamond, three letters ("LIF"), and three numbers ("392"). The target items are interspersed throughout lines of non–target items of the same class. Scoring is based on the total number of seconds taken to complete all three pages and the number of incorrect responses (number of omissions plus number of commissions).

Given the recent evidence that schizophrenics have postmortem changes in the temporal and hippocampal areas of the brain indicative of neurodevelopmental pathology (48) and that MRI studies have also documented reductions in size of the hippocampus, amygdala, and whole temporal lobes in schizophrenic patients (49,50), it would seem logical that schizophrenic patients have memory difficulties since these areas of the brain are crucial to memory functioning. Numerous studies have attempted to elucidate the nature of this dysfunction. Some studies suggest that schizophrenics have difficulty in recall but not recognition (51), whereas others suggest that difficulties in memory are due to organizational deficits present at the time of encoding (52). Chronically ill patients may have deficits in both recognition and recall (53). Some investigators claim that memory dysfunction in schizophrenia is not unlike the classical amnestic syndrome of preserved immediate memory and deficient long-term memory (54) although Paulsen and coworkers (55) would dispute this viewpoint. Her findings using the California Verbal Learning Test demonstrate that schizophrenic patients have adequate retention of previously learned information (savings or storage), but are deficient in initially encoding information (acquisition) and in retrieval (the amount recalled is less than the amount of information recognized). She argues that this pattern of memory functioning is similar to that of patients with subcortical dementias, as opposed to cortical dementias such as Alzheimer's disease.

Some investigators have asserted that schizophrenic patients have a preferential deficit in verbal memory; that is, verbal or semantic memory is relatively more impaired than other cognitive functions (31). Yet, in other studies, schizophrenic patients are equally impaired on recall of both verbal and visual information (56,57). Still other studies find evidence for diffuse impairment across all measured cognitive abilities (12,30,58).

From a clinical standpoint, there are a number of memory measures than can be reliably used in schizophrenic patients. Ideally, memory measures should allow for the measurement of immediate and delayed recall, recognition ability, and assessment of organizational strategies used in the encoding of information. The California Verbal Learning Test (59) yields information on all these components of memory. The test requires the individual to remember a 16-item grocery list, which is repeated five times. A measure of learning slope can be calculated by assessing the amount of additional recall after each subsequent trial. The grocery list has four items in each of four categories: fruits, tools, spices, and clothing. Organizational strategy in encoding can be assessed by the degree to which subjects use the categories to aid in memory. At the end of the fifth trial, a second 16-item grocery list is given for one trial as an interference list. After subjects attempt to recall the second list, they are asked to recall items from the first list (free recall). They are then given the four category names and asked to remember items from each category from the first list (cued recall). After 30 minutes, subjects are asked to recall items from the first grocery list (delayed free recall) and items from each of the categories (delayed cued recall), and are given a list of 64 items in which they must indicate yes or no if the item was on the original grocery list (delayed recognition).

Other verbal memory measures that involve a recognition and recall component are the Logical Memory and Verbal Paired Associates from the Wechsler Memory Scale–III (WMS-III) (46) and previous versions of this test. The former test requires the subject to remember information from two stories read by the examiner (immediate free recall), to recall story details 30 minutes later (delayed free recall), and to answer yes or no questions about the story content (delayed recognition). The second test requires the memory of unrelated word pairs read by the examiner for four consecutive trials (immediate recall and learning slope), as well as delayed recall and recognition of the word pairs 30 minutes later.

Commonly used measures of visual memory are the Visual Reproduction Test from the WMS-III (46), and previous versions of the WMS, and the Benton Visual Retention Test (60). Both require the patient to draw geometric designs on paper after having been shown them on a card for 10 seconds. The Visual Reproduction Test from the WMS-III has an immediate and delayed recall component as well as a recognition and copying component.

Motor Speed, Perceptual-Motor Speed, and Sensory-Perceptual Functioning

Motor dysfunction has long been recognized as a feature of schizophrenic illness. Schizophrenic patients have been noted to have motor incoordination, clumsiness, and soft neurological signs (61). Although many neuroleptics and other psychotropic medications can cause motor slowing, as well as extrapyramidal side effects and tardive dyskinesia, there is also evidence that motor abnormalities can exist in neuroleptic-naive or unmedicated patients (62). In comprehensive reviews of the literature, it has been concluded that both acute and chronic administration of typical neuroleptics can reduce motor dexterity and speed (63,64); however, most cognitive functions, especially attentional measures, are improved or unchanged after chronic neuroleptic treatment (65).

Commonly used measures of motor function include the Finger Tapping Test and Grip Strength (33) and the Purdue Pegboard (66). The Finger Tapping Test requires the patient to tap a small lever with his index finger as many times as possible within a 10-second period. The Purdue Pegboard requires the placement of small pegs into holes on a board as quickly as possible within 30 seconds. Both are timed tests. In the Grip Strength Test, the subject must use each hand to squeeze a hand dynamometer. The force of the squeeze is recorded in milligrams. All these tests allow for comparison of dominant to nondominant hand functioning and inferences about functioning of the contralateral cerebral hemisphere.

Measures of perceptual-motor speed include a perceptual and motor component and are also thought to measure overall information-processing speed or cognitive efficiency. Examples include the Trailmaking Test and the Symbol-Digit Modalities Test (SDMT) (67). These tests also measure attention/concentration, visual tracking, and motor speed. As can be seen, most tests are multifaceted and measure more than one component of cognitive ability. The Trailmaking Test was discussed previously. The SDMT requires the individual to write down, as quickly as possible, numbers that are matched to a symbol in the key at the top of the page. The score is the number of correct answers written in a 90-second period.

Sensory-perceptual functioning can be measured in auditory, visual, or tactile modalities. Our battery includes two measures from the Reitan-Klove Sensory-Perceptual Examination (33), the Tactile Finger Recognition Test, and the Finger-Tip Number Writing Perception Test. The first test is a measure of finger agnosia. It requires the subject to identify which finger has been touched by the examiner without the benefit of sight. The second test is a measure of graphesthesia—the examiner writes with a pencil the numbers 3, 4, 5, or 6 on the subject's fingertips while the subject's eyes are closed. The score for both tests is the number correct out of 20 trials on each hand. Again, this test allows for the comparison of left- and right-hand performances with the possibility of making inferences about contralateral hemispheric functioning. In general, sensory-perceptual functioning is intact in most schizophrenic patients and is impaired only in severely ill, treatment-refractory patients or those with concomitant acquired organic brain dysfunction.

CASE EXAMPLES

Case examples appear in Figure 1. The neuropsychological test data are presented in the form of Z scores, which have been calculated by deriving a Z score for individual tests in each domain based on the means and standard deviations of a normal control group of subjects ($n = 74$) of the same average age and parental social class as our patients. The formula is the raw score minus the control-group mean divided by the standard deviation (SD) of control group. The Z scores for each domain are the summed average of individual Z scores for that domain. Z scores reflect the performance of an individual relative to an average

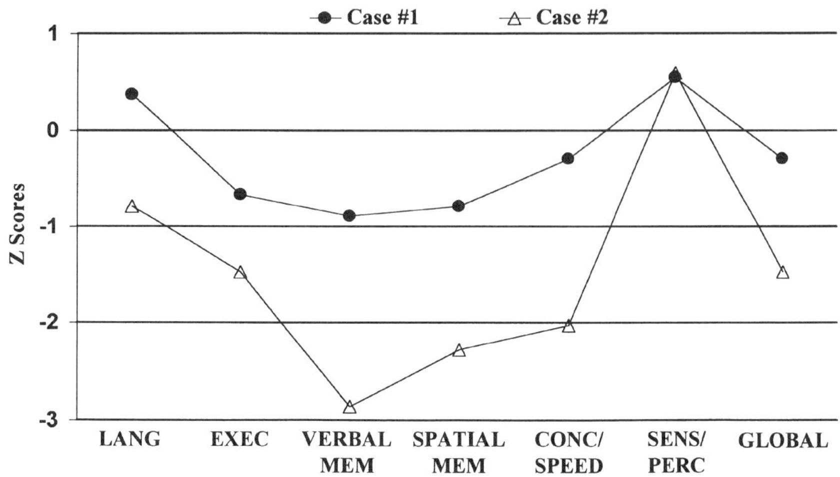

Figure 1 Comparison of two patients with schizophrenia on neuropsychology test battery.

performance of 0 such that minus scores reflect below-average performances and positive scores reflect above-average performances. A standard deviation of –1.0 translates to a percentile rank of 16, and is comparable to an individual who is functioning at the 16th percentile compared to a normal reference group. That is, 84% of average individuals are functioning at a higher level. Tests used for each domain are listed in Table 1. Because the cases are from work done in the late 1980s and early 1990s, the WAIS-R, Wechsler Memory Scale–Revised, and WRAT-Revised are used. For the Verbal IQ, the Satz-Mogel abbreviated version (68) is also used. For additional details regarding the neuropsychological summary scales, see Ref. 12. Tests contributing to each scale are designated.

Case 1

MJ is a 28-year-old, single, left-handed Caucasian male who was an inpatient at Kings Park Psychiatric Center, a state hospital serving the Suffolk County area on Long Island, New York. This was his first psychiatric admission. He was tested after medication stabilization (20 mg haloperidol) approximately four weeks after admission. He had had psychotic symptoms for 18 months prior to admission, and his family had noted a change in behavior (social withdrawal) starting at age 25. As part of our first-episode longitudinal study, he received a diagnosis of DSM-III-R schizophrenia, undifferentiated type, based on the Schedule for Schizophrenia and Affective Disorders–Lifetime (SADS-L) (69), two years after admission. He had had three years of college prior to admission and his total BPRS (70) (1-to-8 score on each item) score at admission was 33, indicating relatively mild symptom severity. His prorated verbal IQ was 110, with a WRAT-Reading IQ equivalent of 114. Review of his summary scale Z scores indicated that his performance was above average on measures of language/verbal ability and sensory-perceptual functioning. His worst performances were on measures of executive and memory functioning, ranging from –0.67 to –0.89 SDs below average, or at the 25th and 19th percentile, respectively. His Global scale—the average of the other six scales—was –0.29 SD below average, or at the 39th percentile. Given his overall premorbid intellectual functioning, his executive and memory functioning are well below expectation and signify a deterioration in cognitive function from premorbid levels.

Case 2

DK is a 44-year-old, left-handed, single male inpatient at Napa State Hospital who was recruited to be part of ongoing studies of neuropsychological function of chronically ill treatment-refractory patients. His age of first hospitalization was 23 years and he had been hospitalized for most of the past 21 years. DSM-III-R diagnosis confirmed by the Structured Clinical Interview for Diagnosis (71) was schizophrenia, paranoid type. He had graduated from college prior to becoming ill. His total BPRS score was 55 at the time of testing, indicating severe psychiatric illness that was chronic and unremitting. He took 750 mg of clozapine daily. His verbal IQ was 98 and his WRAT-Reading IQ equivalent was 99, both in the average range of intellectual functioning. Given his premorbid functioning, one would have expected a higher WRAT-Reading score. His summary Z scores ranged from –0.79 (21%) to –2.86 (0%) SDs below average, with the Global scale being –1.47 (7%). Like MJ, his worst performances were on measures of verbal and spatial memory and executive functioning, but he also had very poor performances on measures of complex attention and perceptual-motor and pure motor speed (CONC/SP). It is difficult to assess how much effect the patient's medications had on his performance. Clozapine has strong anticholinergic properties; however, our group has found that it has a mixed effect on cognitive functioning, with improvement noted on measures of verbal fluency and perceptual-motor and pure motor speed and worse performances on measures of spatial memory and executive functioning compared with typical neuroleptics (72).

Case Analysis

These two cases illustrate that patients with schizophrenia have deficits on measures of verbal and spatial memory, executive functioning, attention/concentration, and perceptual-motor speed. Although these two patients have different levels of illness severity, their pattern of dysfunction was similar. The treatment implications of this neurocognitive dysfunction are that patients are likely to have difficulty in the workforce and at home in areas of functioning that require sustained attention, memory skill, and rapid processing of information. It is important that family members and treating staff develop realistic expectations regarding a patient's true abilities and not attribute failure to laziness or lack of effort. Cognitive dysfunction in schizophrenia is an integral part of the illness and may improve only when effective cognitive rehabilitation and pharmacological strategies have been developed.

POTENTIAL INTERVENTIONS

Because neurocognitive deficits are becoming recognized as core deficits in schizophrenia, there has been a resurgence in interest in designing cognitive rehabilitation programs targeted at this population. That cognitive deficits are a residual part of psychiatric illness and often limit vocational and social choices (73) leads to the conclusion that testing the efficacy of cognitive remediation in schizophrenic illness is a worthwhile goal. A number of investigators have recently made cogent arguments to this effect (74), and a number of groups are attempting programs to target and remediate specific deficits. In targeting attentional processes, some studies have found that schizophrenics can be trained to reduce distraction in reaction time tests (75) and improve on the Continuous Performance Test (a measure of vigilance) and BPRS total score using a computerized program designed for head-injured patients (76). Errorless learning principles (subjects experience no failures) have been successfully utilized in cognitive rehabilitation programs for schizophrenic patients to improve memory (77) and executive functioning (cognitive flexibility, working memory, and planning) (78), although it remains to be seen whether improvements are sustained over time and whether they relate to positive clinical outcome.

Efforts in cognitive rehabilitation of schizophrenic patients are in the infancy stage and much more research will need to be done in this area.

Another approach to the remediation of cognitive deficits is pharmacological. Recent studies suggest that, compared with traditional antipsychotic medication, atypical neuroleptics improve some cognitive functions (reviewed in Refs. 79 and 80). Clozapine improves verbal fluency, attention, and perceptual-motor and pure motor speed, while risperidone improves working memory, secondary memory, selective attention, and executive functions. Olanzapine and quetiapine also improve attention and short-term memory compared with typical neuroleptics. However, although the improvements may be statistically significant, the clinical significance of these improvements has not yet been demonstrated. For example, in a double-blind study, Kern et al. (81) found that patients taking risperidone improved on the California Verbal Learning Test compared with those taking haloperidol. From a practical standpoint, patients improved from a baseline performance that was 4 SDs below the average of normals to a performance 2 SDs below average. Thus, at endpoint, the patient's percentile rank was still 2%, which is a worse performance than 98% of the normal population.

Another potential approach to improving cognitive function is through the use of cognitive enhancers such as those used in the treatment of Alzheimer's disease. While schizophrenia is not thought to be related to a central cholinergic deficiency, cholinomimetics may reverse the effects of anticholinergic properties associated with some neuroleptic and antiparkinsonian medications that may contribute to worse cognitive functioning. A number of research centers are performing double-blind, placebo-controlled studies of adjunctive donepezil (Aricept) in schizophrenic patients. The outcome of these studies is not yet known.

SUMMARY

In summary, cognitive dysfunction in schizophrenia is a core feature of the illness and is strongly related to social, clinical, and occupational outcome. Much of the literature supports the notion of widespread deficits, although some studies suggest that attentional, memory, and executive functions are most impaired. Neuropsychological testing in patients with schizophrenia is an essential tool in developing realistic treatment expectations. It will also be critically important in assessing the efficacy of current and future rehabilitation and psychopharmacological approaches to the treatment of this disorder.

REFERENCES

1. Kraepelin E. Dementia praecox and paraphrenia. Chicago: Chicago Medical Books, 1919.
2. Loebel AD, Lieberman JA, Alvir JMJ, Mayerhoff DI, Geisler SH, Szymanski SR. Duration of psychosis and outcome in first-episode schizophrenia. Am J Psychiatry 1992; 149:1183–1188.
3. Haas GL, Garratt LS, Sweeney JA. Delay to first antipsychotic medication in schizophrenia: impact on symptomatology and clinical course of illness. J Psychiatr Res 1998; 32:3–4.
4. Csernansky JG, Murphy GM, Faustman WO. Limbic/mesolimbic connections and the pathogenesis of schizophrenia. Biol Psychiatry 1991; 30:383–400.
5. Olney JW, Farber NB. Glutamate receptor dysfunction and schizophrenia. Arch Gen Psychiatry 1995; 52:998–1007.
6. Green MF. What are the functional consequences of neurocognitive deficits in schizophrenia? Am J Psychiatry 1996; 153:321–330.
7. Green MF, Nuechterlein KH. Should schizophrenia be treated as a neurocognitive disorder? Schizophr Bull 1999; 25:309–319.
8. Kremen WS, Hoff AL, Wieneke M, DeLisi LE. Individual cognitive profile analysis in sachizophrenia: evidence from a new sample. Biol Psychiatry 2000; 47(8S):32S.
9. Perlick D, Mattis S, Stastny P, Silverstein B. Negative symptoms are related to both frontal and nonfrontal neuropsychological measures in chronic schizophrenia [letter]. Arch Gen Psychiatry 1992; 49:245–246.
10. Liddle PF, Morris DL. Schizophrenic syndromes and frontal lobe performance. Br J Psychiatry 1991; 158:340–345.
11. Hoff AL, Harris D, Faustman WO, Beal M, DeVilliers D, Mone RD, Moses Jr. JA, Csernansky JG. A neuropsychological study of early onset schizophrenia. Schizophr Res 1996; 20:21–28.
12. Hoff AL, Riordan H, O'Donnell D, Stritzke P, Neale C, Boccio A, Anand AK, DeLisi LE. Anomalous lateral sulcus asymmetry and cognitive function in first-episode schizophrenia. Schizophr Bull 1992; 18(2):257–270.
13. Hoff AL, Riordan H, O'Donnell DW, Morris L, DeLisi LE. Neuropsychological functioning of first-episode schizophreniform patients. Am J Psychiatry 1992; 149:898–903.
14. Asarnow R, MacCrimmon D. Attention/information processing, neuropsychological functioning, and thought disorder during the acute and partial recovery phases of schizophrenia: a longitudinal study. Psychiatry Res 1982; 7:301–319.
15. Andreasen NC. Thought, language, and communication disorders. I. Clinical assessement, definition of terms, and evaluation of their reliability. Arch Gen Psychiatry 1979; 36:1315–1321.
16. Faber R, Reichstein M. Language dysfunction in schizophrenia. Br J Psychiatry 1981; 139:519–522.

17. Landre NA, Taylof MA, Kearns KP. Language functioning in schizophrenic and aphasic patients. Neuropsychiatry Neuropsychol Behav Neurol 1992; 5:7–14.
18. Doody GA, Johnstone EC, Sanderson TL, Owens DG, Muir WJ. "*Pfropfschizophrenie*" revisited: schizophrenia in people with mild learning disability. Br J Psychiatry 1998; 173:145–153.
19. Wechsler D. Manual for the Wechsler Adult Intelligence Scale–Revised. San Antonio, TX, Psychological Corporation, 1981.
20. Jastak S, Wilkinson GS. Wide Range Achievement Test–Revised. Wilmington, DE: Jastak Associates, 1984.
21. Woodcock R. Woodcock Reading Mastery Tests. Circle Pines, MN: American Guidance Service, 1973.
22. Goodglass H, Kaplan E. The Assessment of Aphasia and Related Disorders. Philadelphia: Lea & Febiger, 1983.
23. Benton AL, Hamsher KdeS. Multilingual Aphasia Examination. Iowa City: AJA Associates, 1989.
24. Kremen WS, Seidman LJ, Faraone SV, Pepple JR, Lyons MJ, Tsuang MT. The "3 Rs" and neuropsychological function in schizophrenia: application of the matching fallacy to biological relatives. Psychiatry Res 1995; 56:135–143.
25. Miceli G, Caltagirone C, Gainotti G. Neuropsychological correlates of localized cerebral lesions in non-aphasic brain-damaged patients. J Clin Neuropsychol 1981; 3:53–63.
26. Levin S. Frontal lobe dysfunction in schizophrenia. II. Impairments of psychological and brain functions. J Psychiatr Res 1984; 18:57–72.
27. Goldstein K. Functional disturbances in brain damage. In: Arieti S, ed. American Handbook of Psychiatry. New York: Basic Books, 1959:770–794.
28. Weinberger DR, Berman KF, Zec RF. Physiological dysfunction of dorsolateral prefrontal cortex in schizophrenia. I. Regional cerebral blood flow evidence. Arch Gen Psychiatry 1986; 43:114–124.
29. Heaton RK. Wisconsin Card Sorting Test Manual. Odessa, FL: Psychological Assessment Resources, 1981.
30. Braff DL, Heaton R, Kuck J, Cullum M, Moranville J, Grant I, Zisook S. The generalized pattern of neuropsychological deficits in outpatients with chronic schizophrenia with heterogeneous Wisconsin Card Sorting Test results. Arch Gen Psychiatry 1991; 48:891–898.
31. Saykin AJ, Gur RC, Gur RE, Mozley PD, Mozley LH, Resnick SM, Kester B, Stafiniak P. Neuropsychological function in schizophrenia: selective impairment in memory and learning. Arch Gen Psychiatry 1991; 48:618–624.
32. Lezak M. Neuropsychological Assessment. New York: Oxford University Press, 1995.
33. Reitan RR, Wolfson D. The Halstead-Reitan Neuropsychological Test Battery: Theory and Clnical Interpretation. Tucson, AX, Reitan Neuropsychology Laboratory, 1985.

34. Golden CJ. Stroop Color and Word Test: A Manual for Clinical and Experimental Uses. Chicago: Stoelting, 1978.
35. Doty RL, Shaman P, Dann M. Development of the University of Pennsylvania Smell Identification Test: a standardized microencapsulated test of olfactory function. Physiological Behav 1984; 32:489–502.
36. DeFilippis NA, McCampbell E, Rogers P. Development of a booklet form of the Category Test: normative and validity data. J Clin Neuropsychol 1979; 1(4):339–342.
37. Moberg PJ, Agrin R, Gur RE, Gur RC, Turetsky BI, Doty RL. Olfactory dysfunction in schizophrenia: a qualitative and quantitative review. Neuropsychopharmacology 1999; 21:325–340.
38. Goldberg TE, Weinberger DR. Probing prefrontal function in schizophrenia with neuropsychological paradigms. Schizophr Bull 1988:179–183.
39. Atkinson R, Shiffrin R. A proposed system and its control processes. In: Spence K, Spence J, eds. Advances in the Psychology of Learning and Motivation. New York: Academic Press, 1968.
40. Shakow D. Segmental set: a theory of the formal psychological deficit in schizophrenia. Arch Gen Psychiatry 1962; 6:1–17.
41. Kornetsky C, Mirsky A. On certain psychopharmacological and physiological differences between schizophrenics and normal persons. Psychopharmacology (Berl) 1966; 8:309–318.
42. Nuechterlein KH, Dawson ME. Information processing and attentional functioning in the developmental course of schizophrenic disorders. Schizophr Bull 1984; 10:160–203.
43. Asarnow JR, Steffy RA, Mac Crimmon DJ, Cleghorn JM. An attentional assessment of foster children at risk for schizophrenia. In: Wynne LC, Cromwell RL, Matthysse S, eds. The Nature of Schizophrenia: New Approaches to Research and Treatment. New York: Wiley, 1978:339–358.
44. Saccuzzo DP, Braff DL. Information-processing abnormalities: trait- and state-dependent components. Schizophr Bull 1986; 12:447–459.
45. Green MF, Walker E. Symptom correlates of vulnerability to backward masking. Am J Psychiatry 1986; 143:181–186.
46. Wechsler D. Manual for the Wechsler Adult Intelligence Scale. 3rd ed. San Antonio, TX: Psychological Corporation, 1997.
47. Diller L, Ben-Yishay Y, Gerstman LJ. Studies in cognition and rehabilitation in hemiplegia. New York: New York University Medical Center Institute of Rehabilitation Medicine, 1974.
48. Bogerts B, Meertz E, Schonfeldt-Bausch R. Basal ganglia and limbic system pathology in schizophrenia: a morphometric study of brain volume and shrinkage. Arch Gen Psychiatry 1985; 42:784–791.
49. DeLisi LE, Hoff AL, Schwartz JE, Shields GW, Halthore SN, Gupta SM, Henn FA, Anand AK. Brain morphology in first-episode schizophrenic-like psychotic patients: a quantitative magnetic resonance imaging study. Biol Psychiatry 1991; 29:159–175.

50. Shenton ME, Kikinis R, Jolez FA, Pollak SK, LeMay M, Wible CG, Hokama H, Martin J, Metcalf D, Coleman M, McCarley RW. Abnormalities of the left temporal lobe and thought disorder in schizophrenia: a quantitative magnetic resonance imaging study. N Engl J Med 1992; 327:604–612.
51. Koh S. Remembering of verbal materials by schizophrenic adults. In: Schwartz S, ed. Language and Cognition in Schizophrenia. Hillsdale, NJ: Lawrence Erlbaum, 1978:59–99.
52. Calev A, Venables P, Monk A. Evidence for distinct verbal memory pathologies in severely and mildly disturbed schizophrenics. Schizophr Bull 1983; 9:247–264.
53. Calev A. Recall and recognition in mildly disturbed schizophrenics: the use of matched tasks. Psychol Med 1984; 14:425–429.
54. Tamlyn D, McKenna PJ, Mortimer AM, Lund CE, Hammond S, Baddeley AD. Memory impairment in schizophrenia: its extent, affiliations and neuropsychological character. Psychol Med 1992; 22:101–115.
55. Paulsen JS, Heaton RK, Sadek JR, Perry W, Delis DC, Braff D, Kuck J, Zisook S, Jeste DV. The nature of learning and memory impairments in schizophrenia. J Int Neuropsychol Soc 1995; 1:88–99.
56. Calev A, Korin Y, Kugelmass S. Performance of chronic schizophrenics on matched word and design recall tasks. Biol Psychiatry 1987; 22:699–709.
57. Gold J, Randolph C, Carpenter C. The performance of patients with schizophrenia on the Wechsler Memory Scale–Revised. The Clinical Neuropsychologist 1992; 6:367–373.
58. Blanchard JJ, Neale JM. The neuropsychological signature of schizophrenia: generalized or differential deficit? Am J Psychiatry 1994; 151:40–48.
59. Delis D, Kramer J, Kaplan E, Ober B. The California Verbal Learning Test. San Antonio, TX: Psychological Corporation, 1987.
60. Benton AL. The Revised Visual Retention Test. New York: Psychological Corporation, 1974.
61. Green MF, Bracha S, Satz P, Christenson CD. Preliminary evidence for an association between minor physical anomalies and second trimester neurodevelopment in schizophrenia. Psychiatry Res 1994; 53:119–127.
62. Manschreck TC, Maher BA, Waller NG, Ames D, Latham CA. Deficient motor synchrony in schizophrenic disorders: clincial correlates. Biol Psychiatry 1985; 20:990–1002.
63. Cassens G, Inglis AK, Appelbaum PS, Gutheil TG. Neuroleptics: effects on neuropsychological function in chronic schizophrenic patients. Schizophr Bull 1990; 16(3):477–499.
64. Medalia A, Gold J, Merriam A. The effects of neuroleptics on neuropsychological test results of schizophrenics. Arch Clin Neuropsychol 1988; 3:249–271.
65. Spohn HE, Strauss ME. Relation of neuroleptic and anticholinergic medication to cognitive functions in schizophrenia. J Abnorm Psychol 1989; 98:367–380.

66. Tiffin J, Asher EJ. The Purdue Pegboard: norms and studies of reliability and validity. J Appl Psychol 1948; 32:234–247.
67. Smith A. Symbol Digit Modalities Test: Manual. Los Angeles: Western Psychological Services, 1973.
68. Satz P, Mogel S. An abbreviation of the WAIS for clinical use. J Clin Psychol 1962:77–79.
69. Spitzer RL, Endicott J. The Schedule for Affective Disorders and Schizophrenia–Lifetime Version (SADS-L). New York: Biometrics Research Department, New York State Psychiatric Institute, 1978.
70. Overall JE, Gorham DR. The Brief Psychiatric Rating Scale. Psychological Reports 1962; 10:799–812.
71. Spitzer RL, Williams JBW, Gibbon M. Structured Clinical Interview for DSM-III-R–Patient Version. New York: Biometrics Research Department, New York State Psychiatric Institute, 1987.
72. Hoff AL, Faustman WO, Wieneke M, Espinoza S, Costa M, Wolkowitz O, Csernansky JG. The effects of clozapine on symptom reduction, neurocognitive function, and clinical management in treatment-refractory state hospital schizophrenic inpatients. Neuropsychopharmacology 1996:361–369.
73. Goldberg TE, Ragland D, Torrey EF, Gold JM, Bigelow LB, Weinberger DR. Neuropsychological assessment of monozygotic twins discordant for schizophrenia. Arch Gen Psychiatry 1990; 47:1066–1072.
74. Green MF. Cognitive remediation in schizophrenia: is it time yet? Am J Psychiatry 1993; 150:178–187.
75. Hermanutz M, Gestrich J. Computer-assisted attention training in schizophrenia. Eur Arch Psychiatry Clin Neurosci 1991; 240:282–287.
76. Medalia A, M. A, Tryon W, Merriam AE. Effectiveness of attention training in schizophrenia. Schizophr Bull 1998; 24:147–152.
77. O'Carroll RE, Russell HH, Lawrie SM, Johnstone EC. Errorless learning and the cognitive rehabilitation of memory-impaired schizophrenic patients. Psychol Med 1999; 29:105–112.
78. Wykes T, Reeder C, Corner J, Williams C, Everitt B. The effects of neurocognitive remediation on executive processing in patients with schizophrenia. Schizophr Bull 1999; 25:291–307.
79. Keefe RSE, Bollini AM, Silva SG. Do novel antipsychotics improve cognition? A report of a meta-analysis. Psychiatr Ann 1999; 29.
80. Meltzer HY, McGurk SR. The effects of clozapine, risperidone, and olanzapine on cognitive function in schizophrenia. Schizophr Bull 1999; 25:233–255.
81. Kern RS, Green MF, Marshall BD, Jr., Wirshing WC, Wirshing D, McGurk SR, Marder SR, Mintz J. Risperidone versus haloperidol on secondary memory: can newer medications aid learning? Schizophr Bull 1999; 25:223–232.

5

Laboratory Tests to Aid in the Diagnosis of Schizophrenia

Jose Mathews
Metropolitan St. Louis Psychiatric Center
St. Louis, Missouri

John G. Csernansky
Washington University School of Medicine
and Metropolitan St. Louis Psychiatric Center
St. Louis, Missouri

INTRODUCTION

In spite of recent advances in neuroscience, psychiatry relies on a diagnostic system defined by behavioral syndromes and not by a knowledge of etiology and pathophysiological mechanisms. Psychiatry remains the only branch of medicine in which there is a lack of useful laboratory tests to confirm the diagnosis, especially when the clinical symptoms are equivocal.

The *Diagnostic and Statistical Manual of Mental Disorders* (DSM) was developed in 1952 by the American Psychiatric Association as a system of defining and categorizing mental illnesses. It incorporated the dominant psychoanalytical thinking of that time, and the first revision, in 1968, of the DSM (DSM-II), further reflected this philosophy. However, a paradigm shift came in 1980 with the DSM-III, in which the American Psychiatric Association established an empirical system of diagnosis based on research evidence. The current revision, DSM-IV (1), continues this tradition.

A number of studies have convincingly shown that psychiatric patients suffer from undetected physical illnesses that contribute to their psychiatric symptoms. These illnesses are recorded on axes within the DSM-IV nosological system. Hoffman and Koran (2) conducted a detailed literature review and concluded that psychiatric assessments must include a complete medical assessment and that physical illnesses should be in the differential diagnosis when evaluating behavioral symptoms. In fact, the DSM-IV (1) criteria for the diagnosis of schizophrenia include an exclusion criterion of substance abuse/general medical condition (Criterion E). Before making the diagnosis of schizophrenia, it is essential to show that the symptoms are not due to the direct physiological effects of a substance (e.g., a drug of abuse or a prescription medication) or a general medical condition (1).

Unfortunately, there are as yet no biological markers that can be used to confirm the diagnosis of schizophrenia or similar illnesses. In the foreseeable future, with advances in molecular biology and neuroimaging, we may develop biological markers that will identify individuals with specific psychiatric disorders. Ideally, such markers will identify individuals early in the course of their illness and before the most dramatic symptoms of their illness (e.g., psychosis) appear. They may be genetic markers, markers from structural or functional neuroimaging, or the results of detailed cognitive testing. Until then, laboratory tests are best used to exclude general medical conditions or disorders of substance abuse.

DRUG-INDUCED DISORDERS

Several conditions associated with drug abuse or dependence can present with psychotic symptoms such as hallucinations, delusions, and thought disorder. It is important that these conditions be diagnosed as substance-induced psychotic disorder and not as schizophrenia. In general, delirium is likely to be present along with psychosis in disorders associated with drug use. In contrast, disorientation is rare and symptoms do not fluctuate significantly over the course of the day in patients with schizophrenia. Also, auditory hallucinations are more common than visual hallucinations in schizophrenia; the onset of the disturbance is also gradual and prolonged.

As a general rule, patients with atypical presentations of psychosis who are being considered for the diagnosis of a drug-induced mental disorder can benefit from a thorough laboratory evaluation. It is wise to obtain informed consent before ordering laboratory tests and to consult with appropriate specialists when necessary.

The most common drug-induced mental disorders are listed below, along with laboratory tests that can be used to confirm them. The onset of a drug-induced psychosis is usually rapid (within hours to days), often occurring during intoxication, but psychosis may last for several days to weeks following abstinence. However, there is little evidence to support the development of a chronic drug-induced psychosis in individuals with no antecedent psychopathology (3).

Alcohol

Alcohol is the most widely abused drug in the United States. A recent national study of comorbidity reported a lifetime prevalence of alcohol dependence of 20.1% in men and 8.2% in women. About 5% of people with alcohol dependence develop temporary paranoid delusions or auditory hallucinations. These symptoms generally occur in a clear sensorium and are not limited to the period of withdrawal. Usually complete recovery occurs within several days to a month, with no further drinking (3). Although less well described, a similar picture can be expected with the abuse of benzodiazepines, barbiturates, and anxiolytics (3).

Stimulants

Abuse of amphetamine and related compounds, as well as all forms of cocaine, are associated with hypervigilence and suspiciousness. This syndrome often progresses to a condition referred to as stimulant psychosis. Auditory visual or tactile hallucinations and frightening paranoid delusions are common in stimulant psychosis and sometimes result in unprovoked violence. However, the psychosis clears within days to a week of abstinence. There is a high risk of recurrence of stimulant psychosis with repeated drug use (3).

Phencyclidine

Phencyclidine (PCP) was introduced in the 1950s as an anesthetic agent, but was soon abandoned due to the psychosis it caused postoperatively. PCP-induced psychosis is characterized by paranoid delusions, hyperreligiosity, hallucinations, and a thought disorder similar to that seen in schizophrenia. Symptoms usually last 1 to 3 days following drug use, but can persist for 4 to 6 weeks following drug use in some patients. Complete recovery is the rule, although there is a high risk of recurrence with requested drug use (4).

Table 1 Prescription Drugs Reported to Cause Various Psychotic Symptoms

Paranoia and delusions	**Hallucinations**
Acyclovir	Anticholinergic drugs
Amphetamines	Baclofen (on discontinuation)
Anabolic steroids	Calcium-channel blockers
Cephalosporins	Cimetidine
Cimetidine	Dopamine agonists
Corticosteroids	Ethambutol
Cycloserine	5-Flucytosine
Dopamine agonists	Indomethacin
Ethosuximide	Isoniazid
Methylphenidate	Phenytoin
Theophylline	Vincristine
Other unspecified psychotic symptoms	Procaine penicillin
Aminoglycosides	Sympathomimetics
Beta-blockers	Tocainide
Bumetanide	Trimethoprim
Cyclobenzaprine	Vinblastine
Gancyclovir	Zidovudine (AZT)
Hydralazine	
Lidocaine	

Source: Ref. 30.

Hallucinogens

This group of drugs includes lysergic acid diethylamide (LSD), mushrooms (psilocybin), and Ecstasy (methylene dioxymethamphetamine). Hallucinogen-induced psychosis is often marked by visual hallucinations that clear within days following drug use in the absence of preexisting psychotic illness (2).

Cannabinoids

Excessive use of marijuana (tetrahydrocannabinoids) over a short period of time can also cause visual hallucinations and paranoid delusions. Moreover, cannabinoids can precipitate psychotic symptoms in predisposed individuals, for example, patients with idiopathic psychoses such as schizophrenia (5).

Opioids

Opioids generally do not produce psychotic symptoms, except when they are used together with other drugs. "Speedballs"—a combination of heroin and cocaine—can cause paranoid psychosis (2).

In addition to alcohol and the illicit drugs discussed above, certain prescription and over-the-counter drugs can alter an individual's perception of his environment, and occasionally produce psychotic symptoms (see Table 1).

Recommended Lab Tests to Aid Diagnosis

A drug screen can yield invaluable information to aid in the diagnosis of drug-induced mental disorders. The patient's history regarding illicit drug use is often unreliable. Urine and blood are the common sources of specimens used. Several methods can be used for detecting and confirming the presence of an illicit drug. However, gas chromatography–mass spectrometry (GC-MS) is the most sensitive and reliable test. The approximate duration of detectability depends on the amount of drug ingested, the type of compound, and the physical state of the patient (see Table 2).

In the context of alcohol use, a blood-alcohol level or a breath analysis may be needed. However, an alcohol level of zero does not rule out an alcohol-related psychosis because the half-life of alcohol in the body is very short and the psychosis can persist after the cessation of drinking (2). A number of biological markers suggest chronic alcohol use. These markers include GGT, which is a result of direct enzyme induction (Table 3). Liver cell damage results in elevations of SGOT and SGPT blood levels. Carbohydrate-deficient transferrin—an abnormal form of the protein transferrin, which is responsible for iron transport—is also produced after prolonged heavy drinking. Finally, MCV elevations can occur related to folic acid deficiency (2).

Table 2 Toxicology Screens

Drug	Limit of detection (per ml of blood or urine	Approximate duration of detectability (days)
Alcohol	300 μg	1
Amphetamines	500 ng	2
Barbiturates	1000 ng	1–3
Benzodiazepines	300 ng	3
Cocaine	150 ng	2–3
Opiates	300 ng	2
Phencyclidine	25 ng	8
Tetrahydrocannabinol carboxylic acid	<15 ng	3–20

Source: Ref. 31.

Table 3 Biological Markers for Chronic Alcoholism

Marker	Values	Sensitivity and specificity
GGT (gamma glutanyl transaminase)	>30 units/L	70% to 80%
CDT (carbohydrate-deficient transferrin)	>74 mg/L	>80%
MCV (mean corpuscular volume)	>91 μM3	Not known
SGOT (AST) (serum glutamic-oxaloacetic transaminase)	>45 IU/L	Not known
SGPT (ALT) (serum glutamic-pyruvic transaminase)	>45 IU/L	Not known

Source: Ref. 4.

SEIZURE DISORDERS

Historically, there has been a long association between psychosis and epilepsy. Epilepsy patients have a 7% to 12% lifelong prevalence of psychotic disorders, which is higher than in the general population (4). Psychotic symptoms can occur interictally, postictally, or less frequently in association with nonconvulsive status epilepticus. In addition, the prodromes of certain types of seizures, such as partial complex seizures, can resemble hallucinations. Finally, it should be kept in mind that both seizures and and changes in the level of consciousness can be the result of a central nervous system mass lesion. Several clinical features should alert the physician to the possibility of a seizure disorder–related psychosis (Table 4).

In cases of interictal psychosis, the psychotic symptoms are not temporally related to the occurrence of seizures. This syndrome has a typical onset in the third and fourth decade of life, and delusions are usually the first symptom observed (6). There can be a 10- to 15-year latency between the onset of seizures and the development of psychosis.

Table 4 Diagnostic Clues Indicating that Psychosis May Be Due to Seizures

1. Does not meet DSM-IV criteria for schizophrenia
2. Good premorbid social history
3. Abrupt change in personality, mood, or ability to function
4. Rapid fluctuations in mental status
5. Unresponsiveness to usual psychological or biological interventions

Source: Ref. 24.

Also, psychosis is more common among patients with epilepsy of left-temporal-lobe origin (6) (Table 5).

Cases of postictal psychosis are often associated with increases in the number of complex partial seizures. In such cases, seizures can be followed by psychotic symptoms lasting 1 day to 3 months. The psychosis consists predominately of paranoid symptoms and an abnormal mood. Multiple seizure foci and seizure clustering are risk factors for postictal psychosis, which also indicates unfavorable outcome for seizure control. Although the psychosis usually runs a benign course, the condition as a whole has increased morbidity and mortality (7).

Recommended Lab Tests to Aid Diagnosis

An electroencephalogram (EEG) is the diagnostic test of choice for seizures. EEGs measure the electrical activity of the brain recorded from scalp, nasopharynx, or other electrodes. Dysrhythmias and EEG asymmetries generally indicate the presence of a seizure. However, EEGs are not especially sensitive and a normal EEG does not exclude the presence of a seizure disorder. Sleep-deprivation EEGs with nasopharyngial leads, 24-hour ambulatory EEG recording, and video EEG monitoring are more complex techniques, but can be used to extend the sensitivity of EEG as a diagnostic test (Figure 1).

Neuroimaging studies can be done to rule out intracranial pathology, particularly in patients with partial seizures and in patients who develop seizures later in life. Magnetic resonance imaging (MRI) may be superior to computerized tomography (CT) for this use. Also, transient postictal elevations of serum prolactin occur after generalized

Table 5 Features of the Interictal Schizophreniform Psychosis of Epilepsy

Epilepsy characteristics
Complex partial seizures with secondary generalized tonic-clonic seizures
Epilepsy present 11 to 15 years before psychosis
Long interval of poorly controlled seizures
Left temporal focus
Psychosis characteristics
Atypical paranoid psychosis—paranoia with sudden onset
Psychosis alternating with seizures
More positive as opposed to negative symptoms
Few Schneiderian first-rank symptoms

Source: Ref. 4.

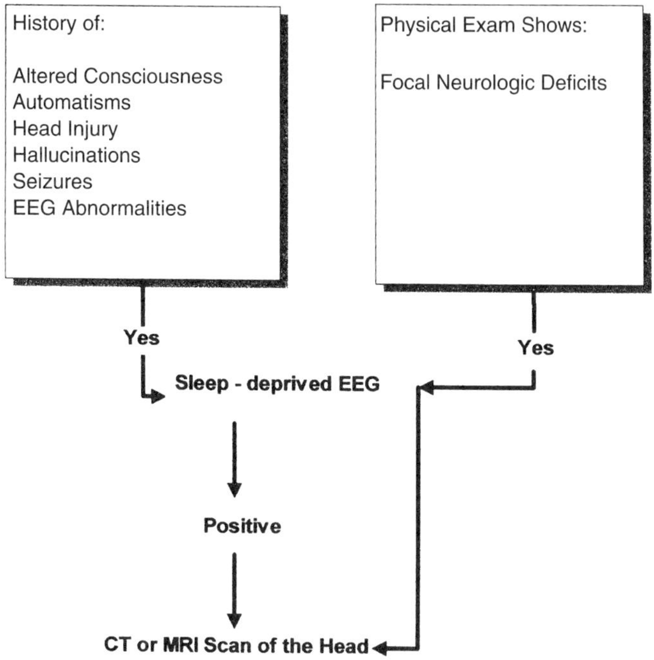

Figure 1 Strategy for obtaining an EEG in a psychiatric patient to rule out epilepsy. MRI may be superior to CT for detecting brain abnormalities related to seizure foci in patients with partial seizure symptoms. (From Ref. 32.)

tonic-clonic and complex partial seizures. However, the high potential for false-positive and false-negative errors limit the usefulness of this test (8).

CNS MASS LESIONS

Brain tumors and other CNS mass lesions can present with psychosis. Keschner at al. (9), in their case series of 530 patients with intracranial lesions confirmed by operation and/or autopsy, found that neuropsychiatric complications were early presenting symptoms in 23% of cases. However, most case reports and uncontrolled studies in this area appeared before the advent of modern neuroimaging techniques.

More recent studies suggest that relatively few patients with brain tumors in various locations within the intracranial space present with psychiatric complaints (10,11). However, in a survey of 18 autopsied

Table 6 Signs and Symptoms Suggestive of a Brain Tumor

1. Seizures, especially new-onset seizures, in adults with a focal or partial pattern.
2. New-onset headache, with a generalized, dull, positional pattern present immediately upon awakening
3. Nausea and vomiting, usually associated with headaches
4. Visual-field defects or diplopia; tinnitus or hearing loss (especially unilateral hearing loss and vertigo)
5. Other focal neurological signs and symptoms, such as ataxia, incoordination, and paraesthesias

Source: Ref. 24.

cases involving intracranial tumors of the limbic system, Malamud (12) found a high incidence of schizophrenia-like illness. Eight patients from this series were first hospitalized at a state mental hospital, and 10 patients had a diagnosis of schizophrenia, and two other patients were diagnosed with psychoneurosis (12).

It should also be kept in mind that, because slow-growing tumors may not cause focal neurological signs and symptoms, syndromes produced by such tumors are more likely to be misdiagnosed as primary psychiatric disorders. A summary of signs and symptoms suggestive of a CNS mass lesion is provided in Table 6.

Recommended Lab Tests to Aid Diagnosis

Neuroimaging has revolutionized the diagnosis of CNS mass lesions. CT scans with contrast enhancement are capable of detecting over 90% of brain tumors (4). MRI, with its higher resolution and superior anatomical definition, can detect the remaining tumors of smaller size (<0.5 cm), especially when they are located in the posterior fossa and the brainstem. Use of paramagnetic agents such as gadolium can further enhance the visualization of brain tumors using MRI. However, compared to MRI, CT scans are quicker, less expensive, and perhaps better at visualizing calcified lesions. CT scans may also be used when MRI is contraindicted (e.g., in a patient who has a pacemaker or aneurysm clips).

CEREBROVASCULAR EVENTS

Psychosis is infrequently reported in the initial presentation of stroke patients. However, this information has been derived mainly from small case series. More recently, a study by Rabins et al. (13) found that five patients who developed psychosis after stroke had right-hemisphere lesions and subcortical atrophy, compared with five patients matched for lesion size who did not develop psychosis. Seizures were also common in this group of patients, especially when the onset of seizures preceded the psychosis. In addition, constructional apraxia has been noted as a consistent neurological finding in stroke patients who develop psychosis (14).

Three factors may be most important in predicting which stroke patients will develop poststroke psychosis: 1) right-hemisphere lesions, 2) presence of seizures, and 3) presence of subcortical atrophy.

Recommended Lab Tests for Diagnosis

CT scanning is the laboratory test of choice in the first 48 hours after stroke, and can also be used to distinguish between infarction and hemorrhage. MRI is the diagnostic modality of choice beyond this period of time. In addition, MRI may be more useful in detecting small infarcts, subcortical infarcts, and early-stage infarcts (6). Special MRI techniques, such as diffusion-weighted imaging and the use of paramagnetic contrast agents, can further enhance the detection of small infarcts.

HUMAN IMMUNOVIRUSES

The rate of new-onset psychotic symptoms in human immunovirus (HIV)-positive patients can range from 0.5 to 15% after one excludes delirium and other confounding syndromes (4). Three of five patients in a case series reported by Halstead et al. (15) presented with psychotic symptoms prior to being diagnosed with HIV. Paranoid delusions, bizarre delusions, and formal thought disorder were prominent in these patients. Halevie-Goldman et al. (16) described auditory hallucinations and bizarre delusions as presenting symptoms in a single-case report.

Direct effects of HIV on the brain and coinfection of the patient with other viruses such as cytomegalovirus may be etiological factors in cases of HIV infection and psychosis. In addition, drug abuse may be involved in the production of psychosis in HIV-positive patients. Sewell et al. (17) reported a higher prevalence of stimulant and sedative/hypnotic abuse or dependence, greater global neuropsychological impairment, and a significantly higher mortality rate in patients with HIV-associated psychosis. Delusions with persecutory or grandiose themes were the most prevalent symptom. Auditory hallucinations were also quite common, along with thought disorder and prominent mood instability.

Recommended Lab Tests for Diagnosis

The diagnosis of HIV infection is based on antibody tests, including enzyme-linked immunosorbent assays (ELISA) and confirmatory Western blot tests. However, these tests should be both preceded and followed by counseling. Counseling is intended to reduce risky behavior and promote help-seeking behavior in persons at risk for HIV infection. A recent meta-analysis examining the effect of HIV counseling and testing on the reduction of sexual-risk behavior found significant reduction in unprotected sex and increased condom use in HIV-positive participants (18).

In addition to laboratory tests to reveal the presence of infection, the CT and MRI scans may reveal nonspecific atrophy of the brain in HIV-positive patients and EEGs may show nonspecific slowing.

NEUROSYPHILIS

Before the availability of penicillin, 5–15% of psychiatric hospitalizations were due to tertiary neurosyphilis (i.e., general paresis of the insane). Fortunately, neurosyphilis is now uncommon. However, there continue to be case reports of atypical cases of neurosyphilis in which psychosis is the presenting symptom (19). Tertiary syphilis can develop months to years after initial infection. Primary syphilis is characterized by the chancre, the genital syphilitic ulcer. Secondary syphilis involves systemic dissemination of the spirochete including a flu-like syndrome, skin rash, mucus lesions, and lymphadenopathy. Untreated, both primary and secondary syphilis resolve as the patient enters the latent period. However, about one-third of patients in the latent stage eventually develop tertiary syphilis (4).

The clinical manifestations of neurosyphilis can include dementia and depression, as well as psychosis. Paranoid delusions, auditory hallucinations, and ideas of reference are the most common symptoms of psychosis in the "paranoid" or "paraphrenic" form of neurosyphilis (6).

Recommended Lab Tests to Aid Diagnosis

The diagnosis of neurosyphilis is based on screening serological tests, including venereal disease research laboratory (VDRL) or rapid plasma reagin (RPR) tests. A positive cerebrospinal (CSF) VDRL test can be diagnostic for tertiary syphilis; however, a positive fluorescent treponemal antibody–absorption (FTA-ABS) test is needed for confirmation. CT or MRI scans may also be useful with diagnosis of tertiary syphilis in that they can show cortical atrophy.

SYSTEMIC LUPUS ERYTHEMATOSUS

Neurological symptoms, including seizures and psychosis, are among the American Rheumatism Association's criteria for systemic lupus erythematosus (SLE). The presence of psychotic symptoms has been reported in about 12% of patients with SLE. Often such symptoms occur in the context of delirium (20).

Recommended Lab Tests to Aid Diagnosis

Serum antinuclear antibody (ANA), anti-DNA antibody, and lupus anticoagulant (LA) are serological tests commonly used to diagnosis SLE. However, there are no specific tests that correlate with the presence of psychiatric symptoms in SLE. There have been reports of a positive association between antibodies to the ribosomal p protein and the psychiatric manifestations of SLE. However, other studies have found no such association, making the use of this assay doubtful.

VITAMIN B_{12} DEFICIENCY

Vitamin B_{12} deficiency can present with psychosis, dementia, mood disorder, and personality changes. Neuropsychiatric impairment is estimated to occur in about 40% of these patients, with about 16% having overt symptoms of psychosis (7). Delusions of persecution, uncharacteristic aggression, mood instability, and delirium are some of the commonly reported symptoms. This condition can also be commonly seen in alcoholics (21). Megaloblastic anemia is a common feature of this condition and can aid in the diagnosis. However, there are also case reports of neuropsychiatric symptoms secondary to vitamin B_{12} in the absence of megaloblastic anemia (22).

Recommended Lab Tests to Aid Diagnosis

A complete blood count that shows a megaloblastic anemia and decreased vitamin B12 levels may be used to suggest the presence of this diagnosis.

In consultation with internists and hematologists, the Schilling test is then used to confirm the diagnosis of B12 deficiency. The Schilling test measures the absorption of orally ingested radiolabeled vitamin B12 with and without the intrinsic factor. This test also reveals the mechanism of the vitamin B12 deficiency in a particular patient.

ACUTE INTERMITTENT PORPHYRIA

Psychosis can be a manifestation of acute intermittent porphyria (AIP), even in the absence of the typical physical manifestations of the disease. These manifestations include abdominal pain, autonomic dysfunction, and motor neuropathy. AIP results from the reduced activity of the heme-synthesizing enzyme porphobilinogen deaminase (PBG-D). In a study by Tishler et al. (23), the overall prevalence of AIP in two state psychiatric hospitals caring for mostly long-term patients was two per 1000. All the patients with AIP met criteria for DSM-III diagnosis of atypical psychosis or schizoaffective disorder (23). Thus, AIP can be difficult to differentiate from idiopathic psychotic illness unless laboratory tests are used.

Recommended Lab Tests to Aid Diagnosis

The laboratory diagnosis of AIP can be made by detecting elevated levels of urine porphobilinogen (PBG), aminolevulinic acid (ALA), and uroporphyrin in a 24-hour urine sample. Quantitative measurement is the recommended test; however, qualitative determination (e.g., the Watson-Schwartz test) can be substituted.

THYROID DISEASE

Hypothyroidism frequently manifests with psychiatric symptoms. Cognitive disturbances and mood disorders are most commonly present. However, in some cases, psychotic symptoms occur comorbidly with mood instability and cognitive symptoms. In unselected hypothyroid populations, only about 5% of patients presenting with psychiatric symptoms have psychosis (24). Several case reports, however, suggest that psychosis may be more common in hypothyroidism (25,26).

Psychosis is uncommon in patients with hyperthyroidism. Older studies report a higher occurrence of psychosis, but they are fraught

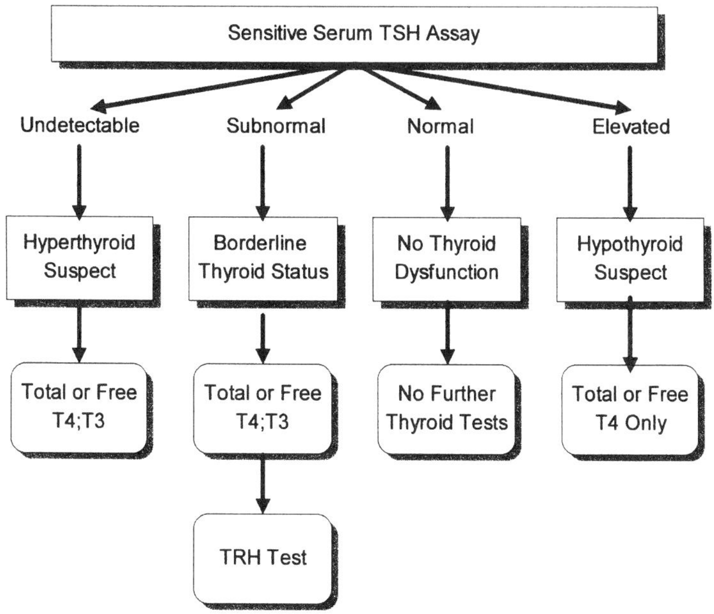

Figure 2 TSH test as a screening tool. (From Ref. 33.)

with diagnostic uncertainties. For example, in 1961, Bursten (27) reported a "manic veneer" in 10 patients with psychotic symptoms and thyrotoxicosis. However, in a more recent study by Trzepacz et al. (28), none of 13 patients with thyrotoxicosis and psychiatric symptoms presented with psychosis.

Recommended Lab Tests to Aid Diagnosis

The assay of thyroid-stimulating hormone (TSH) is the screening test of choice for detecting thyroid disorders. A diagnostic strategy is outlined in Figure 2 for its use. Normal TSH concentrations suggest a normal thyroid function. An elevated TSH level signifies possible hypothyroidism and further testing for total or free T4 (thyroxine) is indicated. Subnormal or undetectable TSH may signify hyperthyroidism and total or free T4 and T3 (triiodothyronine) levels or a thyrotropin-releasing hormone–stimulation (TRH) test can be obtained for diagnostic confirmation.

Table 7 Laboratory Evaluations of First-Episode Patients

First-line
Drug screen
General chemistry screen
Complete blood count
Urinalysis
Second-line
Pregnancy test
Electrocardiogram
MRI or CT scan of the brain
Electroencephalogram
Neuropsychological testing
General psychological testing

Source: Ref. 29.

SUMMARY

There is no agreement on what constitutes "routine" laboratory screening tests for diagnosing schizophrenia. Some researchers recommend a narrow group of tests; others recommend a nonselective, larger number of tests.

As suggested by the information presented in this chapter, laboratory tests are most useful when used to rule out a specific medical condition. However, the Expert Consensus Guideline for the treatment of schizophrenia recommends several laboratory evaluations (Table 7) for first-episode psychosis (29).

Laboratory tests should not be used as a substitute for a thorough history, complete review of systems, careful physical and neurological examination, and mental-status examination. The physician must take into account all aspects of the clinical evaluation, and use sound clinical judgment when ordering a lab test. Clinicians are most likely to select the proper laboratory test when they suspect particular medical conditions based on information obtained from the history and clinical examination. Medical conditions that are likely to present with psychosis as discussed in the text are summarized in Table 8 with the relevant laboratory tests.

Table 8 Medical Conditions That May Present with Psychosis, and Relevant Lab Tests

Condition	Test
Drug-induced conditions	Urine and/or serum drug screen Biologic markers for alcoholism Specific assays for prescription drugs
Seizure disorders	EEG MRI if indicated
Brain tumors	CT scan with contrast MRI
Stroke	CT scan in the first 48 hours MRI
HIV	ELISA and Western blot
Neurosyphilis	VDRL or RPR CSF VDRL FTA-ABS
SLE	Serum ANA (antinuclear antibodies) Serum anti-DNA antibodies LA (lupus anticoagulant)
Thyroid disorders	TSH and other tests per diagnostic strategy
Acute intermittent porphyria (AIP)	Urine PBG (porphobilinogen) Urine ALA (aminolevulinic acid) Uroporphyrin
Vitamin B_{12} deficiency	CBC Vitamin B_{12} levels Schilling test

REFERENCES

1. American Psychiatric Association. Diagnostic and Statistical Manual of Mental Disorders. 4th ed. Washington, DC: American Psychiatric Press, 1994.
2. Hoffman RS, Koran LM. Detecting physical illness in patients with mental disorders. Psychosomatics 1984; 25(9):654–660.
3. Schuckit MA. Drug and Alcohol Abuse. 5th ed. New York: Kluwer Academic/Plenum, 2000.
4. Kaplan HI, Sadock BJ. Comprehensive Textbook of Psychiatry. 7th ed. Baltimore: Williams & Wilkins, 2000.
5. Lowinson JH, Ruiz P, Millman RB. Substance Abuse: A Comprehensive Textbook. 3rd ed. Philadelphia: Lippincott, Williams & Wilkins, 1997.
6. Lishman WA. Organic Psychiatry: The Psychological Consequences of Cerebral Disorder. 3rd ed. London: Blackwell Science, 1998.

7. Stoudemire A, Fogel BS, Greenberg D. Psychiatric Care of the Medical Patient. 2nd ed. New York: Oxford University Press, 2000.
8. Schmidt D, Schachter S. Epilepsy: Problem Solving in Clinical Practice. London: Martin Dunitz, 2000.
9. Keschner M, Bender MB, Strauss I. Mental symptoms associated with brain tumors: a study of 530 verified cases. JAMA 1938; 110:714–718.
10. Roberts JKA, Lishman WA. The use of CAT head scanner in clinical psychiatry. Br J Psychiatry 1984; 145:152–158.
11. Remington FB, Robert SL. Why patients with brain tumors come to a psychiatric hospital: a thirty year survey. Am J Psychiatry 1962; 119:256–257.
12. Malamud N. Psychiatric disorder with intracranial tumors of limbic system. Arch Neurol 1967; 17:113–123.
13. Rabins PV, Starkstein SE, Robinson RG. Risk factors for developing atypical (schizophreniform) psychosis following stroke, J Neuropsychiatry 1991; 3(1):6–9.
14. Levine DN, Finkelstein S. Delayed psychosis after right temporoparietal stroke or trauma: relation to epilepsy. Neurology 1982; 32:267–273.
15. Halstead S, Riccio M, Harlow P, Oretti R, Thompson C. Psychosis associated with HIV infection. Br J Psychiatry 1988; 153:618–623.
16. Halevie-Goldman BD, Potkin SG, Poyourow P. AIDS-related complex presenting as psychosis. Am J Psychiatry 1987; 144(7):964.
17. Sewell DD, Jeste DV, Atkinson JH, Heaton RK, Hesselink JR, Wiley C, Thal L, Chandler JL, Grant I. HIV-associated psychosis: a study of 20 cases. Am J Psychiatry 1994; 151:2:237–242.
18. Weinhardt LS, Carey MP, Johnson BT, Bickham NL. Effects of HIV counseling and testing on sexual risk behavior: a meta-analytic review of published research, 1985–1997. Am J Public Health 1999; 89:1397–1405.
19. Sivakumar K, Okocha CI. Neurosyphilis and schizophrenia. Br J Psychiatry 1992; 161:251–254.
20. Lim L, Ron MA, Ormerod IEC, et al. Psychiatric and neurological manifestations in systematic lupus erythematosus. Q J Med 1988; 66:27–38.
21. Cook CC, Hallwood PM, Thomson AD. B vitamin deficiency and neuropsychiatric syndromes in alcohol misuse. Alcohol Alcohol 1998; 33:317–336.
22. Payinda G, Hansen T. Vitamin B12 deficiency manifested as psychosis without anemia. Am J Psychiatry 2000; 157(4):660–661.
23. Tishler PV, Woodward B, O'Connor J, Holbrook DA, Seidman LJ, Halett M, Knighton DJ. High prevalence of intermittent acute porphyria in a psychiatric patient population. Am J Psychiatry 1985; 142:1430–1436.
24. Yudofsky SC, Hales RE. The American Psychiatric Textbook of Neuropsychiatry. 3rd ed. Washington, DC: American Psychiatric Press, 1997.
25. Easson WM. Myxedema with psychosis, Arch Gen Psychiatry 1966; 14:277–283.
26. Pitts FN, Guze SB. Psychiatric disorders and myxedema. Arch Gen Psychiatry 1961; 142–147.

27. Bursten B. Psychoses associated with thyrotoxicosis. Arch Gen Psychiatry 1961; 4:73–79.
28. Trzepacz PT, McCue M, Klein I, Levey GS, Greenhouse J. A psychiatric and neuropsychological study of patients with untreated Graves' Disease. Gen Hosp Psychiatry 1988; 10:49–55.
29. Expert Consensus Guideline Series. Treatment of schizophrenia. J Clin Psychiatry 1996; 57:31 & 50.
30. Goldman LS, Wise TN, Brody DS. Psychiatry for Primary Care Physicians. American Medical Association and American Psychiatric Press, 1998.
31. Kay J, Tasman A. Psychiatry: Behavioral Science and Clinical Essentials. Philadelphia: WB Saunders, 2000.
32. Rosse RB, Giese AA, Deutsch SI, Morihisa JM. Laboratory Diagnostic Testing in Psychiatry. Washington, DC: American Psychiatric Press, 1989.
33. Klee GG, Hay ID. Assessment of sensitive thyrotropin assays for an expanded role in thyroid function testing: proposed criteria for analytic performance and clinical utility. J Clin Endocrinol Metab 1987; 64:461–471.

6

Treatment of Acute Psychotic Episodes

Michael D. Jibson and Rajiv Tandon
University of Michigan Health System
Ann Arbor, Michigan

INTRODUCTION

The clinical course of schizophrenia typically involves a recurring pattern of acute psychotic episodes, during which the patient experiences significant worsening of positive symptoms, including delusions, hallucinations, thought disorganization, and catatonia. In fact, repeated periods of acute psychosis are among the hallmarks of schizophrenic illness. However, deterioration in the basic realms of life is equally significant in the clinical presentation of schizophrenia. Loss of social, occupational, and personal interests is an important, and potentially devastating, aspect of the illness.

In general, acute episodes of illness are defined by a worsening of active psychotic symptoms, and treatment of an episode focuses on the control of these symptoms. However, optimal treatment of schizophrenia requires attention to all areas of pathology, even during the acute phase. This chapter addresses the treatment of acute episodes of schizophrenia, focusing on the rapid and complete control of psychotic symptoms, but with attention to the implications of such treatment for the longer course of the illness.

BASIC CONCEPTS

A period of acute psychotic illness can herald the diagnosis of schizophrenia, bringing to light both positive and negative symptoms that may have developed over a period of months or years. Although such individuals may be referred to as "first-episode" or "new-onset" schizophrenic patients, it is important to recognize that it may be only the recognition of symptoms that is new; significant psychopathology may have been present for a considerable period (1,2). Left untreated, psychosis tends to worsen in severity and becomes less responsive to treatment, a trend that continues throughout the course of illness (3,4). Although many patients will not fully respond to antipsychotic treatment, a reasonable goal of acute therapy is the total alleviation of active psychotic symptoms.

Negative symptoms, such as blunted affect, alogia, loss of motivation, asociality, anhedonia, and inattention, may also worsen during acute episodes of illness. In contrast to active psychotic symptoms, negative symptoms respond slowly to treatment, and may not return to their previous baseline following an acute episode of illness, even with aggressive medication and psychosocial management. Deterioration in social and occupational function are highly correlated with persistent negative symptoms (5,6), which can progress during acute phases of the illness (7). At present, the most effective intervention to minimize the long-term deterioration in function associated with schizophrenia appears to be prevention of, or early intervention in, acute psychotic episodes (8).

The course of schizophrenia is highly variable (9). Following the initial period of overt illness, only a small number of patients enjoy full recovery, with no subsequent episodes of active illness or significant functional deterioration (10). A larger minority of patients have a more severe course, and experience unremitting psychotic symptoms over many years, with rapid and profound loss of function. Unfortunately, however, a common pattern is a course of gradual deterioration, with periodic exacerbation of psychosis, followed by only partial symptom remission (11). Thus, over the course of illness, acute psychotic symptoms may become less responsive to medications, episodes may take longer to resolve, and functional deterioration progresses in a stepwise fashion with each relapse. Early, aggressive antipsychotic treatment is essential to prevent this from happening (4,12).

CLINICAL ISSUES

Symptoms of Acute Episodes

Psychosis

Active psychosis is the hallmark of an acute schizophrenic episode. Delusions have been reported to occur in 65% of patients with acute symptoms, while hallucinations and thought disorganization each are reported in about 50% of patients. The content of both delusions and hallucinations crosses a wide range of types and subjects. There appears to be little diagnostic or prognostic significance to the content of these phenomena, although patients with persecutory delusions are more likely than others to act on their psychotic thoughts (13). Other psychotic symptoms, such as suspiciousness, unusual thought content, and catatonia, are noted less commonly. More than half of patients experience multiple symptoms (14).

The duration of psychotic symptoms is variable. Among undiagnosed schizophrenic individuals, periods of 1–2 years of active psychotic symptoms have been reported as being typical prior to diagnosis and treatment (1,2). Among patients receiving ongoing treatment, it is expected that worsening of psychotic symptoms will be detected more promptly. More difficult to characterize are patients who drop out of treatment and are lost to follow-up. Such patients may remain without treatment over extended periods, until their symptoms become unendurable to themselves or families, or they come to the attention of public agencies such as community mental health or law enforcement.

Agitation

Agitation is a state of anxiety, heightened emotional arousal, and increased motor activity, not specific to any one psychiatric condition or diagnosis. The agitated patient may be uncooperative with evaluation and treatment, attempt to flee the treatment setting, or become argumentative, hostile, and aggressive when approached.

The causes of agitation are many, and cross numerous psychiatric and medical diagnoses. Drug intoxication, alcohol withdrawal, personality disorders, mood disorders, delirium, hypoxia, endocrine disorders, and impaired cognition are among the more common causes of agitation. A prior diagnosis of schizophrenia should not exclude from consideration other possible causes of agitation, which may occur concurrently.

In conjunction with psychotic symptoms, agitation may arise in response to the disturbing content of delusions or hallucinations. It may also be the product of a deteriorating capacity to maintain an organized and coherent train of thought, or may arise in response to the perceived intrusions of mental health and law enforcement officials offering therapeutic interventions.

Of special note is the apparent similarity of akathisia, which is a subjective sense of restlessness, and occurs as a side effect of antipsychotic medications. The prevalence of akathisia with conventional antipsychotic medications, especially high-potency neuroleptics such as haloperidol or fluphenazine, is high. Rates of akathisia reported with atypical antipsychotic medications are lower, but still clinically significant. Akathisia is strongly associated with premature discontinuation of treatment (15,16). Despite the implications of akathisia for outcome, it often goes unreported by patients and physicians, or may be mistaken for agitation, anxiety, insomnia, or tardive dyskinesia.

Aggression

Threats or acts of violence toward others, self, or inanimate objects are common among untreated schizophrenic patients. Aggression has been found to be positively correlated with active psychosis and with cognitive impairment, both of which may be present in schizophrenia. A comparison of aggressive and nonaggressive schizophrenic patients shows that more severe psychopathology, more active psychotic symptoms, a higher incidence of persecutory delusions, greater thought disorganization, and lower impulse control occur in the aggressive group (17).

The relationship between active psychosis and aggressive behavior suggests that violent threats and acts may be reduced by effective treatment of psychotic symptoms. Although antipsychotic medications have not been found to reduce violence in the nonpsychiatric population, they are effective among schizophrenic patients (18). Additional approaches include reduction in agitation and akathisia, verbal de-escalation, and physical intervention.

Negative Symptoms

Negative symptoms may worsen during acute schizophrenic episodes in conjunction with active psychosis. Increased social isolation and withdrawal, lack of motivation for work and recreation, inattention to social situations and cues, and deficient affective expression are common during acute episodes. Increases in negative symptoms secondary to depression, institutionalization, or side effects of antipsychotic medications may also occur during episodes of active illness. In contrast to psychotic symptoms, negative symptoms do not typically show a rapid or complete response to antipsychotic medications, and may remain at an elevated level indefinitely following an acute episode.

Catatonia

The catatonic symptoms of immobility, mutism, posturing, and waxy flexibility are most often associated with mood and medical disorders (19), but may be seen in patients with schizophrenia. The history may be especially useful to identify the underlying disorder, as catatonic symptoms tend to be recurrent in schizophrenic patients. Catatonia may also be confused with severe medication side effects, such as bradykinesia, acute dystonia, or neuroleptic malignant syndrome.

Precipitating Factors

Although the natural history of schizophrenia includes episodic exacerbation of psychotic symptoms, it is often the goal of treatment to produce a total remission of psychosis. Worsening of psychotic symptoms despite appropriate treatment can occur spontaneously, but is most often the result of specific precipitating factors. Thus, treatment of the acute episode requires attention to these relapse triggers, which are sufficiently common that they should be considered in every acute case.

Treatment Noncompliance

The most common cause of relapse in schizophrenia is the failure to comply with prescribed treatment. Treatment noncompliance increases the risk for relapse fivefold (20), and nearly 20% of relapsing patients have abandoned prescribed treatment within 3 months of discharge (21). It is not surprising, therefore, that nearly 75% of patients with recurrent psychotic symptoms have discontinued antipsychotic medications (22).

Several factors appear to be related to treatment noncompliance, including denial of illness, lack of insight, inadequate family and social support, and side effects. Of these, unacceptable side effects may be most prominent. With conventional neuroleptics, extrapyramidal side effects (EPS) such as akathisia, bradykinesia, rigidity, and dystonia are common. Less conspicuous consequences of EPS, including cognitive dysfunction, dysphoria, and secondary negative symptoms, further contribute to patient dissatisfaction (23). Other side effects of widespread concern to patients include tardive dyskinesia, anticholinergic effects, sexual dysfunction, sedation, and weight gain.

The advent of atypical antipsychotic medications has greatly reduced the side-effect burden faced by schizophrenic patients. Atypical agents are far less likely to cause EPS and tardive dyskinesia than their predecessors; hence, acceptance of these medications is better than with conventional agents. In general, patients have been more willing to continue taking atypical antipsychotics, and their improved compliance has resulted in a reduction in relapse rates and an improvement in the long-term course of illness (8).

Despite their improved side-effect profiles, however, the newer drugs are not totally free of unfavorable side effects. Akathisia, sedation, weight gain, and sexual dysfunction are all noted by patients, and these side effects can also adversely influence patient acceptance of treatment. Even with atypical antipsychotics, side effects remain the leading cause of treatment noncompliance.

Other predictive factors to consider in order to understand patient noncompliance are lack of insight and hostility toward treatment providers (2,22). Patient education, attention to the patient–physician relationship, family support, and psychosocial interventions may be helpful in reducing noncompliance due to these factors.

Substance Abuse

Substance abuse is common among schizophrenic patients (24), and can also play a role in relapse (25,26). Illicit drugs can exacerbate preexisting symptoms, stimulate new symptoms, and lower the threshold for psychotic decompensation. Assessment of the patient's current drug use and risk for subsequent substance abuse is essential. Dual-diagnosis treatment of substance abuse has been recommended as an effective tool to improve outcome in this population, although data to support the effectiveness of these interventions are sparse (27).

Psychosocial Stressors

A relationship between psychosocial stressors and schizophrenic relapse has long been noted (28,29). Vulnerability of schizophrenic patients to the effects of life stress is heightened by their social isolation, limited insight, cognitive impairments, and narrow range of coping skills. The likelihood of relapse in the wake of stressful life events may be reduced by effective antipsychotic treatment, social-skills training, family psychoeducation, and aggressive case management (30).

Depression

The prevalence of depression in the schizophrenic population is high, affecting more than half of patients (31). Depressive symptoms may occur in conjunction with acute episodes of schizophrenia, and are sometimes masked by the more florid symptoms of acute psychosis.

There is also significant overlap in the presentation of the vegetative signs of depression and the negative symptoms of schizophrenia, making the simultaneous diagnosis of both conditions difficult. Negative symptoms further reduce the likelihood that depression will be recognized by the patient or the physician by masking the usual affective presentation of the disorder, and by creating significant limitations in the patient's ability to identify and report mood symptoms.

Medical Illness

At least half of schizophrenic patients have a significant medical condition, yet they present medical complaints to health-care providers at a lower rate than the general population (32). Inattention to self-care, difficulty describing physical complaints, negative reactions from health-care providers, and lack of access to medical care all contribute to a high rate of unrecognized and untreated medical illness (33). As in the case of psychosocial stress, physical illness may predispose an otherwise stable patient to relapse. Attention to medical comorbidity is therefore essential for maintenance therapy, and for the evaluation of relapsing patients.

CLINICAL INTERVENTIONS

Treatment Setting

Not all acutely psychotic patients require inpatient care. With the advent of Assertive Community Treatment (ACT) programs and acute residential facilities, it is possible to treat many patients with escalating symptoms in the community. Factors to consider in the decision of where to treat an acutely psychotic patient include patient safety, safety of others, clarity of diagnosis, degree of patient compliance, prior history of treatment, degree of treatment compliance, and access to clinical care (Table 1). More than one setting may be employed during a single acute psychotic episode, with changes in the level of care provided in response to the patient's improving or deteriorating condition.

Table 1 Criteria for Admission to Various Treatment Settings

Emergency room evaluation	Acute residential treatment	Inpatient hospitalization
Threats or acts of harm to self or others	Inattention to self-care	Dangerousness to self or others
Acute agitation	Need for additional support staff	Severe agitation
Serious medication side effects	Passive noncompliance	Grossly inadequate self-care
Severe medical symptoms		Need for aggressive medication therapy
Rapid escalation of psychotic symptoms		Poor cooperation with treatment
		Significant diagnostic uncertainty
		Lack of alternative community-based services

Emergency Room

With 24-hour operation and access to both inpatient and outpatient services for disposition, hospital emergency rooms are essential clearinghouses for acutely psychotic patients of all types. Most large emergency rooms are able to deal with acutely disturbed and agitated patients more safely than other settings. In addition, a well-staffed emergency room is able to bring medical, as well as psychiatric, expertise to the case quickly and efficiently. Major drawbacks to the use of emergency rooms can be lack of access to the patient's psychiatric records, separation of the patient from usual care providers, limited continuity of care, and uncertain access to a psychiatric specialist.

Appropriate reasons for the use of emergency room services include acute agitation, rapid escalation of psychotic symptoms, threats or acts of harm to self or others, severe medical symptoms, and serious medication side effects. Emergency rooms are not appropriate substitutes for an organized plan of continuing outpatient care.

The goals of emergency room treatment are to assure safety, reduce agitation and aggressiveness, assess the patient's medical condition and psychiatric symptoms, and determine the appropriate setting for the next step in evaluation and treatment. Treatment for acute medical problems and for emergent medication side effects should be administered in the emergency room setting. It is also reasonable to resume a known treatment regimen in a noncompliant patient. In general, initiation of a new treatment plan or of major changes in an existing treatment plan should be deferred to other settings, where the continuity of care can be assured.

Acute Residential Care

Intermediate levels of treatment are available in some communities, with greater staffing, physical security, and physician involvement than is routinely available to the patient in independent living or residential settings (34). These "respite care" or "crisis care" centers feature 24-hour nursing or other mental health staff, and supervision by a psychiatrist. In these settings the patient's symptoms can be monitored closely and medication compliance can be assured. These programs are appropriate for patients whose symptoms require their removal from home but who are able to maintain their safety and appropriate behavior with increased supervision and professional attention. Such settings are ideal for patients who have ceased caring adequately for themselves, who are passively noncompliant, or who benefit from the support of additional staff members. Often these programs are connected with outpatient settings such as community mental health (CMH), so that patients' clinic records may be immediately available. It may also be possible for the patient's regular psychiatrist to continue providing treatment, thereby assuring continuity of care.

Acute residential programs may be an effective and less costly alternative to hospitalization for some patients. Length of stay should be adjusted to assure that the patient's symptoms are under good control before a return to home and standard outpatient care. In cases where the patient's symptoms continue to escalate, hospitalization remains an option.

Inpatient Hospitalization

Dangerousness to self or others, severe agitation, grossly inadequate self-care, poor cooperation with treatment, lack of alternative community-based services, significant diagnostic uncertainty, and the need for aggressive medication therapy are among the reasons for hospital admission.

The hospital setting provides a safe, structured environment ideally suited for the sustained treatment of an acutely psychotic patient. In addition to assuring safety, the inpatient unit is staffed by a treatment team that possesses a range of psychiatric and psychosocial expertise to quickly and effectively diagnose and treat the patient. The primary advantages of hospital-based care over outpatient or intermediate levels of treatment are physical security, high staffing levels, and prompt availability of intensive diagnostic and therapeutic evaluation.

Once hospitalized, the patient should remain under the care of the inpatient treatment team until all acute symptoms either have been adequately controlled or are clearly improving. A workable outpatient treatment plan should be in place prior to discharge. A sufficient supply of medications and adequate supervision of the patient to ensure compliance with the follow-up plan must be provided.

Voluntary vs. Involuntary Treatment

The acutely psychotic patient is often unwilling to accept treatment. All legal jurisdictions in the United States, and most throughout the world, provide for the involuntary hospitalization and treatment of psychotic patients who are dangerous to themselves, dangerous to others, or incapable of providing for their own physical needs, such as food, clothing, or shelter. Specific procedures for civil commitment differ among the states and by country.

The decision to provide involuntary treatment should be based on the degree of danger the psychotic patient presents to self or others, and the likelihood of the patient's voluntarily complying with treatment. Paradoxically, long-term patient compliance may actually be increased by a firm therapeutic stance during such periods of dangerousness, even if the patient initially refuses to cooperate. A majority of patients forced by court order to accept antipsychotic medications against their will later acknowledge the benefits of having been made to do so, and report an increased willingness to remain compliant with treatment (35).

Phases of Treatment

Treatment of an acute psychotic episode may be conceptualized as occurring in three phases. First, active psychosis must be controlled. Second, as much of the patient's normal function as possible must be returned. Third, continuing care must be initiated to maximize maintenance of remission (36,37). Each phase involves specific interventions, and each intervention has implications for the treatment that follows. It is essential that therapeutic decisions made in the initial stages of treatment not compromise later phases of care.

Phase One: Control of Active Psychosis

Rapid control of delusions and hallucinations, particularly if they are accompanied by agitation or aggression, is the essential first step in treatment. This should be done with the fewest possible side effects, and in such a way as to minimize future transitions in treatment. Although high-potency conventional agents, such as haloperidol, may seem desirable at this point, consideration should be given to their implications for later treatment. The risk of early EPS may be a disincentive to patients already ambivalent about treatment, or may discourage patients receiving treatment for the first time. In addition, conventional neuroleptics are not optimal agents for routine long-term care, thus requiring a transition later in treatment to a different antipsychotic. In most instances, immediate initiation of an atypical antipsychotic at this stage of treatment leads most smoothly into successive stages of care.

Phase Two: Restoration of Normal Functions

As acute agitation and psychotic symptoms resolve, it becomes easier to address the negative symptoms and cognitive impairments that generally accompany active psychosis. The goal of treatment at this stage is to return the patient to the highest level of function possible. However, these symptoms resolve slowly (38,39), and much of this phase of treatment usually occurs outside the acute setting. Nonetheless, it is important to ensure treatment compliance by selecting a drug acceptable to the patient at a dose sufficient to minimize the risk of relapse. Active attention to side effects, establishment of a working relationship with the patient, and patient education are also essential components of this phase of treatment.

Phase Three: Maintenance of Remission

Although maintenance of remission is not a part of acute treatment, it has important implications for treatment decisions made throughout the course of the acute episode. The goals of this phase of treatment are continued medication compliance, participation in psychosocial treatments, and establishment of a treatment alliance with outpatient staff. As noted above, early selection of an antipsychotic with a favorable side-effect profile will have major implications for patient compliance during this phase. Additionally, continued attention to development of a working alliance with the patient throughout treatment will enhance the patient's long-term cooperation.

Selection of Medications

Conventional Neuroleptics

For nearly two generations, conventional neuroleptics were the mainstay of treatment for acute psychotic episodes. These agents are dramatically effective in reducing hallucinations, delusions, disorganization, psychotic agitation, and behavioral dyscontrol. They are also readily available, inexpensive, and easy to administer. They come in several convenient forms, including pills, liquid concentrate, and sterile solution for intramuscular or intravenous injection. Two of them, haloperidol and fluphenazine, are available in depot form for long-term administration.

Unfortunately, conventional antipsychotics are limited by their unfavorable side-effect profiles. EPS are frequent and severe, with implications for long-term side effects, such as tardive dyskinesia. EPS contribute to patient discomfort, secondary negative symptoms, the stigma of movement disorders, cognitive impairments, and dysphoria. The frequent outcome of the use of these medications is noncompliance and increased risk of relapse.

Even with these limitations, conventional neuroleptics may be used because of the need for injectable medication, patient preference, prior treatment failure on atypical agents, or anticipation of depot antipsychotic administration.

Atypical Antipsychotic Medications

Atypical antipsychotic medications are the preferred treatment for acute psychosis in both the short and long term. These agents have at least equal efficacy with conventional drugs in the treatment of positive symptoms, and are somewhat more effective against negative symptoms and cognitive impairments. Furthermore, they enjoy a more favorable side-effect profile, especially with regard to EPS. Antipsychotic effectiveness in the absence of EPS is the essence of the atypical drugs. The development of EPS with these medications, or the need to use anticholinergic agents to avoid EPS, constitutes a loss of their atypicality, and merits consideration of a change in medication or dose. EPS are rare at low and moderate doses of risperidone, and at all doses of olanzapine, quetiapine, and ziprasidone. Current evidence suggests that these agents are equally efficacious in treatment of psychotic symptoms, and are equivalent in speed of onset of action. They may differ, however, in pharmacological profile and side-effect patterns.

Although large studies have not conclusively shown that any one of these agents is superior to the others in clinical activity, a growing body of anecdotal evidence suggests that individual patients may respond differently to them. Thus, patients whose symptoms fail to respond adequately to one agent should be treated with a different atypical drug. The question of how many first-line atypical medications should be used before clozapine is tried has not been definitively answered. However, it now appears reasonable to suggest that at least two first-line drugs, and possibly more, should be tried. The question of whether a conventional neuroleptic should also be tried prior to clozapine remains open.

The initial selection of a first-line atypical antipsychotic drug is left to patient and physician preference. A comparison of first-line medications is shown in Table 2. The medication should be rapidly titrated to a full therapeutic dose, but not beyond that. Side effects with the first few doses may resolve spontaneously, but should nevertheless be monitored for the comfort of the patient, and to ensure continued compliance.

If side effects do become limiting, the drug dose may be adjusted downward for a time, followed by a second attempt at upward dose titration. If this fails, a change to another agent may be warranted. At this point in treatment, the physician should be well aware of the side effects most troublesome to the patient, and can select the drug least likely to cause that side effect.

Olanzapine. Olanzapine is a widely used first-line antipsychotic agent with excellent efficacy against positive symptoms and some effectiveness against negative and cognitive symptoms (40). As with all atypical medications, EPS are minimal, with the exception of akathisia, which is reported in a significant number of patients (41). Olanzapine has a relatively long elimination half-time, making it practical for once-daily dosing. The medication is well tolerated, and can be started at the full dose or rapidly titrated without severe side effects in most cases. Long-term compliance tends to be good.

Major side effects of olanzapine include weight gain, sedation, dry mouth, nausea, lightheadedness, orthostatic hypotension, dizziness, constipation, headache, akathisia, and transient elevation of hepatic transaminases. The risk of tardive dyskinesia is low (42). Weight gain can become a problem for a significant portion of patients, and should be monitored periodically.

A typical initial dose of olanzapine is 5 mg b.i.d., followed by titration at a rate of 5–10 mg/day. The average olanzapine dose currently in clinical use is 15–20 mg/day. Also, the manufacturer's recommended maximum dose of 20 mg/day can be exceeded in clinical practice, usually without problems. Although olanzapine is appropriate

Table 2 Dosing Schedules for First-Line Antipsychotic Mediations

	Initial dose (mg b.i.d.)	Rate of titration (mg/day)	Standard dose (mg/day)	Dosing frequency	Maximum recommended dose (mg/day)	Advantages	Disadvantages
Atypical antipsychotics							
Olanzapine	5	10	15–20	q.d.–b.i.d.	40	Well tolerated; stabilizes mood	Weight gain; no liquid form; no injectable form
Quetiapine	25	50–100	400–600	b.i.d.–t.i.d.	800	Well tolerated; lowest EPS risk	Slow titration; sedation; no liquid form; no injectable form
Risperidone	1–2	2	2–6	q.d.–b.i.d.	6–8	Well tolerated; well defined dose range	Dose-dependent EPS; no injectable form
Ziprasidone	40–80	Not reported	80–160	b.i.d.	160	Well tolerated; no weight gain	Limited clinical experience; qT prolongation
Conventional neuroleptics							
Haloderidol	5	10	15–20	q.d.–b.i.d.	30	Injectable	Unfavorable side effects—EPS

for once-daily dosing, it is often initiated on a twice-daily schedule to minimize initial side effects. Olanzapine is not currently available in liquid, injectable, or depot forms.

Quetiapine. Quetiapine is gaining acceptance as a first-line antipsychotic medication with efficacy for positive, negative, and cognitive symptoms comparable to other atypical agents (43). EPS occur rarely, even at the maximum dose of 800 mg/day. A relatively short elimination half-time suggests the need for at least twice-daily dosing, although once-daily dosing has been tried successfully. The medication requires dose titration to avoid initial side effects, after which it is well tolerated.

Major side effects of quetiapine are somnolence, postural hypotension, dizziness, agitation, dry mouth, and weight gain (44). Akathisia occurs rarely, and in some studies was reported at a rate comparable to placebo. Early data on tardive dyskinesia are suggestive of a low incidence.

Most clinical doses of quetiapine are in the 400–600-mg/day range, although doses up to 800 mg/day are well tolerated. Early clinical experience suggests a tendency of physicians to underestimate the effective dose range of quetiapine for many patients, resulting in less than optimal responses. A low threshold for dose titration into the 400–800-mg/day range is recommended to avoid this problem. An initial dose of 25 mg b.i.d., followed by titration in 25–50-mg/day increments, is often useful to minimize sedation and hypotension. Also, these side effects generally resolve within a few days, after which the dose titration can proceed more rapidly (50–200 mg/day), but with some continuing risk of side effects. Quetiapine is not available in liquid, injectable, or depot forms.

Risperidone. Risperidone was the earliest of the first-line atypical antipsychotics to be introduced, giving it the longest period of open clinical experience. The medication shows efficacy equal to that of other first-line atypical drugs against the full range of schizophrenic symptoms (45,46). The medication is well tolerated with once- or twice-daily dosing. Dose titration may be useful to avoid initial side effects, but is not essential. Long-term compliance and rates of relapse are favorable with maintenance treatment.

Common side effects of risperidone include drowsiness, orthostatic hypotension, lightheadedness, anxiety, akathisia, constipation, nausea, nasal congestion, prolactin elevation, and weight gain. At doses up to 6 mg/day, risperidone shows little propensity for EPS, except akathisia, which is common. Above 6 mg/day, dose-dependent EPS become significant. The risk of tardive dyskinesia with risperidone appears to be low.

An initial dose of 1–2 mg b.i.d. tends to be well tolerated. Most patients respond well to maintenance doses of 2–6 mg/day. Although clinical studies show that doses up to 16 mg/day are safe, doses higher than 6 mg/day should be used with caution, because of the risk of EPS. The medication is often initiated on a twice-daily schedule to minimize side effects. Risperidone is available in pill and liquid form, but not as an injectable agent. A depot form is currently in clinical trials.

Ziprasidone. Ziprasidone is now available for clinical use in the United States, having undergone a number of clinical trials demonstrating its safety and efficacy against positive and negative symptoms of schizophrenia (47,48). The medication is administered twice daily, in keeping with a brief elimination half-time. Data on long-term compliance in standard clinical use are not yet available.

The major side effects associated with ziprasidone are headache, somnolence, nausea, dyspepsia, and prolongation of the qT_c interval, with a lower frequency of dizziness, weakness, nasal discharge, orthostatic hypotension, and tachycardia. Ziprasidone is unique among atypical antipsychotic medications in apparently not causing weight gain (49). EPS, including akathisia, also do not appear to be a problem. Preclinical data suggest a low risk of tardive dyskinesia, but no clinical studies are yet available. Prolongation of the qT_c interval occurs with all atypical (and with high doses of conventional) antipsychotic medications, although to a somewhat greater degree with ziprasidone than with the others. Although this finding has generated much discussion and scrutiny of the medication, its clinical significance is unclear.

Doses of 80–160 mg/day have been found to be most effective in clinical trials. Ziprasidone is unique among atypical agents in that an injectable form, as well as pills, is being developed. This may prove to be an especially useful tool in the acute setting.

Clozapine. Clozapine is not a first-line antipsychotic medication, but may be used in the acutely psychotic patient if other agents have proven ineffective. Clozapine remains the only antipsychotic agent proven to be effective in treatment-refractory cases (50). Major disadvantages of clozapine use in these patients include the need for gradual titration, an unfavorable side-effect profile, and the uncertainty that the patient will be sufficiently compliant with blood tests during the maintenance phase of treatment.

Depot Antipsychotic Medications

Only the conventional neuroleptic agents haloperidol and fluphenazine are currently available in decanoate preparations for depot administration. These medications are of proven efficacy in relapse prevention

(51,52), and are particularly useful in patients whose compliance with daily medications is suboptimal. These medications may be considered in the acute phase of illness for patients recently maintained on them or known to be noncompliant with other antipsychotic treatments.

In general, patients should be stabilized on an oral preparation of the drug to be given prior to initiation of depot injections. A useful guideline for estimation of the dose of haloperidol decanoate is 10 times the total daily dose administered every 4 weeks. No similar rule for prediction of fluphenazine decanoate dosing has been suggested.

Antipsychotic Drug Combinations

The simultaneous prescription of more than one antipsychotic medication for schizophrenic patients is common, and may, in fact, be increasing in frequency. This strategy is most often used for treatment-refractory patients who have previously had subtherapeutic responses to single antipsychotic agents. However, routine use of multiple antipsychotic agents in patients who also respond to monotherapy is associated with numerous problems, and has little to recommend it (3).

In the acute phase of treatment, common indications for use of more than one antipsychotic drug are the need to use an injectable agent in a patient already receiving an oral atypical medication, and cross-titration of an ineffective medication with the agent selected to replace it. As noted above, whenever possible, oral administration of antipsychotic drugs is preferable to injection. When oral dosing is not an option, injection of conventional neuroleptics becomes the only available avenue. In these cases, a single conventional agent should be used until it is possible to resume oral dosing with the atypical medication.

Attempts are sometimes made to avoid higher than recommended doses of antipsychotic medications (e.g., >20 mg/day of olanzapine) by addition of a second antipsychotic agent when the maximum dose of the first drug is reached. It should be borne in mind that the most likely basis for antipsychotic activity is dopamine-D_2-receptor blockade, and that the somewhat different receptor profiles of the various typical and atypical drugs do not imply reduced D_2-receptor activity (53). Thus, there is no advantage to the combination of two medications over the use of one drug at a higher dose.

In cases of a transition from one medication to another, it is usual to cross-titrate. This involves the gradual taper of the previous medication with the simultaneous upward titration of the replacement (Figure 1). In high-risk cases, it is often useful to titrate the new

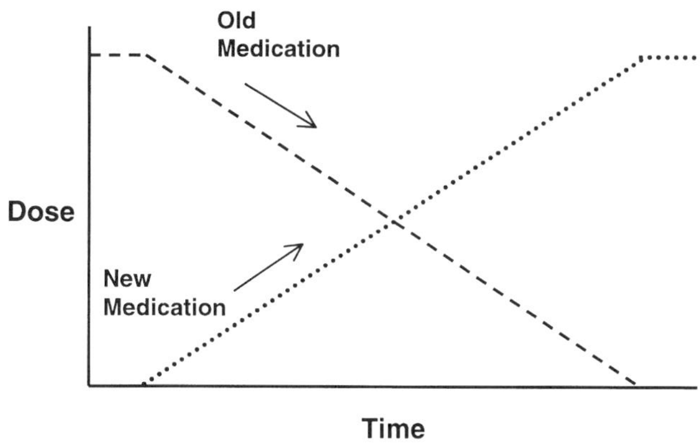

Figure 1 Standard cross-titration of antipsychotic medications. The old medication (dashes) is gradually tapered as the new medication (dots) is simultaneously increased.

medication to its full dose prior to taper of the existing therapy (Figure 2). Although this briefly exposes the patient to full doses of two antipsychotic medications, it ensures that the patient's dosing regimen never falls below a potentially effective level. This procedure is generally well tolerated.

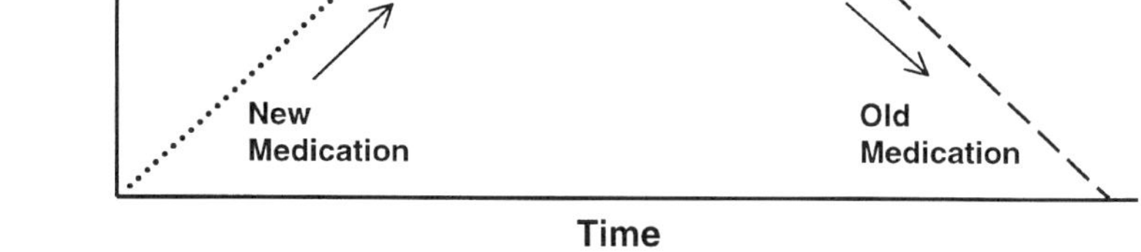

Figure 2 High-risk cross-titration of antipsychotic medications. The new medication (dots) is titrated to its full dose before the old medication (dashes) begins to be tapered.

Benzodiazepines

The use of benzodiazepines, such as lorazepam or clonazepam, to reduce agitation in acutely psychotic patients is well established. Clinical data suggest that the combination of benzodiazepines and antipsychotics given together yields superior results to either agent alone (54). Benefits of benzodiazepines include rapid calming and sedation, decreased anxiety, and reduction of akathisia. Although it was formerly suggested that these drugs might augment the antipsychotic effects of conventional neuroleptics or the newer atypical agents, there is scant evidence to suggest that they have any inherent antipsychotic efficacy.

These medications are most useful in the early days or weeks of treatment. Tolerance to these drugs develops, and they are not as beneficial when continued in the longer term. Indications for the long-term use of benzodiazepines include persistent akathisia and anxiety.

In cases of catatonia or mutism, a single dose of benzodiazepine may bring about dramatic, although often temporary, improvement (55). This is especially useful in patients with symptoms of unknown etiology with whom a diagnostic interview is otherwise difficult or impossible. One dose of benzodiazepine often makes it possible to interview the patient and conduct essential aspects of the mental-status examination that were previously inaccessible. This simple and safe diagnostic procedure has replaced the more complex and hazardous barbiturate infusion ("amytal interview") in most settings. The striking improvement seen in many catatonic or mute patients following this procedure is not usually sustained, however, even with scheduled doses of the medication. Definitive treatment for this condition, such as electroconvulsive therapy, is usually required (56,57).

Anticholinergics

During the era of conventional neuroleptics, the use of anticholinergic agents was almost ubiquitous in treatment regimens. Their capacity to reduce EPS, including bradykinesia, akathisia, and acute dystonic reactions, made them an essential adjunct to antipsychotic treatment. In situations where conventional agents are still given, this remains true. If these drugs are preferred because of the availability of injectable or depot forms, or a history of efficacy in an individual patient, anticholinergic agents should always be available. In patients with recurrent or persistent EPS, even if mild, scheduled anticholinergic treatment is appropriate.

Anticholinergic agents are not without side effects, which must also be monitored. The classic symptoms of dry mouth, constipation, blurred vision, and urinary hesitancy are common. Less obvious consequences of anticholinergic use include cognitive impairment and mild intoxication, hence their potential for abuse by patients and others. The empirical observation that patients who receive higher doses of anticholinergic agents are at increased risk for developing tardive dyskinesia (TD) probably reflects the relationship between EPS and TD, rather than a causative effect of the drugs.

The use of anticholinergic medications in conjunction with atypical antipsychotic drugs is less well established. EPS in the presence of higher doses of risperidone are usually better treated by a dose reduction or by selection of an alternative agent. However, anticholinergic medications may be useful in patients for whom alternatives to high doses of risperidone are limited. A major indication for anticholinergic augmentation with the atypical agents may be akathisia, which remains common even with the newer drugs. Anticholinergic treatment is, however, only one of several options to alleviate akathisia. β-blocking agents, benzodiazepines, and antihistamines are also useful. Finally, sialorrhea associated with clozapine may be reduced by anticholinergic administration, though perhaps at the expense of worsening constipation, blurred vision, and urinary retention.

β-Blockers

β-adrenergic-receptor antagonists are used in psychiatry for the treatment of akathisia, chronic agitation, impulsive aggression, behavioral dyscontrol, performance anxiety, and the somatic component of anxiety disorders. In an acute psychotic episode, they are especially useful for treatment of akathisia (58). They may also be helpful in cases of persistent agitation and behavioral dyscontrol.

However, significant disadvantages of these drugs include hypotension and respiratory difficulties in asthma patients. Hypotension may be worsened by the tendency of most antipsychotic agents, both conventional and atypical, to cause the same effect.

Mood Stabilizers

Although mood stabilizers such as lithium, valproate, and carbamazepine have been used in conjunction with antipsychotic medications for schizophrenic patients, convincing data in support of their use with this population are lacking. Their primary indication appears to be adjunctive treatment in patients with significant mood instability, as in schizoaffective disorder, and in patients with persistent agitation. These medications do not appear to be effective when used alone to treat psychosis in schizophrenic patients.

Conversely, recent evidence has been presented in support of the mood-stabilizing effects of olanzapine (59) and clozapine (60). Additional data support the use of clozapine with or without a mood stabilizer in treatment-refractory bipolar- and schizoaffective-disorder patients. Studies in support of the use of olanzapine as a lone agent in these patients are less compelling. There may, however, be an indication for the use of olanzapine as a preferred treatment in schizophrenic patients with significant mood symptoms. Similar studies with other antipsychotics in this patient population are very limited, but suggest that both conventional and atypical antipsychotics also stabilize mood (61).

Electroconvulsive Therapy

Electroconvulsive therapy (ECT) was among the earliest effective treatments for psychosis, but has fallen from favor since the advent of antipsychotic drugs that require less intensive administration and are of more continuous benefit. ECT remains the preferred treatment for catatonia, but is otherwise relegated to the treatment of refractory patients. ECT has been shown to be safe and effective when used together with antipsychotic drugs, including clozapine (62).

SUGGESTED GUIDELINES FOR CLINICIANS

Assess and Assure Safety

The highest priority in any acute case is to assure the safety of the patient, staff, and others. The patient's degree of dangerousness may be determined by interview of the patient and accompanying individuals, review of documents available at presentation, and observation of the patient's degree of agitation. Specific threats of harm to self or others should be taken seriously, but are not essential to make the judgment that the patient presents a risk of injury. Hostility, anger, depression, hopelessness, extreme suspiciousness, agitation, psychomotor activation, command hallucinations, intoxication, and resistance to verbal interventions all suggest the possibility of dangerousness. The possession of a firearm is strongly associated with risk of both suicide and assault (63,64), and determination of the availability of such weapons to the patient is essential (Table 3). When discrepant information is presented (e.g., a family member reports having been threatened) but the patient denies it, the more cautious position should be assumed.

Steps sufficient to assure safety should be implemented promptly. These may include frequent checks on the patient, the continuous

Table 3 Assessment of Safety

	High risk	Possible risk
Suicide risk	Threats of suicide	Depression
	Active intent	Passive suicidal ideation
	Lethal plan	Intoxication
	Hopelessness	Firearm possession
	Command hallucinations	
Homicide risk	Threats of assault	Hostility
	Assault history	Anger
	Active intent	Agitation
	Specific plan	Suspiciousness
	Command hallucinations	Intoxication
	Persecutory delusions	Firearm possession
	Resistance to verbal interventions	

presence of staff, legal holds (i.e., commitment), use of antipsychotic or sedative medications, room confinement, or physical restraint. Arrangements should be made to remove weapons, particularly firearms, from the home.

Control Agitation and Aggression

When dealing with an agitated or aggressive patient, a sufficient number of staff, which may include law-enforcement or security personnel, must be present to ensure that the patient can be handled without injury to anyone involved (including himself). Verbal de-escalation should be attempted. A period of time in an isolated room with minimal sensory and social stimulation may be useful. In some cases, physical management may be the only option available.

Medication management should include an antipsychotic medication, a sedative agent, or both. The combination of an antipsychotic drug and a benzodiazepine has been shown to be more effective than either agent alone (52). Benzodiazepines have the additional benefit of treating anxiety and the akathisia that may accompany administration of antipsychotic medication. Lorazepam is the only benzodiazepine that is reliably absorbed intramuscularly, if that is the only route available to initiate treatment.

If the patient is cooperative, medication is best administered orally. Liquid concentrates of medications are absorbed more rapidly than pills, and are more difficult for the patient to surreptitiously discard.

Table 4 Medication for Acute Agitation

Oral dosing	
Option 1	Risperidone liquid concentrate 2 mg q2hr x 3
	Lorazepam 2 mg po q2hr x 3
Option 2	Olanzapine 5 mg q2hr x 3
	Lorazepam 2 mg p.o. q2hr x 3
i.m. Dosing	Haloperidol 5 mg q2hr x 3
	Lorazepam 2 mg q2hr x 3

Standard doses of medications should be used, with intervals sufficient to ascertain the effect of each dose (Table 4). Agitation usually responds to medication management within minutes or hours.

Injectable medications may be used if the patient is uncooperative with oral administration. This route of delivery has the advantages of assured compliance and rapid onset. However, these favorable factors come at the expense of increased side effects, reduced treatment alliance, and the likelihood of a need for a different medication or route of administration later in treatment.

Evaluate Presenting Symptoms

The patient should be interviewed promptly to determine the range and depth of symptoms present. Specific attention should be paid to the presence or absence of psychotic, mood, intoxication, and anxiety symptoms. Hallucinations should be characterized as to their sensory modality, frequency, intensity, and the presence or absence of threatening or command voices. Delusions should be explored as to their nature, intensity, duration, and impact on behavior. Mood symptoms may include depression or mania, and should be characterized by duration, course, intensity, and accompanying vegetative signs. Evidence of intoxication or withdrawal should be sought by history, interview, examination, and laboratory studies. This information can then be used to determine the underlying diagnosis, and to identify the symptoms most in need of treatment.

The clinician must be aware of the limitations of diagnostic evaluation in the acute patient. It may be impossible to distinguish with certainty at this stage of illness schizophrenia, schizoaffective disorder, mania, and depression with psychotic features. Such distinctions may require additional information regarding the patient's longitudinal history and development of symptoms.

Identify and Treat Precipitating Factors

Psychological, social, financial, legal, and medical issues are among the things that should be considered in the search for precipitating factors. Medical issues, including intoxication and withdrawal, may be addressed in the acute setting. Other types of stressors may be remediable in the emergency setting, or may require longer-term interventions.

It is essential to determine the patient's recent level of compliance with medications. Evidence of noncompliance should be sought by history, interview, and laboratory studies. Corroborative information from family and caregivers may be especially enlightening. If available, medical records should be reviewed. The decision of whether to immediately administer an antipsychotic medication and, if so, which medication, can sometimes be determined by this information.

Essential medical evaluation should include a medical review of systems, physical examination, and basic screening laboratories. Among the most useful laboratory studies are a toxicology screen, electrolytes, liver enzymes, TSH level, complete blood count, and urinalysis. Additional tests may be indicated by abnormal findings in the history or examination. Brain-imaging studies may be useful if suggestive neurological symptoms are present.

Treat Psychosis

Once a measure of certainty regarding the diagnosis of schizophrenia has been reached, psychotic symptoms should become the focus of treatment. This generally involves initiation of a first-line atypical antipsychotic medication (olanzapine, quetiapine, risperidone, or ziprasidone) at a tolerable initial dose, with prompt titration to a standard effective level (Table 2).

There is no compelling evidence in favor of any one atypical antipsychotic drug as a first-line treatment. For patients receiving medications for the first time, the principal factors to consider in selecting among them are physician preference, patient preference, and anticipated follow-up setting. Even patients without experience taking antipsychotic medications may have preferences. These may be based on, for example, experience of family members, publicity, or education. Compliance will be increased if attention is paid to patient preferences whenever possible. Factors of concern to the physician should include experience accrued with the medications, published studies of efficacy and adverse effects, cost, and availability. Levels of advertising, success in marketing, and availability of samples are not clinically relevant factors.

Issues to consider in the relapsing patient are patient preference, history of side effects, patterns of compliance and noncompliance, history of symptom response, and anticipated follow-up setting. Medications that have previously been effective are likely to be effective again, while patterns of side effects, noncompliance, or nonresponse are also likely to be repeated if the same medication is used. One rational basis for medication choice at this point in treatment is selection of the drug least likely to cause the side effects most troublesome to the patient in the past.

Whenever possible, oral administration is preferred. Several of the first-line atypical drugs are available in liquid form for rapid gastrointestinal absorption and to ensure patient compliance. There is no clear evidence to suggest that one of these agents has a more rapid onset of action or is more efficacious than the others.

If oral administration is refused by the patient, intramuscular injection of a conventional neuroleptic may be the only available choice (injectable forms of atypical drugs are currently in development but are not yet available). High-potency neuroleptics have the advantage of a less extensive side-effect profile, while low-potency agents provide greater sedation. In all cases, anticholinergic medication should be available if needed. A transition to an atypical drug should be arranged as soon as possible.

Even in the acute phase of illness, standard doses of antipsychotic medications should be adequate to assure rapid resolution of psychosis, and there is little evidence to suggest that extremely high doses of these drugs are beneficial. Unusually high doses of medications should be used only in patients known to be rapid metabolizers of a specific drug, or known to respond preferentially to high doses. Below-standard doses of these medications may be indicated in pediatric or geriatric patients, the medically ill, and patients with a known response to low doses of medications.

Once the antipsychotic medication is selected and started, it should be maintained within the standard dose range for at least 4–6 weeks before conclusions are drawn about its efficacy. Side effects should be actively sought and treated, with either dose adjustment or adjunctive medications. In cases of severe or persistent side effects, it may become necessary to change to an alternative medication. In the acute setting, this should be done as rapidly as possible. Frequent dose adjustments and medication changes should otherwise be avoided.

Implement Psychosocial Treatments

As the patient begins to respond to treatment, additional interventions should be initiated. These may include patient and family education, supportive psychotherapy, occupational therapy, and the establishment of case-management services. These interventions may begin in hospital, acute residential, or outpatient settings. They have been shown to contribute significantly to the stability of recovery from the acute episode, and should not be deferred unnecessarily.

Prepare for the Next Phase of Treatment

As early as possible in treatment, the patient should be placed on a scheduled dose of antipsychotic medication. Dosing changes should be limited to situations in which side effects are a problem or there is a clear failure to respond to a specific agent.

The reconstitution and maintenance phases of schizophrenia treatment generally occur in a less intense setting than the acute phase. Transitions in treatment carry increased risk of relapse, and thus should be minimized whenever possible. Unavoidable changes in medication or dose should be made as early in treatment as is practical to avoid disruption of the later stages of care. Introduction of staff who will follow up with the patient is a useful addition to the later part of the acute phase.

In anticipation of maintenance treatment, the patient should be placed on a medication and a dose that will maximize compliance and efficacy. In general, this will involve an atypical antipsychotic at the same dose that was effective to control acute symptoms. The dose may be reduced if necessary to minimize side effects. Although the long-held rule of "lowest effective dose" is essential with conventional antipsychotics, it may not be equally true for all patients on atypical agents. In order to establish the lowest effective dose, it is necessary to reduce the dose of medication until psychotic symptoms are again detected. In some patients these symptoms quickly resolve when the dose is raised, but in others they trigger a full psychotic episode. With atypical antipsychotic medications there is less compelling justification for exposure of patients to the risk of relapse by the automatic reduction of dosage after the acute phase of illness. Clinicians should carefully examine the risks, as well as the benefits, for an individual patient before making changes in medication dose.

A second reason for selection of atypical antipsychotic drugs at this stage of treatment is their improved efficacy against negative and cognitive symptoms. Although no antipsychotic medication has been shown to be dramatically effective in treatment of these symptoms, atypical agents clearly have superior efficacy compared to conventional neuroleptics.

Depot Antipsychotic Medications

For chronically noncompliant patients, depot antipsychotics should be introduced at this point in treatment. At present, the only depot agents available in the United States are the conventional antipsychotic agents haloperidol and fluphenazine. These drugs have proven efficacy in maintenance of remission, and should be considered for any patient who responds to treatment but is unwilling to continue compliance in the long term.

Several procedures have been described to rapidly load haloperidol decanoate in the acute setting. This option is desirable for patients who respond well to conventional antipsychotic treatment but are so consistently noncompliant that even temporary maintenance on oral medications is clinically unmanageable. An accelerated loading procedure minimizes the need for extended hospitalization, with its attendant expense, disruption of life activities, limitation of freedom, and risk of institutionalization.

We recommend the following procedure for patients who are known to tolerate and respond to haloperidol. Such patients are placed on a standard oral dose of the drug, typically 15–20 mg/day, for at least 3 days. On the first day of depot loading, the patient is given an initial dose of 100 mg haloperidol decanoate. The oral haloperidol is continued at its full dose. Two days later (i.e., on day 3 of the procedure) the patient is given haloperidol decanoate at 10 times the daily oral dose. Thus, for a patient receiving 20 mg/day of oral haloperidol, the dose of the decanoate preparation is 200 mg. The oral dose of the medication is then reduced by 50%. Two days later (i.e., on day 5 of the procedure) the patient is again given 10 times the daily oral dose of the decanoate, and the oral medication is discontinued. The patient is then placed on the same dose of haloperidol decanoate every 28 days from the beginning of the loading protocol (Table 5). Clinically stable patients may be discharged to outpatient care after the third loading dose (i.e., on day 5). This procedure has been used at the University of Michigan Hospital for the past 6 years in over 80 patients, with no significant adverse events and no cases of rapid relapse.

Side Effects

Side effects should be addressed aggressively at this stage of treatment. However, to limit transitions in treatment, dose adjustment is preferable

Table 5 Haloperidol Decanoate Loading Procedure for a Patient on Oral Haloperidol 15 or 20 mg/day

	Dose (mg)			
	Day 1	Day 3	Day 5	Day 28
Oral dose	15	7.5	Discontinue	None
Decanoate dose	100	150	150	150
Oral dose	20	10	Discontinue	None
Decanoate dose	100	200	200	200

to medication change to reduce side effects. When a change in medications does need to be made, a gradual cross-titration is preferable to complete discontinuation of one drug followed by titration of another. Although there is little evidence to suggest the superiority of one atypical agent over another in the acute phase of treatment, the different side-effect profiles of the first-line atypical drugs allow for the rational selection of a drug that will minimize the side effects most troublesome to the individual patient.

Psychosocial Issues

Psychosocial issues must again be addressed at this time. Attention to the treatment alliance will improve patient compliance with medications and other treatment. Patient and family education will reduce distress associated with the acute episode and improve later cooperation with treatment. Recommendations for vocational and social rehabilitation programs may also be made at this time.

SUMMARY

Acute psychotic episodes are a core element of schizophrenia, and represent critical periods in the course of illness. These periods represent times of greatest risk for injury to the patient and others, for development of persistent positive and negative symptoms and for deterioration in all aspects of function. The rapid and effective management of acute psychosis has significant consequences for the patient's immediate well-being and long-term condition.

Essential elements of clinical management include assurance of safety, evaluation and treatment of precipitating factors, rapid alleviation of psychotic symptoms, and prompt transition to medications optimal for long-term care. Atypical antipsychotic medications are the mainstay of treatment throughout the course of illness.

Treatment of acute episodes of illness does not occur in isolation, but rather in the context of the patient's individual history, symptom profile, psychosocial situation, and outpatient treatment setting. Attention to each of these factors is essential to a favorable outcome.

REFERENCES

1. Loebel AD, Lieberman JA, Alvir JM, Mayerhoff DI, Geisler SH, Szymanski SR. Duration of psychosis and outcome in first-episode schizophrenia. Am J Psychiatry 1992; 149:1183–1188.
2. Hafner H, Maurer K. Are there two types of schizophrenia? True onset and sequence of positive and negative symptoms prior to first admission. In: Marneros A, Andreason NC, Tsuang MT, eds. Negative Versus Positive Schizophrenia. Berlin: Springer-Verlag, 1991:134–159.
3. Wyatt RJ, Green MF, Turna AH. Long-term morbidity associated with delayed treatment of first admission schizophrenic patients: a reanalysis of the Camarillo State Hospital data. Psychol Med 1997; 27:261–268.
4. DeQuardo JR. Pharmacologic treatment of first-episode schizophrenia: early intervention is the key to outcome. J Clin Psychiatry 1998; 59(suppl 19):9–17.
5. Davidson L, McGlashan TH. The varied outcomes of schizophrenia. Can J Psychiatry 1997; 42:34–43.
6. McGlashan TH, Fenton WS. Subtype progression and pathophysiologic deterioration in early schizophrenia. Schizophr Bull 1993; 19:71–84.
7. Jibson MD, Tandon R. The negative symptoms of schizophrenia. Directions in Psychiatry 1995; 15:1–7.
8. DeQuardo JR, Tandon T. Do atypical antipsychotic medications favorably alter the long-term course of schizophrenia? J Psychiatry Res 1998; 32:229–242.
9. Carpenter WT Jr, Kirkpatrick B. The heterogeneity of the long-term course of schizophrenia. Schizophr Bull 1988; 14:645–652.
10. Breier A, Schreiber JL, Dyer J, Pickar D. National Institute of Mental Health longitudinal study of chronic schizophrenia: prognosis and predictors of outcome. Arch Gen Psychiatry 1991; 48:239–246.
11. Carpenter WT Jr, Buchanan RW. Medical progress: schizophrenia. N Engl J Med 1994; 330:681–690.
12. Lieberman JA. Pathophysiologic mechanisms in the pathogenesis and clinical course of schizophrenia. J Clin Psychiatry 1999; 60(suppl 12):9–12.
13. Appelbaum PS, Robbins PC, Roth LH. Dimensional approach to delusions: comparison across types and diagnoses. Am J Psychiatry 1999; 156:1938–1943.

14. Breier A, Berg PH. The psychosis of schizophrenia: prevelance, response to atypical antipsychotics, and prediction of outcome. Biol Psychiatry 1999; 46:361–364.
15. Miller CH, Mohr F, Umbricht D, Woerner M, Fleischhacker WW, Lieberman JA. The prevalence of acute extrapyramidal signs and symptoms in patients treated with clozapine, risperidone, and conventional antipsychotics. J Clin Psychiatry 1998; 59:69–75.
16. Van Putten T, Marder SR, Mintz J. A controlled dose comparison of haloperidol in newly admitted schizophrenia patients. Arch Gen Psychiatry 1990; 47:754–758.
17. Glazer WM, Dickson RA. Clozapine reduces violence and persistent aggression in schizophrenia. J Clin Psychiatry 1998; 59(suppl 3):8–14.
18. Keck PE Jr, Strakowski SM, McElroy SL. The efficacy of atypical antipsychotics in the treatment of depressive symptoms, hostility, and suicidality in patients with schizophrenia. J Clin Psychiatry 2000; 61(suppl 3):4–9.
19. Abrams R, Taylor MA. Catatonia: a prospective clinical study. Arch Gen Psychiatry 1976; 33:579–581.
20. Robinson D, Woerner MG, Alvir JM, Bilder R, Goldman R, Geisler S, Koreen A, Sheitman B, Chakos M, Mayerhoff D, Lieberman JA. Predictors of relapse following response from a first episode of schizophrenia or schizoaffective disorder. Arch Gen Psychiatry 1999; 56:241–247.
21. Olfson M, Mechanic D, Hansell S, Boyer CA, Walkup J, Weiden PJ. Predicting medication noncompliance after hospital discharge among patients with schizophrenia. Psychiatr Serv 2000; 51:216–222.
22. Ayuso-Gutierrez JL, del Rio Vega JM. Factors influencing relapse in the long-term course of schizophrenia. Schizophr Res 1997; 28:199–206.
23. Jibson MD, Tandon R. New atypical antipsychotic medications. J Psychiatr Res 1998; 32:215–228.
24. McPhillips MA, Kelly FJ, Barnes TR, Duke PJ, Gene-Cos N, Clark K. Detecting comorbid substance misuse among people with schizophrenia in the community: a study comparing the results of questionnaires with analysis of hair and urine. Schizophr Res 1997: 25:141–148.
25. Swofford CD, Kasckow JW, Scheller-Gilkey G, Inderbitzin LB. Substance use: a powerful predictor of relapse in schizophrenia. Schizophr Res 1996; 20:145–151.
26. Olfson M, Mechanic D, Boyer CA, Hansell S, Walkup J, Weiden PJ. Assessing clinical predictions of early rehospitalization in schizophrenia. J Nerv Ment Dis 1999; 187:721–729.
27. Drake RE, Mercer-McFadden C, Mueser KT, McHugo GJ, Bond GR. Review of integrated mental health and substance abuse treatment for patients with dual disorders. Schizophr Bull 1998; 24:589–608.
28. Leff J, Kuipers L, Berkowitz R, Vaughn C, Sturgeon D. Life events, relatives' expressed emotion and maintenance neuroleptics in schizophrenic relapse. Psychol Med 1983; 13:799–806.

29. Nuechterlein KH, Dawson ME, Gitlin M, Ventura J, Goldstein MJ, Snyder KS, Yee CM, Mintz J. Developmental processes in schizophrenic disorders: longitudinal studies of vulnerability and stress. Schizophr Bull 1992; 18:387–425.
30. Liberman RP. Psychosocial treatments for schizophrenia. Psychiatry 1994; 57:104–114.
31. Hirsch SR, Jolley A, Barnes T. Are depressive symptoms part of the schizophrenic syndrome? In: DeLisi L, ed. Depression in Schizophrenia. Washington, DC: American Psychiatric Press, 1990:25–37.
32. Jeste DV, Gladsjo JA, Lindamer LA, Lacro JP. Medical comorbidity in schizophrenia. Schizophr Bull 1996; 22:413–430.
33. Goldman LS. Medical illness in patients with schizophrenia. J Clin Psychiatry 1999; 60(suppl 21):10–15.
34. Weisman GK. Crisis-oriented residential treatment as an alternative to hospitalization. Hosp Commun Psychiatry 1985; 36:1302–1305.
35. Greenberg WM, Moore-Duncan L, Herron R. Patients' attitudes toward having been forcibly medicated. Bull Am Acad Psychiatry Law 1996; 24:513–524.
36. Marder SR. Management of schizophrenia. J Clin Psychiatry 1996; 57(suppl 3):9–13.
37. Jibson MD, Tandon R. Treatment of schizophrenia. Psychiatry Clinics of North America Annual of Drug Therapy 2000; 7:83–113.
38. Sweeney JA, Haas GL, Keilp JG, Long M. Evaluation of the stability of neuropsychological functioning after acute episodes of schizophrenia: one-year follow-up study. Psychiatry Res 1991; 38:63–76.
39. Jibson MD, Tandon R. A summary of new research findings on the new antipsychotic drugs. Essential Psychopharmacol 1996; 1:27–37.
40. Beasley CM, Jr, Hamilton SH, Crawford AM, Dellva MA, Tollefson GD, Tran PV, Blin O, Beuzen JN. Olanzapine versus haloperidol: acute phase results of the international double-blind olanzapine trial. Eur Neuropsychopharmacol 1997; 7:125–137.
41. Tran PV, Dellva, MA, Tollefson, Beasley CM Jr, Potvin JH, Kiesler GM. Extrapyramidal symptoms and tolerability of olanzapine versus haloperidol in the acute treatment of schizophrenia. J Clin Psychiatry 1997; 58:205–211.
42. Tollefson GD, Beasley CM Jr, Tamura RN, Tran PV, Potvin JH. Blind, controlled, long-term study of the comparative incidence of treatment-emergent tardive dyskinesia with olanzapine or haloperidol. Am J Psychiatry 1997; 154:1248–1254.
43. Borison RL, Arvanitis LA, Miller BG. ICI 204,636, an atypical antipsychotic: efficacy and safety in a multicenter, placebo-controlled trial in patients with schizophrenia. J Clin Pharmacol 1996; 16:158–169.
44. Small JG, Hirsch SR, Arvanitis LA, Miller BG, Link CG. Seroquel Study Group. Quetiapine in patients with schizophrenia: a high- and low-dose

double-blind comparison with placebo. Arch Gen Psychiatry 1997; 54:549–557.

45. Marder SR, Meibach RC. Risperidone in the treatment of schizophrenia. Am J Psychiatry 1994; 151:825–835.
46. Peuskens J. Risperidone in the treatment of patients with chronic schizophrenia: a multinational, multicentre, double-blind, parallel-group study versus haloperidol. Br J Psychiatry 1995; 166:712–726.
47. Keck P Jr, Buffenstein A, Ferguson J, Feighner J, Jaffe W, Harrigan EP, Morrissey MR. Ziprasidone 40 and 120 mg/day in the acute exacerbation of schizophrenia and schizoaffective disorder: a 4-week placebo-controlled trial. Psychopharmacology 1998; 140:173–184.
48. Daniel DG, Zimbroff DL, Potkin SG, Reeves KR, Harrigan EP, Lakshminarayanan M. Ziprasidone Study Group. Ziprasidone 80 mg/day and 160 mg/day in the acute exacerbation of schizophrenia and schizoaffective disorder: a 6-week placebo-controlled trial. Neuropsychopharmacology 1999; 20:491–505.
49. Allison DB, Mentore JL, Heo M, Chandler LP, Cappelleri JC, Infante MC, Weiden PJ. Antipsychotic-induced weight gain: a comprehensive research synthesis. Am J Psychiatry 1999; 156:1686–1696.
50. Kane J, Honigfeld G, Singer J, Meltzer H. Clozapine for the treatment-resistant schizophrenic: a double-blind comparison with chlorpromazine. Arch Gen Psychiatry 1988; 45:789–796.
51. Youssef HA. Duration of neuroleptic treatment and relapse rate: a 5-year follow-up study with haloperidol decanoate. Clin Neuropharmacol 1991; 14(suppl 2):S16–23.
52. Carpenter WT Jr, Buchanan RW, Kirkpatrick B, Lann HD, Breier AF, Summerfelt AT. Comparative effectiveness of fluphenazine decanoate injections every 2 weeks versus every 6 weeks. Am J Psychiatry 1999; 156:412–418.
53. Seeman P. Dopamine receptor sequences: therapeutic levels of neuroleptics occupy D2 receptors, clozapine occupies D4. Neuropsychopharmacology 1992; 7:261–284.
54. Battaglia J, Moss S, Rush J, Kang J, Mendoza R, Leedom L, Dubin W, McGlynn C, Goodman L. Haloperidol, lorazepam, or both for psychotic agitation? A multicenter, prospective, double-blind, emergency department study. Am J Emerg Med 1997; 15:335–340.
55. Rosebush PI, Hildebrand AM, Furlong BG, Mazurek MF. Catatonic syndrome in a general psychiatric inpatient population: frequency, clinical presentation, and response to lorazepam. J Clin Psychiatry 1990; 51:357–362.
56. Ungvari GS, Leung CM, Wong MK, Lau J. Benzodiazepines in the treatment of catatonic syndrome. Acta Psychiatr Scand 1994; 89:285–288.
57. Bush G, Fink M, Petrides G, Dowling F, Francis A. Catatonia. II. Treatment with lorazepam and electroconvulsive therapy. Acta Psychiatr Scand 1996; 93:137–143.

58. Zubenko GS, Lipinski JF, Cohen BM, Barreira PJ. Comparison of metoprolol and propranolol in the treatment of akathisia. Psychiatry Res 1984; 11:143–149.
59. Tohen M, Sanger TM, McElroy SL, Tollefson GD, Chengappa KN, Daniel DG, Petty F, Centorrino F, Wang R, Grundy SL, Greaney MG, Jacobs TG, David SR, Toma V. Olanzapine HGEH Study Group. Olanzapine versus placebo in the treatment of acute mania. Am J Psychiatry 1999; 156:702–709.
60. Green AI, Tohen M, Patel JK, Banov M, DuRand C, Berman I, Chang H, Zarate C Jr, Posener J, Lee H, Dawson R, Richards C, Cole JO, Schatzberg AF. Clozapine in the treatment of refractory psychotic mania. Am J Psychiatry 2000; 157:982–986.
61. Segal J, Berk M, Brook S. Risperidone compared with both lithium and haloperidol in mania: a double-blind randomized controlled trial. Clin Neuropharmacol 1998; 21:176–180.
62. Kales HC, DeQuardo JR, Tandon R. Combined electroconvulsive therapy and clozapine in treatment-resistant schizophrenia. Prog Neuropsychopharmacol Biol Psychiatry 1999; 23:547–556.
63. Wintemute GJ, Parham CA, Beaumont JJ, Wright M, Drake C. Mortality among recent purchasers of handguns. N Engl J Med 1999; 341:1583–1589.
64. Azrael D, Hemenway D. "In the safety of your own home": results from a national survey on gun use at home. Soc Sci Med 2000; 50:285–291.

7

Maintenance Treatment for Schizophrenia Patients

John G. Csernansky
Washington University School of Medicine
and Metropolitan St. Louis Psychiatric Center
St. Louis, Missouri

INTRODUCTION

In almost all patients who suffer from schizophrenia, it is a lifelong disorder. After the resolution of an acute episode of psychotic symptoms, treatment must be continued to prevent such episodes in the future. Furthermore, negative symptoms and cognitive deficits often remain after the resolution of a psychotic episode, and become the focus of efforts at rehabilitation. Relapse prevention, the mitigation of negative symptoms, and at least the recognition of cognitive deficits are all essential to improve the quality of life for patients with schizophrenia. The major goal of this chapter is to review current knowledge about maintenance drug treatment for schizophrenia patients and to extract simple principles from this literature as a guide for clinicians.

Today, clinicians and their patients have more and better drugs to choose from in designing their strategies for maintenance treatment. In the United States, the use of clozapine, risperidone, olanzapine, quetiapine and other second-generation drugs has surpassed the use of the first-generation antipsychotic drugs, such as haloperidol, thiothixene, and fluphenazine. Second-generation antipsychotic drugs have been shown to have advantages in the inpatient treatment setting, including improved efficacy and reduced extrapyramidal side effects, and their use during maintenance treatment also offers many advantages over the older antipsychotic drugs.

This discussion of maintenance drug treatment for schizophrenia patients is organized around three key issues: 1) prevention of psychotic relapse, 2) minimization of side effects during long-term administration of antipsychotic drugs, and 3) treatment of negative symptoms, depression, and cognitive deficits in stabilized patients. Comparisons of second-generation and older drugs will be made whenever data are available. In addition, strategies for combining psychosocial rehabilitation with such drug treatments to enhance relapse prevention and the quality of life for patients are reviewed.

PREVENTION OF PSYCHOTIC RELAPSE

Prevention of Psychotic Relapse Using First-Generation Antipsychotic Drugs

First-generation antipsychotic drugs, such as haloperidol and fluphenazine, were shown to be highly effective in preventing psychotic relapse many years ago (1,2). However, given the potentially serious side effects of first-generation antipsychotic drugs used over prolonged periods of time (e.g., tardive dyskinesia), relapse-prevention studies using such drugs soon began to focus on finding lowest effective doses (3). Two first-generation antipsychotic drugs—fluphenazine and haloperidol—are available in depot form in the United States and, because the administration of such can be ensured, they were often used in such studies. Although the usual doses of fluphenazine decanoate and haloperidol decanoate are 25 mg every 2 weeks and 200 mg every 4 weeks, respectively, fluphenazine doses as low as 5–10 mg every 2 weeks (4–6) and haloperidol doses as low as 50 mg every 4 weeks (7) have been shown to prevent psychotic relapse in schizophrenia patients. However, in the most detailed comparison of several doses of haloperidol decanoate, gradually increasing relapses were seen with lower drug doses (7). Specifically, in groups of subjects treated with 25 mg, 50 mg, 100 mg, or 200 mg of haloperidol decanoate every 4 weeks, relapse rates after 1 year were 63%, 25%, 23%, and 15%, respectively. Thus, it may be difficult to define an absolute dose threshold for first-generation antipsychotic drugs above which relapse prevention is optimally achieved.

As an alternative means of lowering the doses of first-generation antipsychotic drugs used during maintenance treatment, the intermittent dosing of such drugs has been explored (8). In this strategy for maintenance treatment in patients with schizophrenia, drug treatment is stopped when the symptoms of an acute psychotic relapse have resolved, and resumed when the earliest symptoms of an impending psychotic relapse are noticed by the patient, his or her caregiver, or the treating clinician. While some studies suggest that this strategy can work (9,10), others suggest that it is associated with a greater risk of relapse than conventional, continuous dosing (11–13). Finally, the combination of low-dose maintenance drug therapy with intermittent increases in drug doses triggered by symptom worsening has been proposed as a strategy for relapse prevention (6). However, the practicality of all intermittent treatment strategies may be limited, because many patients do not have caregivers and their insight into the need for treatment may be limited, especially early in the course of a psychotic relapse. Also, prodromal symptoms may not always reliably predict impending psychotic relapse (14,15).

While these studies suggest that first-generation antipsychotic drugs do prevent relapse in patients with schizophrenia, they also illustrate the limitations of these older drugs. Although many patients with schizophrenia are not compliant with treatment because they lack insight into their illness (16), anyone might be reluctant to continue treatment with such drugs after the acute symptoms of illness have subsided, because of the side effects usually encountered with long-term use (e.g., pseudoparkinsonism, akathisia, and tardive dyskinesia) (17). As reviewed above, attempts at dose reduction to minimize side effects while maintaining the efficacy of such drugs have had only limited success. Fundamentally better drugs are needed.

Preventing Psychotic Episodes Using Second-Generation Antipsychotic Drugs

Second-generation antipsychotic drugs have a broader therapeutic index than first-generation antipsychotic drugs. This means that the doses required for second drugs to be effective are more widely separated from (i.e., lower than) the doses likely to cause acute neurological side effects, such as pseudoparkinsonism and akathisia (18,19), compared to first-generation drugs. In addition, the results of some clinical trials suggest that second-generation antipsychotic drugs are more effective for the treatment of both positive and negative symptoms than first-generation antipsychotic drugs (19,20). Given the reduced side effects of such drugs at a wider range of doses and improved efficacy, they would seem to be ideal for use as maintenance treatments for schizophrenia patients.

Although originally developed in the 1960s, clozapine remains the prototype for second-generation antipsychotic drugs. Because of the ability of clozapine to cause agranulocytosis, this drug was first tested in patients known to be refractory to treatment with first-generation antipsychotic drugs. In this group of patients, a substantial minority (30%) appear to respond after several weeks (20). Other studies suggest that after several months of use, the percentage of patients who respond to clozapine may be even higher (i.e., 60%) (21). Breier and his colleagues (22)—the first to compare clozapine to haloperidol in outpatients being treated for schizophrenia—found that clozapine was superior to haloperidol both for the control of psychotic symptoms and for improving patients' quality of life. Thus, both acute and long-term studies of clozapine suggest that this drug may have superior efficacy. Further, because the degree of efficacy may grow with the passage of time, the benefits of the drug may best emerge during maintenance treatment.

Risperidone was the first second-generation antipsychotic drug introduced in the United States following clozapine. During acute treatment of schizophrenia patients, the efficacy of this drug for psychotic symptoms and negative symptoms has been shown to be superior to that of first-generation antipsychotic drugs, especially when it is used within the dose range of 4–6 mg/day (19,23,24). Further, Lindstrom and colleagues (25) showed in an open study that switching schizophrenia patients from first-generation antipsychotic drugs to risperidone during the maintenance phase of treatment resulted in fewer relapses and rehospitalizations. More recently, a 1–2-year, double-blind comparison of risperidone and haloperidol in outpatients with schizophrenia was conducted (26). In this study, risperidone was associated with a substantially lower risk of relapse (23% for risperidone and 35% for haloperidol after 1 year of treatment). This lower risk of relapse was associated both with better control of psychotic and negative symptoms and with lower rates of neurological side effects. However, somewhat contrary to expectations, the difference in relapse rates between subjects treated with risperdone and haloperidol could not be explained by differences in compliance. This study represents the only comparison to date of a first- and second-generation antipsychotic drug for relapse prevention in schizophrenia.

Olanzapine was introduced after risperidone in the United States, and it too has enjoyed wide acceptance and use. In a 1-year, double-blind comparison of two different doses of olanzapine (i.e., 5–15 versus 1 mg/day) and placebo, usual doses of olanzapine (5–15 mg/day) were found to be superior to both the low dose of olanzapine and placebo for relapse prevention (27). Recently, a direct comparison of risperidone and olanzapine was undertaken in both inpatients and outpatients with schizophrenia over 6 months (28). In this study, olanzapine was found to have long-term benefits compared to risperidone in patients who achieved a significant acute reduction of symptoms. While this study was not a relapse-prevention study per se, it does suggest that significant clinical differences between second-generation antipsychotic drugs may exist that are relevant for the maintenance treatment of schizophrenia patients.

In addition to clozapine, risperidone, and olanzapine, other second-generation antipsychotics are now available. These drugs represent both chemical analogs of clozapine (e.g., quetiapine) and compounds with distinct chemical structures (e.g., ziprasidone). While the acute efficacy of these drugs has been well demonstrated (29), data are lacking related to their capacity to prevent relapse, particularly in comparison to first-generation antipsychotics or other second-generation antipsychotics, such as clozapine, risperidone, and olanzapine. Some indication of the efficacy of such drugs can be appreciated from so-called continuation studies, that is, the continuation of treatment in subjects who were randomized during more acute phases of their illness. However, more prospectively designed relapse-prevention trials are needed to fully demonstrate the efficacy of second-generation antipsychotic drugs for maintenance treatment. In particular, comparisons among the second-generation drugs are needed, since these drugs are now widely accepted as first-line treatments for acute psychotic episodes.

Before leaving the topic of relapse prevention, a word of caution is needed. Given the relative lack of studies comparing the relative efficacy for second-generation drugs for relapse prevention, it is tempting to make comparisons among these drugs by comparing relapse rates across studies. However, to do so could be highly misleading, since the risk of relapse can be determined by the characteristics of the particular subjects included in a clinical trial as well as the treatments used. For example, the presence of symptoms of tardive dyskinesia have been shown to predict psychotic relapses when drug treatment is withdrawn (30). However, while this information may be useful in patients treated with typical antipsychotic drugs, it has much more limited value in patients treated with atypical drugs associated with a lower risk of acute neurological side effects. In addition, common sense suggests that patients with higher rates of relapse in the past or more refractory symptoms are likely to be at higher risk for future relapse regardless of the treatment selected.

Table 1 Efficacy of Second-Generation Antipsychotic Drugs for Relapse Prevention

Drug	Efficacy vs. no treatment	Efficacy vs. first-generation drug
Clozapine	Yes	More effective
Risperidone	Yes	More effective
Olanzapine	Yes	Unknown
Quetiapine	Yes	Unknown

Guidelines for Clinicians

Substantial work has been done to establish optimal doses for first-generation antipsychotic drugs for relapse prevention. However, at least some second-generation antipsychotics been shown to be superior to first-generation drugs for relapse prevention (see Table 1). More research is needed to establish relative advantages and disadvantages among second-generation antipsychotic drugs for the maintenance treatment of patients with schizophrenia. However, in the meantime, the clinician should select the antipsychotic drug best able to induce a remission of acute psychosis in the patient being treated, and use the lowest dose of this drug possible. Especially when using second-generation antipsychotic drugs, a dose should be found that is effective in preventing relapse, yet below that which produces unwanted neurological side effects.

The impact of reducing relapse rates in patients with schizophrenia cannot be overestimated. Repeated relapses can lead to progressive clinical deterioration and disability. Only when patients are free of the interruptions in living caused by psychotic episodes can progress be made toward resumption of school or work activities. Moreover, the patient's family can be severely affected by psychotic relapses, particularly when the patient's behavior is frightening or dangerous. Finally, from the viewpoint of society, relapse often triggers rehospitalization, which is widely acknowledged to be the most costly phase of treatment. Thus, relapse prevention is essential for the patient, his family, and the social service agencies that often bear the cost of intensive treatment.

MANAGEMENT OF DRUG SIDE EFFECTS DURING MAINTENANCE TREATMENT

Side effects can seriously undermine the efficacy of maintenance antipsychotic drug treatment. Some side effects increase with increasing doses of drug (i.e., they are dose-dependent) and so prevent patients from taking the drug doses needed to optimally treat their symptoms. Other side effects, such as akathisia, can be so distressing to patients that they become unwilling to continue with treatment. For a more detailed discussion of the side effects of antipsychotic drugs, see Chapter 10. However, because of relationships between drug side effects and noncompliance during maintenance treatment, the topic is also be presented here.

Neurological Side Effects

Of the neurological side effects of antipsychotic drugs, pseudoparkinsonism (i.e., tremor, masked facies, and festination) is perhaps most common. However, akathisia (i.e., a subjective or objective sense of motor restlessness) is also common and can more often be the cause of noncompliance (31,32). A large body of research has shown that schizophrenia patients who experience such side effects have a poorer outcome of treatment (33–35). Therefore, to optimize the outcome of patients with schizophrenia in the long term, such side effects should be minimized.

The severity of pseudoparkinsonism and akathisia is dose-related (33,34), and so reductions in antipsychotic drug dose may be used to mitigate such side effects. Unfortunately, while the efficacy of first-generation antipsychotic drugs has been associated with approximately 70% occupancy of brain dopamine receptors (D_2), the threshold for drug-induced side effects, such as pseudoparkinsonism, appears to be only slightly higher (approximately 80%) (36). These results are discouraging in that it appears that the doses of typical antipsychotic drugs needed for efficacy and the doses that produce side effects are nearly the same. However, similar studies of second-generation drugs, such as clozapine, suggest a wider separation between the doses required for symptom efficacy and those likely to produce neurological side effects (36). This wider window appears to be due to the fact that clozapine is effective even at doses at which relatively fewer brain dopamine receptors are blocked.

There appear to be important relationships between the severity of schizophrenia symptoms and neurological side effects. Thus, the minimization of such side effects may also help the clinician to optimize the efficacy of maintenance treatment. Relationships between schizophrenia symptoms and drug side effects may occur on a variety of levels. For example, neuroleptic-induced pseudoparkinsonism or sedation may make it difficult to assess the negative symptoms of schizophrenia, such as avolition and flat affect (17,37). In addition, other negative symptoms, such as avolition, may be related to the features of depression, such as decreased work and activities, motor retardation, and decreased libido (38). Until the exact nature of such relationships can be clarified, negative symptoms that appear to overlap with other psychopathological syndromes should not be considered primary.

Relationships have also been reported between antipsychotic-drug-induced akathisia and the severity of psychotic symptoms in schizophrenia patients undergoing maintenance treatment with antipsychotic drugs (36). Moreover, suicidal (39) and violent (40) behavior has been linked to such akathisia. The results of these studies are consistent with observations made long ago by clinicians that akathisia induced by treatment with antipsychotic drugs can be mistaken for an "agitated depression" (41) and warnings that akathisia can be associated with a poorer clinical outcome overall (42,43).

Finally, the so-called "tardive" side effects of antipsychotic drugs deserve special consideration during the maintenance phase of treatment. Various movement disorders occur with differing frequencies after the long-term use of antipsychotic drugs (18). Of these movement disorders, tardive dyskinesia appears to be most common, with an annual incidence rate of 3–5%. Other movement disorders may also appear after a delay, such as tardive dystonia and tardive akathisia, but much less commonly. Fortunately, the second-generation antipsychotic drugs appear to have a substantially lower risk of such delayed side effects, which is in keeping with their lower risk of acute neurological side effects (26).

Side Effects of Antipsychotic Drugs on Other Systems (e.g., Agranulocytosis, Hyperprolactinemia, Hypotension, Weight Gain, and Insulin Resistance)

Given recent trends in favor of the use of second-generation antipsychotic drugs, concern about the neurological side effects of antipsychotic drugs has been fading. However, because of the tendency of second-generation antipsychotic drugs to act on neurotransmitter systems other than dopamine, concern about other types of side effects is on the rise. Such effects can occur because of unwanted adrenergic-receptor blockade, disturbances of neuroendocrine and metabolic systems, and the idiosyncratic actions of some drugs on the synthesis of white blood cells.

Many first- and second-generation antipsychotic drugs are antagonists at α_1-noradrenergic receptors. This drug action can cause orthostatic hypotension, which can lead to falls in elderly or medically ill patients. All first-generation antipsychotic drugs and some second-generation ones (especially risperidone and ziprasidone) cause elevations in plasma prolactin concentrations, via blockade of dopamine D_2 receptors in the pituitary gland (36). Increases in plasma prolactin concentrations are of clinical importance, since they may lead to loss of libido and, more rarely, galactorrhea.

Weight gain has been reported as a side effect of many first- and second-generation antipsychotic drugs, although the latter now appear to be more likely to cause this problem (18). During long-term maintenance therapy, many patients experience weight gain in excess of 10% of their usual body weight, which can raise serious medical concerns. Because of the likelihood that maintenance treatment will be indefinite, substantial weight gain may place the patient at increased risk for heart disease and diabetes mellitus. Moreover, new-onset cases of diabetes mellitus have been reported during treatment with second-generation antipsychotic drugs even in the absence of weight gain. Many clinics are now developing routine guidelines to monitor glucose and lipid regulation in patients with schizophrenia who are undergoing maintenance treatment with all antipsychotic drugs. Unfortunately, of all antipsychotic drugs, only molindone has been shown to be associated with weight loss.

With the recent introduction of the second-generation drug ziprasidone in the United States, concern about the cardiac side effects of antipsychotic drugs has again increased. Ziprasidone, along with many other antipsychotic drugs, may cause a delay in the repolarization of the heart (i.e., QT prolongation) (44). It is notable that the development of another second-generation antipsychotic drug, sertindole, was discontinued, and the package labeling for the first-generation drug thioridazine was recently altered, because of this side effect. All first- and second-generation antipsychotic drugs are capable of causing this side effect, although most are less likely to do so than ziprasidone and thioridazine. In otherwise healthy individuals, this effect can be associated with potentially fatal arrythmias of the heart and sudden death. Such disasters are more common in individuals with a pre-existing history of heart disease. In addition, antipsychotic drugs that are anticholinergic can also cause cardiac side effects, because of their tendency to increase the heart rate.

Finally, treatment with clozapine requires monitoring of white blood cell (WBC) count, because of the unlikely but potentially fatal possibility of agranulocytosis (18). During the first 6 months of clozapine treatment, WBC should be checked every week, and thereafter

Table 2 Drug Side Effects of Special Concern During Maintenance Treatment

Delayed neurological side effects (tardive dyskinesia, tardive dystonia, tardive akathisia)
Haloperidol = fluphenzine = thiothixene > risperidone = olanzapine = quetiapine > clozapine
Metabolic side effects (weight gain, diabetes mellitus)
Clozapine > olanzapine = quetiapine > risperidone = ziprasidone > haloperidol > molindone
Cardiac side effects (repolarization arrhythmias)
Ziprasidone = thioridazine > risperidone = olanzapine = quetiapine = haloperidol

= and > represent the relative risks for various drugs.

every 2 weeks. The requirement for WBC monitoring during long-term clozapine can be a serious disincentive for patients to continue therapy with this agent.

Guidelines for Clinicians

Side effects of special concern during maintenance treatment with antipsychotic drugs are summarized in Table 2. While second-generation antipsychotic drugs have lower risks for neurological side effects, their effects on other physiological systems should not be overlooked. In this latter group of side effects, those related to metabolism (i.e., weight gain and diabetes) need to be more fully evaluated. As new antipsychotic drugs are developed, emphasis should be given to drugs that lack these additional problems.

NEGATIVE SYMPTOMS, DEPRESSION, AND COGNITIVE DEFICITS

Helping patients with schizophrenia resume their lives in a way that is satisfying to them and their families requires more than the prevention of psychotic relapses. Recent studies have shown that the persistence of other types of symptoms, especially negative symptoms, depression, and cognitive deficits can prevent patients from returning to school or work. Therefore, the treatment of these other symptom domains should be the major focus for our efforts, especially during the maintenance phase of treatment.

Treatment of Negative Symptoms, Depression, and Cognitive Deficits Using First-Generation Antipsychotic Drugs

The efficacy of first-generation antipsychotic drugs for the treatment of negative symptoms is probably related to the degree to which such drugs cause acute neurological side effects. In other words, first-generation drugs capable of causing substantial pseudoparkinsonsim are unlikely to have any efficacy for the treatment of negative symptoms (35,45). As pointed out above, the neurological side effects of first-generation drugs can be mitigated by lowering the dose of the drug, and, in some cases, cautious lowering of drug doses can improve a patient's affect and motivation. However, relatively little research has addressed the question of whether first-generation antipsychotic drugs are effective for the treatment of negative symptoms that are not correlated with drug side effects or other confounding factors (e.g., primary negative symptoms) during maintenance treatment. Some early studies indicated that the negative symptoms of schizophrenia respond poorly to typical antipsychotic drugs (46,47). However, the results of many of these studies are difficult to interpret because of inadequate sample size, the use of rating instruments insensitive to negative symptoms, and the inclusion of patients with few negative symptoms prior to treatment (48). Literature reviews have provided some evidence that first-generation antipsychotic drugs are effective for the treatment of negative symptoms, although the magnitude of this effect is small compared to their efficacy for positive symptoms (49).

Unfortunately, first-generation antipsychotic drugs have not been shown to be effective for the treatment of depression or cognitive deficits in schizophrenia patients undergoing maintenance treatment (50). Again, the propensity of such drugs to cause such side effects as pseudoparkinsonism and akathisia may be related to this failure. Moreover, anticholinergic drugs are often coprescribed with first-generation antipsychotic drugs, and such drugs are well known to cause mild cognitive impairment in otherwise healthy individuals and to worsen cognitive impairment when it is already present. Fortunately, recent studies of second-generation antipsychotic drugs now suggest that such drugs may be superior to the first-generation antipsychotic drugs in regard to their efficacy for depression (51,52) and at least some cognitive deficits found in patients with schizophrenia (53).

Treatment of Negative Symptoms, Depression, and Cognitive Deficits Using Second-Generation Antipsychotic Drugs

Clozapine, the prototypical second-generation drug, has been clearly shown to be effective for the treatment of negative symptoms that occur together with psychosis in both treatment-responsive (54) and treatment-resistant patients (20). However, in a study of outpatients undergoing maintenance treatment, clozapine had only a modest advantage over haloperidol for the treatment of negative symptoms (20,55). In a group of Veteran outpatients with schizophrenia, similar results were obtained (56). Somewhat in contradiction to these findings, however, clozapine treatment in outpatients with schizophrenia has been shown to improve quality of life, work ability, and interpersonal relationships (21). The apparent discord between these two types of studies may reflect limitations in our understanding of negative symptoms, and how such symptoms correlate with "real-life" phenomena, such as capacities for interpersonal relationships and employment. The presence or absence of negative symptoms may contribute to such capacities, but may not totally determine them.

Other second-generation antipsychotic drugs also appear to be more effective than typical antipsychotic drugs for the treatment of negative symptoms (see Table 3 for summary). Risperidone, when administered within its optimal dose range (i.e., 4–6 mg/day), has been shown to be superior to haloperidol for this purpose (23,24). Similarly, olanzapine has been shown to be superior to haloperidol for the treatment of negative symptoms in acute schizophrenia inpatients (57). Moreover, olanzapine's efficacy for negative symptoms was associated with a significant improvement in patients' quality of life (58). Unfortunately, quetiapine, administered in a range of doses (75–750 mg/day), has not been shown to be superior to haloperidol (12 mg/day) for the treatment of negative symptoms (29). Given the lack of pseudoparkinsonism and other neurological side effects with quetiapine, this finding suggests that the mere absence of such side effects is not sufficient to bring about improvement in negative symptoms.

The effectiveness of second-generation antipsychotic drugs for the treatment of depressive symptoms in patients with schizophrenia has

Table 3 Comparative Efficacy of First- and Second-Generation Antipsychotic Drugs for Negative Symptoms, Depression, and Cognitive Deficits

Syndrome	First-generation drugs	Second-generation drugs
Negative symptoms (2°)	Questionably effective	Effective
Negative symptoms (1°)	Not effective	Questionably effective
Depression	Not effective	Effective
Cognitive deficits	Not effective	Effective

become the topic of much recent research. A trial in acutely psychotic patients showed olanzapine to be superior to haloperidol for the treatment of depressive symptoms. Furthermore, this effect could not be attributed to olanzapine's effects on positive or general negative symptoms or to the absence of neurological side effects (28,51,52). The antidepressant efficacy of second-generation antipsychotic drugs may be related to their blockade of brain 5-HT2 receptors, since other, more selective, antagonists at these receptors (e.g., trazodone, nefazadone) have also been shown to have antidepressant effects.

Evaluating the efficacy of atypical antipsychotic drugs for the cognitive deficits of schizophrenia (e.g., impairments in attention, working memory, and executive function) has been of increasing interest in recent years, in large part because their presence has been linked to poor outcome (59). Treatment with clozapine has been associated with improvements in performance on tests of memory (60) and verbal fluency (55), but not necessarily on other cognitive tests, including tests of executive function (e.g., the Wisconsin Cart Sort Test) (60). When patients with schizophrenia were switched from first-generation antipsychotic drugs to clozapine, incremental improvements in verbal fluency and motor speed, but deleterious effects on executive function, were found (61). These results suggest that clozapine may be effective for cognitive deficits in schizophrenia, but that such benefits are limited to a subset of cognitive functions.

The effects of other atypical antipsychotic drugs on cognitive function are now under intense investigation. Acute risperidone treatment has recently been shown to improve performance on verbal memory tasks (53). In a longer-term (12-month) comparative study of risperidone, olanzapine, and haloperidol, both risperidone and olanzapine were shown to produce greater benefits for cognition than haloperidol did (62). Finally, preliminary reports of quetiapine's beneficial effects on cognitive performance are beginning to appear. Thus, it appears that second-generation antipsychotic drugs as a group may have at least limited benefits for cognition in patients with schizophrenia during maintenance treatment, especially in comparison to the effects of first-generation drugs.

Guidelines for Clinicians

Table 3 presents a summary of the comparative benefits of first- and second-generation antipsychotic drugs for negative symptoms, depression, and cognitive deficits in patients with schizophrenia. While there is much yet to achieve, it is also clear that we have taken a major step forward with the development of second-generation drugs. Successful treatment of these symptom domains are of special importance during the maintenance phase of treatment for schizophrenia, because these symptoms appear to correlate better than psychotic symptoms with the patient's capacity for interpersonal interaction and work.

When selecting an antipsychotic drug for maintenance treatment, improvement in negative symptoms, depression, and cognitive function should be carefully monitored, just as one monitors the patient for relapse. Instruments to assess these symptoms exist, and can be found in other chapters in this book. Moreover, the clinician should work with each patient to translate improvements in these symptom domains to achieving goals selected by the patient related to work, housing, or social contact.

COMBINING ANTIPSYCHOTIC DRUGS AND PSYCHOSOCIAL TREATMENTS

The efficacy of psychosocial treatments for schizophrenia is not the central topic of this chapter. However, a patient's compliance with maintenance drug treatment often depends on how much attention the clinician pays to psychosocial variables (63). Psychosocial treatments can also alter the environment to reduce the risk of relapse and offer opportunities to improve the patient's quality of life. The informal combination of drug treatments and psychosocial interventions is carried out on an everyday basis in most outpatient clinics. Thus, a review of this literature is included in this chapter.

Effectiveness of Psychosocial Interventions in Schizophrenia Patients During Maintenance Treatment

Relationships between environmental stresses and symptom exacerbation in patients with schizophrenia have been observed for many years (64). High levels of interpersonal stress within the patient's immediate interpersonal environment, sometimes referred to as high "expressed emotion," have been linked to higher rates of relapse in outpatients with schizophrenia. Moreover, educating family members about the treatment of schizophrenia in such a way that interpersonal criticism is diminished has lowered the risk of relapse during maintenance treatment with antipsychotic drugs (65,66). Follow-up studies of the efficacy of psychosocial interventions in patients with schizophrenia and their families suggest that the effects of such interventions on relapse rates can be long-lasting (67).

Psychosocial treatment may also help to decrease negative symptoms and enhance quality of life. For example, in schizophrenia patients undergoing maintenance treatment, specific social-skills training techniques improved social adjustment and lowered rates of relapse and rehospitalization (63). Again, improvements in the symptoms of schizophrenia and social functioning have been observed long after the psychosocial treatment was completed (68).

Combining Drug Treatments and Psychosocial Interventions

Relatively few research studies have carefully assesssed the interactive effects of psychosocial interventions and drug treatments. In one study (4), the effects of a psychosocial treatment program were assessed in outpatients treated with either a standard or low dose of fluphenazine decanoate. Patients who were in contact with a high "expressed-emotion" environment (i.e., no psychosocial intervention) showed higher rates of relapse, but only when they were being treated with low doses of fluphenazine decanoate. This study has important implications for clinicians who provide maintenance treatment for patients with schizophrenia, because it suggests that special attention should be given to a patient's interpersonal environment when attempting to reduce the dose of a maintenance antipsychotic drug.

Perhaps the most comprehensive study of the interactions between drug treatment and psychosocial intervention was undertaken in the multicenter Treatment Strategies in Schizophrenia Study (69,70), although it had disappointing results. In this clinical trial, fluphenazine decanoate in two dosing ranges (2.5–10 mg every 2 weeks and 12.5–50 mg every 2 weeks) were compared with an intermittent dosing regimen in combination with one of two possible psychosocial interventions—a psychoeducational program to reduce family conflict and increase understanding of the illness (monthly group meetings and home sessions) or nonspecific supportive family therapy (monthly group meetings alone). The results of this study revealed that standard-dose treatment was superior to lower-dose treatment, and that lower-dose treatment was superior to intermittent dosing treatment with regard to the prevention of psychotic relapses. In contrast, however, negative symptoms were best treated using the intermittent dosing regimen; of the two "constant" dosing regimens, lower-dose treatment was superior to standard-dose treatment.

Unfortunately, neither of the psychosocial interventions tested in this study appeared to add to the efficacy of any of the antipsychotic drug therapy to prevent relapse. Therefore, the results of this study cannot be used to support the superiority of one type of psychosocial intervention over another, or even of either form of intervention compared to contacts that ordinarily occur between professionals and their patients.

As mentioned above, psychosocial interventions may be especially useful in improving compliance with antipsychotic-drug treatment. For example, a behaviorally oriented program for teaching medication compliance has been shown to be effective for improving treatment compliance in a large urban care-delivery system (71).

Guidelines for Clinicians

Further research is needed to determine the best ways for antipsychotic drug treatments and psychosocial interventions to be combined in patients with schizophrenia undergoing maintenance treatment. It would seem that the clinician should combine psychosocial treatments with the most effective and best-tolerated antipsychotic drugs available. Much other evidence suggests that second-generation drugs would again be the drugs of choice for this purpose. Moreover, drug treatments with benefits for cognitive function might enhance a patient's capacity to acquire and retain social skills learned through a series of specific interventions. Careful studies are urgently needed in this area to better guide clinical practice.

REFERENCES

1. Davis JM. Maintenance therapy and the natural course of schizophrenia. J Clin Psychiatry 1985; 11:18–21.
2. Kane JM, Lieberman JA. Maintenance pharmacotherapy in schizophrenia. In: Meltzer HY, ed. Psychopharmacology, The Third Generation of Progress: The Emergence of Molecular Biology and Biological Psychiatry. New York: Raven Press, 1987:1103–1109.
3. Schooler NR. Maintenance medication for schizophrenia: strategies for dose reduction. Schizophr Bull 1991; 17:311–324.
4. Hogarty GE, McEvoy JP, Munetz M, et al. Dose of fluphenazine, familial expressed emotion, and outcome in schizophrenia. Arch Gen Psychiatry 1988; 45:797–805.
5. Kane JM, Rifkin A, Woerner M, et al. Low-dose neuroleptic treatment of outpatient schizophrenics: I. Preliminary results for relapse rates. Arch Gen Psychiatry 1983; 40:893–896.
6. Marder SR, Van Putten T, Mintz J, Lebell M, McKenzie J, May PRA. Low- and conventional-dose maintenance therapy with fluphenazine decanoate: two-year outcome. Arch Gen Psychiatry 1987; 44:518–521.

7. Kane JM, Davis JM, Schooler NR, Marder SR, Brauzer B, Casey DE. A one-year comparison of four dosages of haloperidol decanoate. Schizophr Res 1993; 9:239–240.
8. Herz MI, Melville C. Relapse in schizophrenia. Am J Psychiatry 1980; 137:801–805.
9. Carpenter WT Jr, Heinrichs DW, Hanlon TE. A comparative trial of pharmacologic strategies in schizophrenia. Am J Psychiatry 1987; 144:1466–1470.
10. Herz MI, Szymanski HV, Simon JC. Intermittent medication for stable schizophrenic outpatients: an alternative to maintenance mediation. Am J Psychiatry 1982; 139:918–922.
11. Carpenter WT Jr, Hanlon TE, Heinrichs DW, et al. Continuous versus targeted medication in schizophrenic outpatients: outcome results. Am J Psychiatry 1990; 147:1138–1148.
12. Jolley AG, Hirsch SR, Morrison E, McRink A, Wilson L. Trial of brief intermittent neuroleptic prophylaxis for selected schizophrenic outpatients: clinical and social outcome at two years. Br Med J 1990; 301:837–842.
13. Müller P, Bandelow B, Gaebel W, et al. Intermittent medication, coping and psychotherapy interactions in relapse prevention and course modification. Br J Psychiatry 1992; 161(suppl 18):140–144.
14. Herz MI, Lamberti JS, Schwarzkopf SB, Crilly JF. Prodromal symptoms in schizophrenia: a prospective study and review. Schizophr Res 1993; 9:266.
15. Johnston-Cronk K, Marder SR, Wirshing WC, et al. Prediction of schizophrenic relapse using prodromal symptoms. Schizophr Res 1993; 9:259.
16. Van Putten T, Crumpton E, Yale C. Drug refusal in schizophrenia and the wish to be crazy. Arch Gen Psychiatry 1976; 33:1443–1446.
17. Van Putten T. Why do schizophrenic patients refuse to take their drugs? Arch Gen Psychiatry 1974; 31:67–72.
18. American Psychiatric Association. Practice guidelines for the treatment of patients with schizophrenia. Am J Psychiatry 1997; 154 (April suppl).
19. Marder SR, Meibach RC. Risperidone in the treatment of schizophrenia. Am J Psychiatry 1994; 151:825–835.
20. Kane J, Honigfeld G, Singer J and Meltzer H. Clozapine for the treatment-resistant schizophrenic: a double-blind comparison with chlorpromazine. Arch Gen Psychiatry 1988; 45:789–796.
21. Meltzer HY, Burnett S, Bastani B, Ramirez LF. Effects of six months of clozapine treatment on the quality of life of chronic schizophrenic patients. Hosp Comm Psychiatry 1990; 41:892–897.
22. Breier A, Buchanan RW, Kirkpatrick B, et al. Clozapine in schizophrenic outpatients: efficacy, long-term outcome, and relationship to prefrontal cortex. Schizophr Res 1993; 9:257–258.
23. Chouinard G, Jones B, Remington G, et al. A Canadian multicenter placebo-controlled study of fixed doses of risperidone and haloperidol in the treatment of chronic schizophrenic patients. J Clin Psychopharmacol 1993; 13:25–40.

24. Claus A, Bollen J, De Cuyper H, et al. Risperidone versus haloperidol in the treatment of chronic schizophrenic inpatients: a multi-center double-blind comparative study. Acta Psychiatr Scand 1992; 85:295–305.
25. Lindstrom E, Eriksson B, Hellgren A, von Knorring L, Eberhard G. Efficacy and safety of risperidone in the long-term treatment of patients with schizophrenia. Clin Therapeutics 1995; 17:402–412.
26. Csernansky JG, Okamoto A. A long-term double-blind comparison of risperidone and haloperidol in stable outpatients with schizophrenia or schizoaffective disorder. Int J Psychopharmacol 2000; 3(suppl 1):S155.
27. Dellva MA, Tran P, Tollefson GD, Wentley AL, Beasley CM Jr. Standard olanzapine versus placebo and ineffective-dose olanzapine in the maintenance treatment of schizophrenia. Psychiatric Services 1997; 48:1571–1577.
28. Tollefson GD, Sanger JM, Lu Y, Thieme ME. Depressive signs and symptoms in schizophrenia: a prospective trial of olanzapine and haloperidol. Arch Gen Psychiatry 1988; 55:250–258.
29. Arvanitis L, Miller BG, Seroquel Trial 13 Study Group. Multiple fixed doses of "Seroquel" (quetiapine) in patients with acute exacerbation of schizophrenia: a comparison with haloperidol and placebo. Biol Psychiatry 1997; 42:233–246.
30. Lieberman JA, Kane JM, Sarantakos S, et al. Prediction of relapse in schizophrenia. Arch Gen Psychiatry 1987; 44:597–603.
31. Adler LA, Angrist B, Reiter S, Rotrosen J. Neuroleptic-induced akathisia: a review. Psychopharmacology 1989; 97:1–11.
32. Braude WM, Barnes TRE, Gore SM. Clinical characteristics of akathisia. Br J Psychiatry 1983; 143:134–150.
33. Levinson DF, Simpson GM, Singh H, et al. Fluphenazine dose, clinical response, and extrapyramidal symptoms during acute treatment. Arch Gen Psychiatry 1990; 47:761–768.
34. Newcomer JW, Miller LS, Faustman WO, Wetzel MW, Vogler GP, Csernansky JG. Correlations between akathisia and residual psychopathology: a by-product of neuroleptic-induced dysphoria. Br J Psychiatry 1994; 164:834–838.
35. Van Putten T, Marder SR, Mintz J. A controlled dose comparison of haloperidol in newly admitted schizophrenic patients. Arch Gen Psychiatry 1990; 47:754–758.
36. Farde L, Nordstrom A-L, Wiesel F-A, Pauli S, Halldin C, Sedvall G. Positron emission tomographic analysis of central dopamine receptor occupancy in patients treated with classical neuroleptics and clozapine: relation to extrapyramidal side effects. Arch Gen Psychiatry 1992; 49:538–544.
37. Carpenter WT Jr, Heinrichs DW, Wagman AM. Deficit and nondeficit forms of schizophrenia: the concept. Am J Psychiatry 1988; 145:578–583.
38. Prosser ES, Csernansky JG, Kaplan J, Thiemann S, Becker TJ, Hollister LE. Depression, parkinsonian symptoms, and negative symptoms in schizophrenics treated with neuroleptics. J Nerv Ment Dis 1987; 175:100–105.

39. Drake RE, Erhlich J. Suicide attempts associated with akathisia. Am J Psychiatry 1985; 142:499–501.
40. Keckica WA. Violence as a manifestation of akathisia. J Am Med Assoc 1978; 240:2185.
41. Kalinowsky LB. Appraisal of the "tranquilizers" and their influence on other somatic treatments in psychiatry. Am J Psychiatry 1958; 115:294–300.
42. Singh MM. Dysphoric response to neuroleptic treatment in schizophrenia and its prognostic significance. Dis Nerv Syst 1976; 37:191–196.
43. Van Putten T, May PRA. Subjective response as a predictor of outcome in pharmacotherapy. Arch Gen Psychiatry 1978; 35:477–480.
44. Daniel DG, Copeland LF. Ziprasidone: comprehensive overview and clinical use of a novel antipsychotic. Exp Opin Invest Drugs 2000; 9:819–828.
45. Van Putten T, Marder SR, Mintz J, Poland RE. Haloperidol plasma levels and clinical response: a therapeutic window relationship. Am J Psychiatry 1992; 149:500–505.
46. Angrist B, Rotrosen J, Gershon S. Differential effects of amphetamine and neuroleptics on negative vs. positive symptoms in schizophrenia. Psychopharmacology 1980; 72:17–19.
47. Johnstone EC, Frith CD, Gold A, Crow TJ. The outcome of severe acute schizophrenic illnesses after one year. Br J Psychiatry 1979; 134:28–33.
48. Meltzer HY. Dopamine and negative symptoms in schizophrenics: critique of the type I–type II hypothesis. In: M. Alpert, ed. Controversies in Schizophrenia: Changes and Constancies. New York: Guilford Press, 1985:110–136.
49. Goldberg SC. Negative and deficit symptoms in schizophrenia do respond to neuroleptics. Schizophr Bull 1985; 11:453–456.
50. Faustman WO, Hoff AL. Effects of antipsychotic drugs on neuropsychological measures. In: Csernansky JG, ed. Antipsychotics: Handbook of Experimental Pharmacology. Vol 120. Berlin: Springer-Verlag, 1996:445–478.
51. Tollefson GD, Sanger TM, Beasley CM, Tran PV. A double-blind, controlled comparison of the novel antipsychotic olanzapine versus haloperidol or placebo on anxious and depressive symptoms accompanying schizophrenia. Biol Psychiatry 1998; 43:803–810.
52. Tran PV, Hamilton SH, Kuntz AJ, Potvin JH, Andersen SW, Beasley C Jr, Tollefson GD. Double-blind comparison of olanzapine versus risperidone in the treatment of schizophrenia and other psychotic disorders. J Clin Psychopharmacol 1997; 17:407–418.
53. Green MF, Marshall BD, Wirshing WC, et al. Does risperidone improve verbal working memory in treatment-resistant schizophrenia? Am J Psychiatry 1997; 154:799–804.
54. Claghorn J, Honigfeld G, Abuzzahab F, et al. The risks and benefits of clozapine versus chlorpromazine. J Clin Psychopharmacol 1987; 7:377–384.
55. Buchanan RW, Breier A, Kirkpatrick B, Ball P, Carpenter WT. Positive and negative symptom response to clozapine in schizophrenic patients with and without the deficit syndrome. Am J Psychiatry 1998; 155:751–760.

56. Rosenheck R, Dunn L, Peszke M, et al. Impact of clozapine on negative symptoms and on the deficit syndrome in refractory schizophrenia. Am J Psychiatry 1999; 156:88–93.
57. Tollefson GD, Beasley CM Jr, et al. Olanzapine versus haloperidol in the treatment of schizophrenia and schizoaffective and schizophreniform disorders: results of an international collaborative trial. Am J Psychiatry 1997; 154:457–465.
58. Hamilton SH, Revicki DA, Genduso LA, Beasley CM Jr. Olanzapine versus placebo and haloperidol: quality of life and efficacy results of the North American double-blind trial. Neuropsychopharmacology 1998; 18:41–49.
59. Green MF. What are the consequences of neurocognitive deficits in schizophrenia? Am J Psychiatry 1996; 153:321–330.
60. Hagger C, Buckley P, Kenny JT, et al. Improvement in cognitive functions and psychiatric symptoms in treatment-refractory schizophrenic patietns receiving clozapine. Biol Psychiatry 1993; 34:702–712.
61. Hoff AL, Faustman WO, Wiencke M, et al. The effects of clozapine on symptom reduction, neurocognitive function, and clinical management in treatment-refractory state hospital schizophrenic inpatients. Neuropsychopharmacology 1996; 15:361–369.
62. Purdon SE, Jones BD, Stip E, Labelle A, Addington D, David SR, Breier A, Tollefson GD. The Canadian Collaborative Group for Research in Schizophrenia. Neuropsychological change in early phase schizophrenia during 12 months of treatment with olanzapine, risperidone, or haloperidol. Arch Gen Psychiatry 2000; 57:249–258.
63. Liberman RP, Mueser KT, Wallace CJ. Social skills training for schizophrenic individuals at risk for relapse. Am J Psychiatry 1986; 143:523–526.
64. Vaughn CE, Leff JP. The influence of family and social factors on the course of psychiatric illness: a comparison of schizophrenic and depressed neurotic patients. Br J Psychiatry 1976; 129:125–137.
65. Falloon IRH, Boyd JL, McGill CW, et al. Family management in the prevention of morbidity of schizophrenia: clinical outcome of a two-year longitudinal study. Arch Gen Psychiatry 1985; 42:887–896.
66. Tarrier N, Barrowclough C, Vaughn C, Bamrah JS, Porceddu K, Watts S, Freeman H. The community management of schizophrenia: the controlled trial of a behavioral intervention with families to reduce relapse. Br J Psychiatry 1988; 153:532–542.
67. Hogarty GE, Anderson CM, Reiss DJ, et al. Family psychoeducation, social skills training, and maintenance chemotherapy in the aftercare treatment of schizophrenia. II. Two-year effects of a controlled study on relapse and adjustment. Arch Gen Psychiatry 1991; 48:340–347.
68. Bellack AS, Turner SM, Hersen M, Luber RF. An examination of the efficacy of social skills training for chronic schizophrenic patients. Hosp Commun Psychiatry 1984; 35:1023–1028.
69. Schooler NR, Keith SJ, Severe JB, et al. Treatment Strategies in Schizophrenia Collaborative Study Group. Acute treatment response and short term

outcome in schizophrenia: first results of the NIMH treatment strategies in schizophrenia study. Psychopharmacol Bull 1989; 25:331–335.

70. Schooler NR, Keith SJ, Severe JB, Matthews SM. Treatment strategies in schizophrenia: effects of dosage reduction and family management on outcome. Schizophr Res 1993; 9:260.
71. Eckman TA, Liberman RP, Phipps CC, Blair KE. Teaching medication management skills to schizophrenic patients. J Clin Psychopharmacol 1990; 10:33–38.

8

Management of Treatment-Refractory Patients

Robert R. Conley
University of Maryland School of Medicine
and Maryland Psychiatric Research Center
Baltimore, Maryland

INTRODUCTION

A systematic approach to the evaluation and characterization of patients refractory to treatment with conventional antipsychotic drugs has become increasingly important since the introduction of clozapine, risperidone, and olanzapine. The need for accurate evaluation will increase further with the introduction of other new-generation antipsychotic medications. People with schizophrenia may manifest a poor response to drug therapy secondary to intolerance of medication, poor compliance, or inappropriate dosing. In addition, the nature of some patients' illness may account for their resistance to antipsychotic drug therapy. As clinicians face the decision of when to change from one antipsychotic to another, a clear understanding of the appropriate length of a trial and of what target symptoms should respond to antipsychotics is critical for maximizing response in patients with refractory symptoms.

One-fifth to one-third of all patients with schizophrenia have significant refractory symptoms. This finding has been consistent over time (1–3). Treatment of patients in this group has remained a persistent public health problem. These patients are highly symptomatic and require extensive periods of hospital care (4), and their care comprises a disproportionately high share of the total cost of treating schizophrenia (5). These facts may help to explain the enthusiasm of clinicians to use clozapine in treatment-refractory inpatients. However, clozapine treatment carries with it significant morbidity from serious side effects, the need for continual weekly blood monitoring, and a high cost. Now that many new antipsychotics are available, it is important to reevaluate this problem.

BASIC CONCEPTS

Definition of Therapy-Refractory Schizophrenia

The most accepted criteria for treatment-refractory schizophrenia were first widely used by Kane et al. (6) and collaborators in the Multicenter Clozapine Trial (MCT). Originally, these criteria were:

1. Persistent positive psychotic symptoms: item score ≥4 (moderate) on at least two of four positive-symptom items (rated on a 1–7 scale) on the Brief Psychiatric Rating Scale (BPRS) (99)—hallucinatory behavior, suspiciousness, unusual thought content, and conceptual disorganization
2. Current presence of at least a moderately severe illness as rated by the total BPRS score (score ≥45 on the 18 item scale) and a score of ≥4 (moderate) on the Clinical Global Impression (CGI) (100)
3. Persistence of illness: no period of good social and/or occupational functioning within the last 5 years
4. Drug-refractory condition: at least three periods of treatment in the preceding 5 years with conventional antipsychotics (from at least two chemical classes) at doses ≥1000 mg per day of chlorpromazine for 6 weeks, each without significant symptom relief, and failure to improve by at least 20% in total BPRS score or intolerance to a 6-week prospective trial of haloperidol at a dose of 10–60 mg per day

These criteria have face validity for many clinicians because they indentify patients with persistent illness with continuing positive symptomatology in the face of adequate current treatment. Their usefulness was shown in the MCT, where subjects who met them and were then randomized to chlorpromazine treatment showed only a 4% rate of response and no significant changes on total BPRS score or positive symptoms. Clozapine's superior efficacy has been repeatedly demonstrated using similar criteria (7,8).

Defining the Adequacy of Previous Drug Trials

The fourth criterion for resistance, regarding drug trials, has been modified somewhat since it was first proposed. The fact that there was only a 3% response rate to prospective haloperidol treatment and a 4% response rate to double-blind chlorpromazine treatment in the MCT led to the belief that two retrospective drug trial failures would be as effective as three in screening. Kane's group showed that subjects not responsive to two adequate antipsychotic trials (one retrospective and one prospective) have less than a 7% chance of responding to another trial (9) and they now use two prospective drug trials to determine treatment resistance (10). The FDA guidelines for clozapine's use, as reflected in the product labeling for Clozaril (11), state that people should fail to respond to two separate trials of antipsychotics before being treated with clozapine. Thus, two drug-trial failures as a criterion for treatment-refractory schizophrenia are now generally accepted (12). The evidence that second-generation antipsychotics are somewhat more effective than conventional antipsychotics has reopened the question of the type of drug a patient should fail. Clinicians now agree that a failure to respond to second-generation antipsychotics should precede a clozapine trial (13). However, this standard is different from the original, and this must be recognized when populations are described.

There have been other changes regarding the definition of an adequate drug trial. It is generally recognized that a 4- to 6-week period (rather than strictly a 6-week one) is adequate for a treatment trial of an antipsychotic (14). Recommended dosages have also been revised. Doses used during conventional antipsychotic trials were first proposed to be at least 1000 mg per day of chlorpromazine, or their equivalent. However, doses of >400 mg per day of chlorpromazine have been shown to be adequate to block 80–90% of dopamine receptors (thought to be the target of this drug action) (15). Higher doses produce no direct therapeutic benefit even in patients not responsive to therapy (9,16) and do not have greater efficacy in acute treatment than lower doses (17–19). Therefore, a 4- to 6-week trial of 400–600 mg of chlorpromazine is now accepted as a standard for an adequate trial (12,20). These modified criteria have been used to define treatment-refractory schizophrenia in recent clinical trials (10,21). They are also the basis for a recently proposed clinical treatment strategy that allows a clear progression of drug therapy in any patient with schizophrenia to optimize the likelihood of response (20,22). Issues of dosing are also certainly crucial to defining adequate trials of second-generation therapy. An optimal trial of risperidone should be in the range of 2 to 6 mg per day (23); optimal doses of olanzapine and quetiapine are less clear.

Neurobiology of Treatment-Refractory Schizophrenia

Until the establishment of standardized criteria for defining the treatment-refractory state, research into the neurobiological nature of the problem had been scant (24). Recently, however, with the use of more objective criteria, some consistent findings have been seen. People with treatment-refractory schizophrenia appear to have increased cortical atrophy on MRI compared to those with responsive illness (25,26). This is particularly true if they have predominant negative symptoms (27). People with persistent negative symptoms also have a tendency to demonstrate abnormal cell migration in their prefrontal cortex (28). From a clinical point of view, lack of response to early treatment is also predictive of nonresponse (25,29). Delay in first treatment may also be associated with a higher likelihood of refractory symptoms (30).

An intriguing finding related to predicting which new drugs may be effective in treatment-refractory schizophrenia has been the fact that these people appear to have lower catecholamine levels in the CSF (31). Because clozapine response has been associated with low ratios of CSF homovanillic acid to 5-hydroxy-indoleacetic acid (32), drugs with low dopamine antagonism and high serotonergic antagonism may be useful in treatment-refractory schizophrenia.

Prevalence of Treatment-Refractory Schizophrenia

Two independent groups have recently estimated the prevalence of treatment-refractory patients in current treatment populations. Juarez-Reyes et al. (33) used a broad interpretation of the FDA-approved Clozaril package insert to determine treatment-refractory rates in a county mental health system in California. They sampled a random, stratified group of people with schizophrenia (n = 293) consisting of all those served by a county mental health system in 1991 (inpatients and outpatients). Patients were considered treatment-refractory if they were older than 16, had a diagnosis of schizophrenia or schizoaffective disorder, had failed two previous 4-week drug trials at 600 or more mg per day, or had tardive dyskinesia, and had a Global Assessment of Functioning score of less than 61. The estimated proportion of treatment-refractory patients based on these broad criteria was 42.9 ±

5.9%. However, this estimate was lowered to 12.9 ± 2.7% when the criteria of Kane et al. (6) were used, primarily because of a lack of ability to document three previous drug-trial failures. Essock et al. (3) used the criteria of failure of two previous 6-week drug trials of 1000-mg/day chlorpromazine equivalents, inpatient status of at least 4 months and a total length of hospitalization of at least 24 months in the preceding 5 years. They estimated that 48% of all Connecticut state-hospital inpatients with a diagnosis of schizophrenia or schizoaffective disorder were treatment-refractory, from a total sample of 803 inpatients. These estimates of the proportion of treatment-refractory patients are similar to those made when clozapine was first marketed (34). They extrapolate to a total of 200,000–500,000 people with treatment-refractory schizophrenia currently living in the United States.

CLINICAL DESCRIPTIONS OF TREATMENT-REFRACTORY SCHIZOPHRENIA

Chronic Hospitalization vs. Poor Symptom Response

Studies of treatment-refractory schizophrenia have long been hampered by a lack of consistency in definition. Commonly, treatment resistance was considered roughly equivalent to chronic or frequent hospitalization (2). However, current and persistent positive symptoms of psychosis and at least moderate overall severity of illness should be present in order for treatment resistance to be diagnosed (35,36), since chronic hospitalization can occur despite low levels of symptoms (4). Moreover, many patients with presistent psychosis may not meet hospitalization criteria in some communities. It is now generally recognized that chronic hospitalization alone may not accurately in predict the likelihood of response to an antipsychotic trial (37,38).

For various reasons, many people with schizophrenia who have been chronically hospitalized may not be truly refractory to drug treatment. Inadequate psychosocial programming, poor compliance with prescribed drug therapy, or a history of committing violence (38) are all risk factors for chronic hospitalization. Therefore, optimized medication and treatment trials should be employed before a patient's illness is considered nonresponsive. In addition, the effects of drug noncompliance and extrapyramidal side effects (EPS) can both mimic treatment resistance (10,21). A course of at least 1 to 2 years of unambiguous and persistent positive symptoms should be one of the criteria for treatment-refractory schizophrenia.

Negative Symptoms

While most definitions of treatment-refractory schizophrenia have focused on the persistence of positive symptoms of psychosis, there has been a growing awareness of the problems presented by persistent negative symptoms. Moreover, lozapine and other second-generation antipsychotics have all been shown to have superior efficacy in reducing negative-symptom ratings in double-blind clinical trials (6,39–41). There is some controversy as to whether these drugs treat primary negative symptoms or whether their effect is due to secondary benefits (8,42,43). However, categorizing as refractory the illness of patients who have persistent negative symptoms may be clinically useful, because these patients often benefit from a change in their drug therapy to a new antipsychotic.

Violence Associated with Treatment-Refractory Schizophrenia

Violence in schizophrenia has long been considered a problem (44). People with schizophrenic symptoms have a markedly higher rate of perpetrating serious violence toward others (45). Patients with refractory schizophrenia are also more likely to be victims of violence, probably because of their tendency to be chronically hospitalized (46).

There has recently been some therapeutic optimism regarding this problem. Clozapine is more effective than traditional antipsychotic therapy in reducing violent behavior and hostility (47,48). Risperidone treatment has also been seen to decrease hostility (49). This raises the question of whether effectiveness against hostility, rather than being a particular property of clozapine, may be a phenomenon of the reduced EPS liability or other effects shared by the second-generation antipsychotics. It has been recognized that treatment with low-potency conventional antipsychotics that have reduced EPS liability is associated with improvement in violent behavior rates compared with haloperidol therapy (44). However, this finding may have been due to the increased sedation seen with these drugs.

TREATMENTS

Drug Therapy for Treatment-Refractory Schizophrenia

Historically, drug therapy for treatment-refractory schizophrenia has been centered on the use of different dose strategies of conventional antipsychotics or the use of adjunct agents such as lithium, β-blocking drugs, anticonvulsants, and benzodiazepines. These strategies have been well reviewed elsewhere, and none has been shown to be dramatically effective (14). Since the arrival of clozapine, attention in the field has shifted to a greater focus on the use of new antipsychotics for treatment-refractory symptoms in schizophrenia.

Conventional Antipsychotic Drugs

Conventional antipsychotic drugs had long been the first-line drug therapy for treating schizophrenia. However, evidence was always lacking to support the rationale of trying a second conventional drug after a patient had failed treatment with the first drug. These drugs were considered interchangeable in terms of efficacy—in over 100 studies comparing them in treatment of schizophrenia, only one showed a differential effect (50). In controlled trials in people with treatment-refractory symptoms, fewer than 5% responded after having their drug therapy changed from one conventional antipsychotic to another (6). The primary rationale for selecting any particular drug was to reduce side effects and to provide different dosing strategies. High-potency drugs such as haloperidol and fluphenazine have high EPS but cause less sedation and postural hypertension than low-potency drugs such as chlorpromazine and thioridazine. Haloperidol and fluphenazine are the only two conventional antipsychotics available as injectable depot medication, a formulation that can sometimes assure drug delivery and optimize response. This strategy can be useful in patients who show a lack of response, but it is important to note that, unless the patient has a positive therapeutic effect from a drug and associates the drug with that effect, the likelihood of long-term therapeutic benefit and compliance is low.

New-Generation Drugs

Novel antipsychotics are effective as first-line therapy (with the exception of clozapine, because of its serious side effects). Four drugs—risperidone, olanzapine, quetiapine, and clozapine—are reviewed here, primarily because they are currently available in the United States for the treatment of schizophrenia.

Clozapine

Clozapine was approved for use by the Food and Drug Administration in 1990 for the treatment of patients whose symptoms do not adequately respond to conventional antipsychotic therapy, either because therapy was not effective or because it could not be continued secondary to intolerable side effects. It is still the only drug with proven efficacy in rigorously defined treatment-refractory schizophrenia. Clozapine has also been useful in reducing violent behavior (51), tardive dyskinesia (52), and the risk of suicide (43). Despite this efficacy profile, clozapine has been relatively underused (53).

The relative underusage of clozapine is probably due to the costs and complexities of clozapine therapy. These arise from the need for long-term hematological monitoring for agranulocytosis and persistent serious side effects, such as weight gain, sialorrhea, and sedation. Despite the robust clinical effects of clozapine in long-term use (54), benefits that translate into improved living situations and decreased cost of care have not always been shown in large public-health-sector populations (55), particularly in the first year of use (3,56). Perhaps this is because clozapine is reserved for the most difficult to treat segment of the population with schizophrenia (57) or is being used by only a select subset of clinicians comfortable with the drug. With longer-term follow-up, clozapine benefits become more evident to patients, health-care providers, and families (58).

The optimal dose strategy for clozapine is slow dose escalation. Patients should be evaluated for response at dose plateaus of 200–400 mg per day and 500–600 mg per day. People who show clinically detectable improvement in positive symptoms, negative symptoms, or EPS should be continued on clozapine for 4 to 6 months before increases in dosages are considered. This is because continued improvements are frequently seen after even small initial improvement, and many of the serious side effects of clozapine therapy are dose-related.

Only patients with few side effects to clozapine should be titrated to doses higher than 600 mg per day. Patients should not be titrated to a higher dose of clozapine if myoclonus is present, as this side effect may precede the development of seizures. Patients who respond to clozapine will usually begin to respond within 8 weeks of reaching their response dose (59). However, since patients may respond over a wide range of doses, it is important to ensure that an adequate trial of clozapine is given before it is considered a failure.

Risperidone

Risperidone has been approved for use in schizophrenia since 1994. It is indicated for the treatment of positive and negative symptoms of the disorder.

There were early reports of patients with poorly responsive schizophrenia who showed some improvement with risperidone (60,61), but these studies were open-labeled, retrospective, or not controlled. There is one well-controlled double-blind study of risperidone vs. haloperidol in this group (62). Risperidone was more effective and better tolerated than haloperidol in this study, but the differential efficacy was not as large as what was seen with clozapine. There are two studies in which risperidone shows efficacy similar to that of clozapine in chronic poorly responsive schizophrenic patients (63,64). However, in these studies the patients were not categorized by typical treatment-refractory criteria and the study designs were not optimal to truly test a noninferiority hypothesis. Also, in one open study, risperidone therapy was shown to be more effective than prior conventional therapy, but not as effective as clozapine in well-categorized patients (65). In contrast, it has been widely recognized that risperidone treatment is usually not an adequate substitute for clozapine responders (66, 67).

Olanzapine

Olanzapine was approved for the treatment of schizophrenia in 1996. Its chemical structure and receptor-binding profile are very similar to those of clozapine, leading to hopes that it would show similar efficacy. There were several open reports of possible efficacy in this group (68,69). Also, analysis of double-blind comparative data showed that olanzapine had a better effect than haloperidol in people with poorly responsive schizophrenia (70), but this effect was not as great as one would have expected with clozapine. This was confirmed by several other studies. Conley et al. (71), in a double-blind trial, and Sanders and Mossman (72), in an open study, both failed to demonstrate a clozapine-like effect in well-characterized patients with treatment-refractory illness. Furthermore, the olanzapine-refractory patients from the Conley trial (71) did respond to a subsequent trial of clozapine at about the rate that would have been expected in a treatment-refractory group (73). As with risperidone, there is some question of whether the most effective dose of this drug was used. The dose range used in most recent studies has been 10–25 mg per day, which is close to the current recommended dose for unselected groups of patients. There are some preliminary reports that olanzapine might be more effective in higher doses (74,75), which need confirmation under more controlled conditions.

Quetiapine

Quetiapine has been shown to be effective in treatment-responsive schizophrenia (41). It has a pharmacological profile that includes high serotonin (5-HT_{1A})-receptor affinity compared to dopamine-receptor affinity. However, it is a low-potency antipsychotic compound. The most effective doses in clinical studies are 300 mg to 450 mg per day, suggesting a potency similar to that of clozapine. Moreover, there has been no difference between placebo and quetiapine in the amount of EPS or akathisia in published trials to date. There have been a few open-label case reports of beneficial effects of quetiapine in treatment-refractory patients (76,77), but no published controlled trials to date. Until clear evidence from controlled studies is available, this drug should not be considered for usual therapy in this group.

Alternative Therapies

If patients remain refractory to treatment after a clozapine trial or cannot take clozapine, alternative therapies should be considered. These include adjunct medication, reserpine, and electroconvulsive therapy (ECT). The data concerning the efficacy of these therapies are limited, but they may be of use in some patients.

Lithium

Several years ago, adjunct lithium therapy was found to be beneficial in some patients with treatment-refractory schizophrenia (78). These patients were not defined by the rigorous criteria of more recent studies, however. If lithium is tried, a 4-week trial of medication appears to be adequate to define response. The response seen may be more prominent in patients with affective symptoms, but patients who do respond appear to have benefits in areas of functioning other than in the affective domain (79). There are also reports that lithium may be helpful in reducing hostility in people with treatment-refractory schizophrenia (38).

The published trials of adjunct lithium, although positive, have been conducted with small numbers of patients, and often the criteria for defining the treatment-refractory state were not clear, or were overinclusive. The extent of the clinical effect in these trials was limited. Therefore, definitive evidence of the benefit of lithium is not yet available (80). Lithium should be used with caution in combination with conventional antipsychotics or clozapine because of the recognized dangers of delirium, encephalopathy, and neurotoxicity that have been reported (81,82).

Anticonvulsants

Carbamazepine and valproic acid have been observed to be effective in bipolar affective disorder (83), and are often considered as an adjunct therapy in patients with schizophrenia. There have been several controlled trials in schizophrenia using carbamazepine as an adjunct to a conventional antipsychotic. These trials have been consistently positive (84,85); however, they have had relatively few subjects. The positive effects seen have been modest and usually involved nonspecific improvement in areas such as behavior and social adjustment.

Carbamazepine needs to be used with caution because of reports of disorientation and ataxia associated with its use (86,87). It can also reduce the blood level of haloperidol by as much as 50% (88). Valproic acid should be used with caution because of the possibility of hepatic and pancreatic toxicity.

Benzodiazepines

There have been several reports on the use of adjunct benzodiazapines in treatment-refractory schizophrenia. Results have been mixed, with some double-blind studies showing a treatment effect (89) while other studies are negative (90). Given that patients with schizophrenia often have anxiety and irritability, it is not surprising that benzodiazapines are useful. However, there is no firm evidence for a specific adjunct antipsychotic effect with these agents. They should be used with caution because of the risks of chronic sedation, fatigue ataxia, and dependence. There are some reports of behavioral disinhibition (90) with these drugs, and the possibility of synergistic toxicity with clozapine (91). Although these reports have not been systematically confirmed, they suggest that caution should be used with this drug combination.

Electroconvulsive Therapy

There have been no controlled studies of ECT in treatment-refractory schizophrenic patients. Before the use of clozapine, there was some evidence from uncontrolled trials that ECT provided benefit for treatment-refractory patients, but usually the effect of ECT was most robust in patients with a short duration of illness (92). There have been two open trials of ECT added to clozapine in patients who had an inadequate clozapine response (93,94). Both trials showed some benefit from ECT. Also there have been reports of maintenance ECT continuing efficacy and preventing relapse in refractory patients (95). Controlled studies are needed in this area before ECT can be considered recommended.

Sulpiride

Sulpiride is an effective antipsychotic that is used widely, but not marketed in the United States. It belongs to the same drug class as remoxipride, a drug that may have been effective in treatment-

Table 1 Guidelines for Clinicians

1. Identify target symptoms. Antipsychotics are most helpful for the positive symptoms of psychosis: hallucinations, delusions, and thought disorder. Newer medications may also be helpful in reducing negative symptoms, such as poor socialization, withdrawal, and affective blunting, particularly if these are secondary to EPS of conventional antipsychotics. Clozapine has been shown to be effective in hostile, aggressive psychotic patients. Selecting target symptoms for a specific drug trial will allow for greater clarity in defining the parameters of success and failure.
2. Systematically use drugs at appropriate dosages and for a sufficient duration to establish efficacy. This is particularly critical before adjunct drugs are used since these may complicate the therapeutic situation and undermine efforts to define the optimal drug treatment for a patient.
3. Medication intolerance, noncompliance, inadequate social support, and inadequate psychosocial treatment may create the appearance of treatment-refractory symptoms. Consideration of these factors should precede the declaration of any drug therapy to be a failure. Although therapeutic ranges of most antipsychotics are not well established, measuring blood levels may be useful to establish compliance and to rule out poor medication absorption.
4. Exhaust the utility of single agents before using multiple agents. There is tremendous pressure for the clinician to find a drug to rapidly treat every psychological problem manifest in a patient. However, no adjunct agent has been shown to robustly improve antipsychotic response. Hostility, irritability, insomnia, and withdrawal can all be secondary to psychosis and may resolve only after a patient has had a good antipsychotic drug effect.
5. Aggressively prevent EPS through the appropriate choice of primary therapy. Antipsychotic agents that are clearly effective at doses that do not produce extrapyramidal symptoms in the vast majority of patients should allow the clinician to eliminate persistent side effects as a reason for therapeutic failure.
6. Maintain a positive therapeutic attitude. There are more choices than ever for antipsychotic therapy, and new drugs are appearing annually. Patients should be encouraged to think that there is good reason to be optimistic that some therapy will be found that will be beneficial to them, even if they have had a history of severe illness.

refractory schizophrenia (96). One well-controlled double-blind study has shown a positive effect of adjunct sulpiride in clozapine partial responders (97). A separate open study also suggested efficacy in olanzapine partial responders (98). These findings should be more fully explored.

Other Therapies

Although there are historical studies suggesting that β-blockers and reserpine may be useful in refractory schizophrenia, there are no available controlled studies, with current diagnostic criteria. Evidence is very limited that long-term therapy with either of these strategies is beneficial.

SUGGESTED GUIDELINES FOR CLINICIANS

A systematic approach to patients with treatment-refractory schizophrenia is critical. The practices outlined in Table 1 maximize the likelihood of a successful outcome. The most important concept for the clinician here is the need for consistent successive attempts to reverse targeted symptoms while a positive therapeutic attitude is maintained.

SUMMARY

Since antipsychotic drugs being used today may have mechanisms of action different from those of conventional antipsychotics and one another, clinicians should explore the possibility of response with each of these new agents in turn. To date, however, clozapine is the only mediation with demonstrated efficacy in well-defined treatment-refractory schizophrenia. Second-generation drugs may not be as effective as clozapine, but are more effective than conventional antipsychotics. They should be tried before clozapine in almost all patients. The differential efficacy of new drugs in treatment-refractory schizophrenia will be clear only when well-designed double-blind studies using rigorous entry criteria are completed.

Summary of Main Points

1. Treatment-refractory symptoms are common in schizophrenia: 10–30% of treated patients have a poor therapeutic response to medication.
2. Clinicians must consider poor compliance, medication intolerance, and appropriate drug dose and duration, and also define target symptoms, before considering a patient medication-refractory.
3. Second-generation antipsychotics are more effective than traditional antipsychotics, but patients may be refractory to either type of medication.

4. Clozapine is effective in about 40–60% of patients refractory to other antipsychotics. Its use is limited by its toxicity.
5. There is little evidence that adjunct medication is effective for refractory symptoms. The weight of evidence suggests that trying another antipsychotic after one trial has clearly failed is the most effective clinical course.
6. A consistent positive therapeutic attitude is important in providing the best outcome for refractory patients.

REFERENCES

1. Prien RF, Cole JO. High dose chlorpromazine therapy in chronic schizophrenia. Arch Gen Psychiatry 1968; 18(4):482–495.
2. Davis JM, Casper, R. Antipsychotic drugs: clinical pharmacology and therapeutic use. Drugs 1977; 12:260–282.
3. Essock SM, Hargreaves WA, Dohm FA, Goethe J, Carver L, Hipshman L. Clozapine eligibility among state hospital patients. Schizophr Bull 1996; 22(1):15–25.
4. McGlashan TH. A selective review of recent North American long-term follow-up studies of schizophrenia. Schizophr Bull 1988; 14(4):515–542.
5. Revicki DA, Luce BR, Weschler JM, Brown RE, Adler MA. Economic grand rounds: cost-effectiveness of clozapine for treatment-resistant schizophrenic patients. Hosp Commun Psychiatry 1990; 41(8):850–854.
6. Kane J, Honigfeld G, Singer J, Meltzer H, and the Clozaril Collaborative Study Group. Clozapine for the treatment-resistant schizophrenic. Arch Gen Psychiatry 1988; 45:789–796.
7. Pickar D, Owen RR, Litman RE, Konicki E, Gutierrez R, Rapaport M.H. Clinical and biologic response to clozapine in patients with schizophrenia: crossover comparison with fluphenazine. Arch Gen Psychiatry 1992; 49(5):345–353.
8. Buchanan RW, Breier A, Kirkpatrick B, Ball P, Carpenter WT Jr. Positive and negative symptom response to clozapine in schizophrenic patients with and without the deficit syndrome. Am J Psychiatry 1998; 155(6):751–760.
9. Kinon B, Kane JM, Perovish R, Ismi M, Koreen A. Influence of neuroleptic dose and class in treatment-resistant schizophrenia relapse. 32nd Annual Meeting of the New Clinical Drug Evaluation Unit, Key Biscayne, FL, May 1992.
10. Kinon BJ, Kane JM, Johns C, Perovish R, Ismi M, Koreen A, Weiden P. Treatment of neuroleptic-resistant schizophrenia relapse. Psychopharmacol Bull 1993; 29:309–314.
11. Physicians' Desk Reference. Montvale, NJ: Medical Economics Data Production, 1999.
12. Barnes TRE, McEvedy CJB. Pharmacological treatment strategies in the non-responsive schizophrenic patient. Int Clin Psychopharmacol 1996; 11(2):67–71.

13. Smith TE, Docherty JP. Standards of care and clinical algorithms for treating schizophrenia. Psychiatr Clin North Am 1998; 21(1):203–220.
14. Kane JM, Marder SR. Psychopharmacologic treatment of schizophrenia. Schizophr Bull 1993; 19(2):113–128.
15. Farde L, Norstrom AL, Wiesel FA, Pauli S, Haldin C, Sedval G. Positron emission tomographic analysis of central D1 and D2 dopamine receptor occupancy in patients treated with classical neuroleptics and clozapine: relation to extrapyramidal side effects. Arch Gen Psychiatry 1992; 49:538–544.
16. Wolkin A, Barouche F, Wolf AP, Rotrosen J, Fowler JS, Shiue CY, Cooper TB, Brodie JD. Dopamine blockade and clinical response: evidence for two biological subgroups of schizophrenia. Am J Psychiatry 1989; 146:905–908.
17. Rifkin A, Quitkin F, Rabiner CJ, Klein DF. Fluphenazine decanoate, fluphenazine hydrochloride given orally, and placebo in remitted schizophrenics. I. Relapse rates after one year. Arch Gen Psychiatry 1977; 34(1):43–47.
18. Baldessarini RJ, Cohen BM, Teicher M. Significance of neuroleptic dose and plasma level in the pharmacological treatment of psychoses. Arch Gen Psychiatry 1988; 45:79–91.
19. Van Putten T, Marder SR, Mintz J. A controlled dose comparison of haloperidol in newly admitted schizophrenic patients. Arch Gen Psychiatry 1990; 47:754–758.
20. Dixon LB, Lehman AF, Levine J. Conventional antipsychotic medications for schizophrenia. Schizophr Bull 1995; 21(4):567–577.
21. Shalev A, Hermesh H, Rothberg J, Munitz H. Poor neuroleptic response in acutely exacerbated schizophrenic patients. Acta Psychiatr Scand 1993; 87:86–91.
22. Frances A, Docherty JP, Kahn DA. The expert consensus guideline series: treatment of schizophrenia. J Clin Psychiatry 1996; 57(12B):11–50.
23. Love RC, Conley RR, Kelly DL, Bartko JJ. A dose-outcome analysis of risperidone. J Clin Psychiatry 1999; 60(11):771–775.
24. Dencker SJ, Kullhanet F, eds. Treatment Resistance in Schizophrenia. Braunschweig/Wiesbaden: Vieweg Verlag, 1988.
25. Stern RG, Kahn RS, Davidson M. Predictors of response to neuroleptic treatment in schizophrenia. Psychiatr Clin North Am 1993; 16(2):313–338.
26. Bilder RM, Wu H, Chakos MH, Gogerts B, Pollack S, Aronowitz J, Ashtari M, Degreef G, Kane JM, Lieberman JA. Cerebral morphometry and clozapine treatment in schizophrenia. J Clin Psychiatry 1994; 55(suppl B):53–56.
27. Ota P, Maeshiro H, Ishido H, Shimizu Y, Uchida R, Toyoshima R, Ohshima H, Takazawa A, Motomura H, Noguchi T. Treatment resistant chronic psychophathology and CT scans in schizophrenia. Acta Psychiatr Scand 1987; 75:415–427.
28. Kirkpatrick B, Conley RR, Kakoyannis A, Reep RL, Roberts RC. Interstitial cells of the white matter in the inferior parietal cortex in schizophrenia: an unbiased cell-counting study. Synapse 1999; 34(2):95–102.

29. Lieberman JA. Prediction of outcome in first-episode schizophrenia. J Clin Psychiatry 1993; 54(13):7.
30. Edwards J, Maude D, McGorry PD, Harrigan SM, Cocks JT. Prolonged recovery in first-episode psychosis. Br J Psychiatry 1998; suppl 172(33):107–116.
31. Van Kammen DP, Schooler N. Are biochemical markers for treatment-resistant schizophrenia state dependent or traits? Clin Neuropharmacol 1990; 13(1):516–528.
32. Pickar D, Breier A, Keisoe J. Plasma homovanillic acid as an index of central dopaminergic activity: studies in schizophrenic patients? Ann NY Acad Sci 1988; 527:339–346.
33. Juarez-Reyes MG, Shumway M, Battle C, Bacchetti P, Hansen MS, Hargreaves WA. Effects of stringent criteria on eligibility for clozapine among public mental health clients. Psychiatr Serv 1995; 46(8):801–806.
34. Terkelsen KG, Grosser RC. Estimating clozapine's cost on the nation. Hosp Commun Psychiatry 1990; 41(8):863–869.
35. Conley RR, Buchanan RW: Evaluation of treatment-resistant schizophrenia. Schizophr Bull 1997; 23(4)663–674.
36. Meltzer HY. Commentary: defining treatment refractoriness in schizophrenia. Schizophr Bull 1990; 16(4):563–565.
37. Brenner HD, Dencker SJ, Goldstein MJ, Hubbard JW, Keegan DL, Kruger G, Kullanek F, Liberman RP, Malm U, Midha KK. Defining treatment refractoriness in schizophrenia. Schizophr Bull 1990; 16(4):551–561.
38. Christison GW, Kirch DG, Wyatt RJ. When symptoms persist: choosing among alternative somatic treatments for schizophrenia. Schizophr Bull 1991; 17(2):217–245.
39. Marder SR, Meiback RC. Risperidone in the treatment of schizophrenia. Am J Psychiatry 1994; 151:825–835.
40. Beasley CM Tollefson G, Tran P. Olanzapine versus placebo and haloperidol. Neuropsychopharmacology 1996; 14:111–123.
41. Arvanitis LA, Miller BG. The Seroquel Trial 13 Study Group. Multiple fixed doses of "Seroquel" (quetiapine) in patients with acute exacerbation of schizophrenia: a comparison with haloperidol and placebo. Biol Psychiatry 1997; 42(4):233–246.
42. Carpenter WT, Conley RR, Buchanan RW, Breier A, Tamminga CA. Patient response and resource management: another view of clozapine treatment of schizophrenia. Am J Psychiatry 1995; 152:6.
43. Meltzer HY, Okayli G. Reduction of suicidality during clozapine treatment in neuroleptic-resistant schizophrenia: impact on risk-benefit assessment. Am J Psychiatry 1995; 152:182–190.
44. Herrera JN, Sramek JJ, Costa JF, Roy S, Heh CW, Nen BN. High potency neuroleptics and violence in schizophrenics. J Nerv Ment Dis 1988; 176(9):558–561.
45. Eronen M, Hakola P, Tiihonen J. Mental disorders and homicidal behavior in Finland. Arch Gen Psychiatry 1996; 53:497–501.

46. Malone ML, Thompson L, Goodwin JS. Aggressive behavior among the institutionalized elderly. J Am Geriatr Soc 1993; 41(8):853–856.
47. Breier A, Buchanan RW, Irish D, Carpenter WT Jr. Clozapine treatment of outpatients with schizophrenia: outcome and long-term response patterns. Hosp Commun Psychiatry 1993; 44(12):1145–1149.
48. Wilson WH. Clinical review of clozapine treatment in a state hospital. Hosp Commun Psychiatry 1992; 43:700–703.
49. Czobor P, Volavka J, Meibach RC. Effect of risperidone on hostility in schizophrenia. J Clin Psychopharmacol 1995; 15(4):243–249.
50. Klein DF, Davis JM. Diagnosis and drug treatment of psychiatric disorders. Baltimore: Williams & Wilkins, 1969.
51. Mallya AR, Roos PD, Roebuck-Colgan K. Restraint, seclusion, and clozapine. J Clin Psychiatry 1992; 53:395–397.
52. Tamminga CA, Thaker GK, Moran M, Kakigi T, Gao XM. Clozapine in tardive dyskinesia: observations from human and animal model studies. J Clin Psychiatry 1994; 55(suppl B): 102–106.
53. Bustillo JR, Lauriello J, Keith SJ. Schizophrenia: improving outcome. Harv Rev Psychiatry 1999; 6(5):229–240.
54. Rosenheck R, Evans D, Herz L, Cramer J, Xu W, Thomas J, Henderson W, Charney D. How long to wait for a response to clozapine: a comparison of time course of response to clozapine and conventional antipsychotic medication in refractory schizophrenia. Schizophr Bull 1999; 25(4):709–719.
55. Zito JM, Volavka J, Craig TJ, Czobor P, Banks S, Vitrai J. Pharmacoepidemiology of clozapine in 202 inpatients with schizophrenia. Ann Pharmacother 1993; 27:1262–1269.
56. Rosenheck R, Cramer J, Allan E, Erdos J, Frisman LK, Xu W, Thomas J, Henderson W, Charney D. Department of Veterans Affairs Cooperative Study Group on Clozapine in Refractory Schizophrenia. Cost-effectiveness of clozapine in patients with high and low levels of hospital use. Arch Gen Psychiatry 1999; 56(6):565–572.
57. Safferman A, Lieberman JA, Kane JM, Szymanski S, Kinon B. Update on the clinical efficacy and side effects of clozapine. Schizophr Bull 1991; 17(2):247–261.
58. Rosenheck R, Cramer J, Jurgis G, Perlick D, Xu W, Thomas J, Henderson W, Charney D. Clinical and psychopharmacologic factors influencing family burden in refractory schizophrenia. J Clin Psychiatry 2000; 61(9):671–676.
59. Conley RR, Carpenter WT, Tamminga CA. Time to response and response-dose in a 12-month clozapine trial. Am J Psychiatry 1997; 154(9):1243–1247.
60. Chouinard G, Vainer JL, Belanger MC, Turnier L, Beaudry P, Roy JY, Miller R. Risperidone and clozapine in the treatment of drug-resistant schizophrenia and neuroleptic-induced supersensitivity psychosis. Prog Neuropsychopharmacol Biol Psychiatry 1994; 18(7):1129–1141.

61. Keck PE Jr, Wilson DR, Strakowski SM, McElroy SL, Kizer Dl, Balistreri TM, Holtman HM, DePriest M. Clinical predictors of acute risperidone response in schizophrenia, schizoaffective disorder, and psychotic mood disorders. J Clin Psychiatry 1995; 56(10):455–470.
62. Wirshing DA, Marshall BD Jr, Green MF, Mintz J, Marder SR, Wirshing WC. Risperidone in treatment-refractory schizophrenia. Am J Psychiatry 1999; 156(9):1374–1379.
63. Klieser E, Lehmann E, Kinzler E, Wurthmann C, Heinrich K. Randomized, double-blind, controlled trial of risperidone versus clozapine in patients with chronic schizophrenia. J Clin Psychopharmacol 1995; 1(suppl 1):45S–51S.
64. Bondolfi G, Dufour H, Patris M, May JP, Billeter U, Eap CB, Baumann P. The Risperidone Study Group. Risperidone versus clozapine in treatment-resistant chronic schizophrenia: a randomized double-blind study. Am J Psychiatry 1998; 155(4):499–504.
65. Flynn SW, MacEwan GW, Altman S, Kopala LC, Fredrikson DH, Smith GN, Honer WG. An open comparison of clozapine and risperidone in treatment-resistant schizophrenia. Pharmacopsychiatry 1998; 31(1):25–29.
66. Lacey RL, Preskorn SH, Jerkovich GS. Is risperidone a substitute for clozapine for patients who do not respond to neuroleptics? [letter]. Am J Psychiatry 1995; 152(9):1401.
67. Shore D. Clinical implications of clozapine discontinuation: report of an NIMH workshop. Schizophr Bull 1995; 21(2):333–337.
68. Thomas SG, Labbate LA. Management of treatment-resistant schizophrenia with olanzapine. Can J Psychiatry 1998; 43(2):195–196.
69. Tollefson GD, Kuntz AJ. Review of recent clinical studies with olanzapine. Br J Psychiatry Suppl 1999; (37):30–35.
70. Breier A, Hamilton SH. Comparative efficacy of olanzapine and haloperidol for patients with treatment-resistant schizophrenia. Biol Psychiatry 1999; 45(4):403–411.
71. Conley RR, Tamminga CA, Bartko JJ, Richardson C, Peszke M, Lingle J, Hegerty J, Love R, Gounaris C, Zaremba S. Olanzapine compared with chlorpromazine in treatment-resistant schizophrenia. Am J Psychiatry 1998; 155(7):914–920.
72. Sanders RD, Mossman D. An open trial of olanzapine in patients with treatment-refractory psychoses. J Clin Psychopharmacol 1999; 19(1):62–66.
73. Conley RR, Tamminga CA, Kelly DL, Richardson CM. Treatment-resistant schizophrenic patients respond to clozapine after olanzapine non-response. Biol Psychiatry 1999; 46(1):73–77.
74. Reich J. Use of high-dose olanzapine in refractory psychosis. Am J Psychiatry 1999; 156(4):661.
75. Dursun SN, Gardner DM, Bird DC, Flinn J. Olanzapine for patients with treatment-resistant schizophrenia: a naturalistic case-series outcome study. Can J Psychiatry 1999; 44(7):701–704.

76. Szigethy E, Brent S, Findling RL. Quetiapine for refractory schizophrenia. J Am Acad Child Adolesc Psychiatry 1998; 37(11):1127–1128.
77. Reznik I, Benatov R, Sirota P. Seroquel in a resistant schizophrenic with negative and positive symptoms. Harefuah 1996; 130(10):675–677.
78. Growe GA, Crayton JW, Klass DB, Evans H, Strizich M. Lithium in chronic schizophrenia. Am J Psychiatry 1979; 136:454–455.
79. Delva NJ, Letemendia FJ. Lithium treatment in schizophrenia and schizo-affective disorders. In: Kerr A, Snaith P, eds. Contemporary Issues in Schizophrenia. London: Royal College of Psychiatrists, 1986:381–396.
80. Johns CA, Thompson JW. Adjunctive treatments in schizophrenia: pharmacotherapies and electroconvulsive therapy. Schizophr Bull 1995; 21:607–619.
81. Cohen WJ, Cohen NH. Lithium carbonate, haloperidol and irreversible brain damage. JAMA 1974; 230:1283–1287.
82. Miller F, Menninger J. Lithium-neuroleptic neurotoxicity is dose-dependent. J Psychopharmacol 1987; 7:89–91.
83. Post RM. Non-lithium treatment for bipolar disorder. J Clin Psychiatry 1990; 51(suppl):9–16.
84. Schulz SC, Kahn Em, Baker RW, Conley RR. Lithium and carbamazepine augmentation in treatment-refractory schizophrenia. In: Angrist B, Schulz SC, eds. The Neuroleptic-Nonresponsive Patient: Characterization and Treatment. Washington, DC: American Psychiatric Press, 1990:109–136.
85. Simhandl C, Meszaros K. The use of carbamazepine in the treatment of schizophrenia and schizoaffective psychosis: a review. J Psychiatry Neurosci 1992; 17:1–14.
86. Kanter GL, Yerevsanian BI, Ciccone JR. Case report of a possible interaction between neuroleptics and carbamazepine. Am J Psychiatry 1984; 14:1101–1102.
87. Yerevanian BI, Hodgman CH. A haloperidol-carbamazepine interaction in a patient with rapid-cycling bipolar disorder. Am J Psychiatry 1985; 142:785–786.
88. Kahn EM, Schulz SC, Perel JM, Alexander JE. Change in haloperidol level due to carbamazepine: a complicating factor in combined medication for schizophrenia. J Clin Psychiatry 1990; 10:54–57.
89. Wolkowitz OM, Turetsky N, Reus VI, Hargreaves WA. Benzodiazepine augmentation of neuroleptics in treatment-resistant schizophrenia. Psychopharmacol Bull 1992; 28:291–295.
90. Pato CN, Wolkowitz OM, Rapaport M, Schulz SC, Pickar D. Benzodiazepine augmentation of neuroleptic treatment in patients with schizophrenia. Psychopharmacol Bull 1989; 25:263–266.
91. Meltzer HY. New drugs for the treatment of schizophrenia. Psychiatr Clin North Am 1993; 16:365–385.
92. Small JG. Efficacy of electroconvulsive therapy in schizophrenia, mania, and other disorders. I. Schizophrenia. Convuls Ther 1985; 1:263–270.

93. Benatov R, Sirota P, Megged S. Neuroleptic-resistant schizophrenia treated with clozapine and ETC. Convuls Ther 1996; 12(2):117–121.
94. Remington GJ, Addington D, Collins EJ, Jones BD, Lalonde P, MacCrimmon DJ, MacEwan GW. Clozapine: current status and role in the pharmacotherapy of schizophrenia. Can J Psychiatry 1996; 41(3):161–166.
95. Chanpattana W. Maintenance ECT in treatment-resistant schizophrenia. J Med Assoc Thai 2000; 83(6):657–662.
96. Conley RR, Tamminga CA, Nen JA. Clinical action of remoxipride. Arch Gen Psychiatry 1994; 51(12):1001.
97. Shiloh R, Zemishlany Z, Aizenberg D, Radwan M, Schwartz B, Dorfman-Etrog P, Modai I, Khaikin M, Weizman A. Sulpiride augmentation in people with schizophrenia partially responsive to clozapine: a double-blind, placebo-controlled study. Br J Psychiatry 1997; 171:569–573.
98. Raskin S, Durst R, Katz G, Zislin J. Olanzapine and sulpiride: a preliminary study of combination/augmentation in patients with treatment-resistant schizophrenia. J Clin Psychopharmacol 2000; 20(5):500–503.
99. Overall JE, Gorman DE. The Brief Psychiatric Rating Scale. Psychology 1961; 10:799–812.
100. Guy W. ECDEU Assessment Manual for Psychopharmacology. US Department of Health and Human Services publication (ADM) 1976; 76(338):534–535.

9

Psychosocial and Cognitive Rehabilitation

Gitry Heydebrand
Washington University School of Medicine
St. Louis, Missouri

INTRODUCTION

The image of Phillipe Pinel removing the chains from "lunatics" in a Paris asylum at the end of the 18th century can be seen as a symbol for the beginning of the era of "modern" rehabilitation for mentally ill patients. Pinel may or may not have actually gone around striking shackles off of people, but the painting as a representation of enlightenment and reformation marks the beginning of a coherent, organized movement in the treatment of people with mental illness.

The reform movement coalesced with the notion of "moral treatment," typified as a model community in which the mentally ill could relearn life skills in an atmosphere free of tension and chaos. This process was compared to child-rearing, based on the belief that patients could develop behavioral self-control through a corrective relationship with a benign authority figure. In the mid-1800s, this model appeared to be very successful, accounting for a high discharge rate and low rates of readmission. However, the "treatment" relied to a significant extent on the personal charisma and skill of the asylum superintendent, who often established a personal relationship with each patient under his care. The number of patients requiring hospitalization increased dramatically at the beginning of the 20th century, with a corresponding increase in the cases with severe psychiatric disorders (see Ref. 1 for a discussion of the various factors involved in this trend). The solution to this problem was the creation of the large state hospital to house the chronically mentally ill.

Conditions in many state hospitals were poor almost from the outset, but it was not until the 1960s that the next cycle of reform developed, spurred to a large extent by the development of antipsychotic drugs such as chlorpromazine. The new psychotropics gave hope that mentally ill patients could be maintained in the community, and a grand plan for deinstitutionalization was developed. However, while discharging patients from hospitals where they had lived for decades was achieved fairly rapidly, the community mental health centers that were supposed to provide psychiatric care and psychosocial training in the skills necessary to live in the world were not always sufficiently funded, which resulted in a marginal existence for many chronically mentally ill people.

With the advent of atypical antipsychotic drugs, as well as increased understanding of the neuropsychological deficits associated with schizophrenia, rehabilitation of mentally ill individuals has undergone yet another cycle of development. A number of models and programs have been developed over the past 10 years, using a variety of approaches and with various degrees of success.

Psychosocial rehabilitation for persons with schizophrenia refers to programs and treatment interventions that are intended to provide knowledge and teach skills and behaviors for "living in the world." This includes work and social skills, education about the disease, medications, symptom management, and relapse prevention. Some models also offer psychotherapy focusing on how to cope with the trauma of a debilitating mental illness. While rehabilitation generally refers to "living skills," several programs of this type also attempt to target some of the apparent deficits in cognition that appear to interfere with general functioning. Spaulding et al. (2), for example, was able to show that procedures targeting cognitive impairments in schizophrenia can enhance patients' response to standard psychiatric rehabilitation, particularly in the domain of social competence. *Cognitive rehabilitation*, therefore, consists of treatment that addresses specific deficits in neuropsychological function, such as attention and information processing. In contrast, *cognitive-behavioral treatment* relies on learning principles to effect changes in behavioral response.

The notion that patients with schizophrenia can significantly improve their level of functioning is crucial to the paradigm of recovery. A longitudinal study (3) comparing patients who participated in a "meds, maintenance, and stabilization" program vs. a bio-psycho-social rehabilitation program after being discharged from a state hospital in the late 1950s showed that, 30 years later, those who had been in the rehabilitation program had far fewer symptoms of schizophrenia, had a greater percentage in the workforce, and had better community adjustment. The patients had been carefully matched on a large number of variables, suggesting that the rehabilitation program accounted for the significant difference in outcome. Several other studies have demonstrated similar results, indicating that the assumption of poor prognosis in schizophrenia may to some extent be due to self-fulfilling-prophecy factors (e.g., the expectations of mental health professionals) and political influences (e.g., lack of funding for comprehensive programs) rather than biological destiny.

This chapter provides brief descriptions of the key words in psychiatric rehabilitation to guide the clinician in evaluating patient needs and program components. Although it is not intended to be a do-it-yourself manual—rehabilitation has been found to be most successful as a team effort—it may increase awareness of types of possible interventions and direction for treatment.

BASIC CONCEPTS

Rehabilitation

Theories on the causes, mechanisms, and symptoms of schizophrenia reflect specific paradigms that have direct implications in selecting treatment interventions. If, for example, psychotic behavior is "un-understandable" (4) and delusions are therefore "empty speech acts, whose informational content refers to neither world or self" (5), then alleviation of psychosis should result in a return to the level of functioning prior to onset (similar to treating an infection with antibiotics). However, there appears to be broad agreement that outcome in schizophrenia is multidimensional, based largely on several studies by Strauss and Carpenter (6,7) demonstrating only modest correlation across symptomatic, social, and vocational domains and with considerable variations in overall levels of functioning.

Much of the "neuropsychology of schizophrenia" literature suggests that schizophrenia involves multiple discrete impairments, making the scope of dysfunction so extensive that any attempt at cognitive training to improve everyday function would have to address complex cognition systems. However, not all researchers agree with this position. For example, Bellak et al. (8) suggests that the actual deficit pattern observed in schizophrenia may result from a smaller number of specific impairments (e.g., working memory) with broad implications. This possibility would point to the formulation of a rehabilitation approach that is more focused; e.g., rather than trying to teach a person to utilize a "problem-solving approach," Bellak proposes that clinicians focus on the specific skills needed for successful functioning in a given situation (e.g., what ability or skill is required for a designated job?).

Just as the clinician must make a careful and informed decision in the selection of the most appropriate antipsychotic medication in treating a schizophrenic patient, there is also a wide range of choices concerning interventions and rehabilitation programs:

Cognitive/neuropsychological: interventions designed to improve information processing and responses as understood from a neurological model

Cognitive/behavioral: treatment that shapes behavior and teaches patients to cope with symptoms as manifestations of physiological abnormalities

Psychosocial: programs that rely on a skills-deficit model and provide both direct and explicit training in day-to-day-functioning (e.g., how to ride a bus or apply for a job) as well as modeling and social support to assist with living in the world

Some comprehensive treatment programs incorporate aspects of all three models. For example, a patient's daily activities might include playing computer games (cognitive training), attending one-on-one or small-group sessions on how to deal with delusions and hallucinations (cognitive/behavioral), and field trips to the zoo or the employment office to practice specific skills (psychosocial). Outcome studies that have demonstrated the success of such "day programs" have not identified one particular component or factor that accounts for improvement, but have supported the conclusion that comprehensive, multifaceted interventions are most effective in reducing recidivism and improving overall functioning.

Cognitive/Neuropsychological Interventions

At the turn of the 20th century, Kraepelin and his contemporaries postulated a biological basis for schizophrenia to explain the higher-order neurological deficits of aphasia, agnosia, apraxia, etc., that they observed. However, only in the past 30 years has a useful paradigm for the neuropsychology of schizophrenia been developed, due in part to advances in neuroscience and neuroimaging. Corresponding efforts began in the early 1970s to apply principles of rehabilitation based on cognitive deficits, e.g., teaching patients with schizophrenia to use "self-talk" in order to solve problems (9). However, outcome studies of these techniques were unable to demonstrate substantial enhancement in daily community functioning.

Fortunately, later studies (10) provided support for the conclusion that cognitive remediation is helpful but not essential; many researchers in this area therefore determined that although *restoration* of cognitive functioning in schizophrenic patients does not appear possible, *compensation* (development of adaptive skills) can be achieved. The model used in rehabilitation medicine (e.g., learning to use a prosthesis after amputation) appears to be effective for psychiatric interventions as well (8).

As described in other chapters, researchers in the area of the neuropsychology of schizophrenia have identified several areas of cognitive deficits:

Attention and information processing
Working memory (and other aspects of memory function)
Visuospatial skills
Executive function

These functions are briefly reviewed below.

Attention is a complex system that affects all other aspects of processing and response since it is the "input" point for cognition. Attention includes:

Active exploration
Systematic exploration
Focus on both the whole and parts of a stimulus field
Simultaneous consideration of sources of information
Sustaining focus of attention
Screening multiple sources of stimulation (suppression)
Shifting focus

These functions may also tap aspects of working memory and executive function (see below).

Working memory refers to the capacity to hold and manipulate information (e.g., doing arithmetic in one's head, keeping track of a phone number long enough to punch the buttons, etc.). Thus, it involves concentration, rehearsal, and short-term encoding. Working-memory tasks may call on visual memory function (picturing numbers on a blackboard) and strategizing (muttering words or numbers to oneself) in order to complete a given task. People with schizophrenia appear to have impairments in working-memory function that are distinct from attentional impairments and psychosis, and they also tend to be slower to learn new material. Therefore, successful training programs must incorporate awareness of these cognitive deficits.

Impairment of *visuospatial skills* has been shown to be another neuropsychological deficit in schizophrenia. This area of function includes being able to use conceptualization and reasoning for nonverbal tasks (e.g., reproducing designs, putting together pieces of something), and its disruption may interfere with activities such as reading a map and following directions, referring to a diagram (as in assembling a bicycle), or scanning an area systematically and effectively to detect an item. Clearly, strong attentional demands are related to visuospatial responses, with additional demands related to the areas of the cortex that regulate visual and visuospatial responses.

Deficits in *executive function* present the greatest challenge for adaptive and independent daily living. Impaired executive abilities, which implicate frontal-lobe dysfunction, refer to the capacity to integrate and analyze incoming information accurately and to formulate appropriate responses. The frontal lobes have been described as the "chairman of the board," as the final destination for all sensory input and the source for outgoing actions/responses, responsible for understanding the world and being able to organize information and initiate a plan accordingly. The "negative symptoms" seen in schizophrenia have been attributed in part to deficits in executive function, particularly what is seen as "lack of motivation." However, amotivation has increasingly been understood as lack of initiation (no "spark" or signal to "go") rather than a psychologically based apathy. To understand the complexity of "executive function," it may be useful to consider the many components of information processing (see Table 1).

The therapist attempting to remediate executive-function deficits may focus on individual components of processing, or may aim for teaching global strategies that incorporate many of the functions described above. Selection of treatment goals may be guided by a number of factors, including:

Severity of deficits: The degree of impairment may be mild to profound; in the latter case, a clinician would not try to teach step-by-step problem solving until and unless the patient could demonstrate the ability to recognize and discriminate between a relevant and irrelevant cue.

Learning capacity: Some individuals with a very concrete thinking style may have limitations in their ability to develop a capacity for abstraction due to below-average intelligence.

Table 1 Components of Executive Function

Discrimination	Recognition of critical distinguishing features
	Distinguishing between relevant and irrelevant cues
	Association, clustering, and detecting patterns of organization
Problem solving	Identifying and defining a problem
	Inferential, hypothetical thinking and testing
	Systematic approach to problems
	Prediction of consequences
	Error detection
	Reflection; incorporation of feedback
Organization	Planning
	Flexibility and reversibility of thinking
	Prioritization of information
Abstraction	Comprehension of symbols and concepts
	Comparison of similarities and difference
Goals	Generating realistic goals
	Anticipation of future goals
Self-control	Frustration tolerance
	Awareness of task difficulty and one's own capabilities

Behavior: Frequent impulsive and/or dysfunctional behavior would suggest a need to prioritize the development of prediction of consequences and perhaps frustration tolerance.

Goals: The patient (and family) may have specific goals in mind, such as being able to live independently or to work. These goals would then prompt the clinician to focus on relevant functions. For example, if helping someone to prepare for work as a cashier, "error detection" might be crucial; living in an apartment might require development of "planning" capabilities (budgeting, etc.).

Cognitive-Behavioral Interventions

Aaron Beck first proposed the use of cognitive therapy with schizophrenics in the 1950s, suggesting that if the manifestation of schizophrenia is seen primarily as a disturbance in thinking, then cognitive interventions to "correct" the thought disorder would be an obvious solution (35). While psychotic symptoms are now understood to be caused by physiological dysfunction, and are effectively treated with medication, work has also been done—primarily in England—to develop cognitive-behavioral interventions to combat psychotic symptoms (11,12,36). These can be particularly helpful with mildly refractory or "breakthrough" psychotic symptoms (e.g., provoked by a stressful situation), to increase a sense of self-efficacy in the patient and avoid overmedication.

A central assumption of cognitive-behavioral interventions for schizophrenia is that disordered thought generates anxiety due to the nature of the percepts (persecution, etc.) and to impaired functioning, which further interferes with accurate processing of "reality." If the disruption of thought processes associated with schizophrenia is seen as an illogical association between events that most people would not see as connected, then the point of intervention is the illogical nature of the assumption. Treatment should therefore focus on developing the necessary self-control skills to change thought patterns for more effective reality processing. Within this framework, several groups of strategies have been developed that are designed to cope with psychotic symptoms, including behavior change (e.g., seeking out social interaction as a buffer against intrusive hallucinations), relaxation techniques to decrease physiological arousal, and cognitive coping methods such as ignoring symptoms or "diversionary" activities (13). As with cognitive therapy for other types of disorders, the greatest challenge is helping patients accept the notion that there are alternative explanations for their perceptions and experiences, sometimes called "taking the role of the other" (14). Thus, while the emphasis in cognitive-behavioral therapy is to some extent on teaching fairly specific strategies and encouraging logical thinking, factors such as the therapeutic alliance are crucial to successful outcome.

Psychosocial Interventions

A number of studies have indicated that cognitive improvements may occur in response to psychosocial treatment (see Ref. 15 for a review of this literature).

Whether the changes are due to stimulation and rebuilding of damaged cortical pathways, learned behavior, or prosthetic mechanisms (new skills replacing impaired abilities), these findings offer strong support for comprehensive, skill-based training programs.

The emphasis in psychosocial rehabilitation is on teaching patients how to access resources and adjust to and maintain community living as independently as possible. Programs may range from providing such basics as meals and housing assistance to enrichment and self-development classes.

The Clubhouse Model

In the same era as deinstitutionalization, and partly in response to the perceived need for community support, the clubhouse model emerged in the 1970s. Often referred to as the Fountain House model, named after the first facility established in New York City in 1948, this type of program emphasizes the importance of a supportive social milieu, with integrated services for housing, employment, and counseling. There is a strong focus on self-help and avoidance of the stigma of mental illness, and a built-in expectation for achieving maximum potential. By the mid-1980s, there were 180 clubhouses in the United States patterned after the original Fountain House model. Such models have repeatedly been shown to be highly successful (i.e., they reduce recidivism and therefore save money in treatment costs, which is of course the most important concern) but remain underfunded (16).

The role of social support in buffering stress has been well established, as has the correlation between higher levels of stress and more severe psychopathology (e.g., 17–19). Thus, one of the most important roles of clubhouses has been to provide a "safe place." However, many such programs have also incorporated supported- or independent-living programs, employment programs, and specific interventions to address the needs of chronically mentally ill patients. Staff members either directly or indirectly provide feedback and guidance on appropriate behavior and effective communication. Programs may also include focused classes or groups on social skills, symptom management, resource utilization, etc. Some also include programs for families, to provide education about schizophrenia and thereby also assist them in providing a therapeutic (or at least low-stress) environment at home.

CLINICAL DESCRIPTIONS

Cognitive Rehabilitation Techniques

The necessary first step in developing a cognitive rehabilitation treatment plan—assessment—is best completed by a qualified neuropsychologist familiar with the profile of deficits seen in schizophrenia. Treatment interventions to improve cognitive functioning tend to consist of training modules or programs administered either individually or in small group settings. Although computer-based remediation appeared promising at first, investigators found that while performance improved on the particular task presented by a computer program, generalization did not occur (e.g., a patient's response time and ability to maintain attention to a flashing target improved, but this did not "translate" to improved day-to-day functioning). Training sequences with goals such as improving social interaction have demonstrated success in teaching patients to attend to specific stimuli (e.g., whether a prospective social partner appears friendly) and then building on this foundation to improve social interaction in real-life situations.

Attention

The goal in rehabilitation of attention deficits is not merely to "pay attention" but to increase attention span while improving the efficiency of information processing. This involves not just maintaining an attentional set but making an ongoing active evaluation of the information presented and responding appropriately to selected items. The task consists of being able to shift and scan for relevant details within the "stimulus field," to suppress extraneous input (i.e., to not be distracted), and to inhibit a response until all pertinent information has been considered. Recognition of the components of attention involved in completion of any type of task points to the "units" or training modules that may be developed to improve processing capacity.

Successful strategies for attention deficits in schizophrenia should emphasize reducing demands on verbal memory and vigilance (rather than trying to "restore" working-memory function) and relying on compensatory techniques such as overlearning skills (20). As noted above, training in attention may also be used to improve specific behaviors ("is the other person smiling?") and specific skills ("a smile = go—start the conversation!").

There are several software programs designed to remediate attention deficits associated with brain injury or dysfunction. Ben-Yishay and Diller (21) developed an Orientation Remediation Module that includes exercises such as improving reaction time to auditory stimuli (Attention Reaction Conditioner), spatial focusing with visual cues (Zero Accuracy Conditioner), and temporal vigilance with auditory and visual cues (Time Estimates). Bracy (22) developed an extensive set of computer programs that include attentional demands, such as divided-attention tasks requiring vigilance (watching three dials and responding when one drops below a certain line, as in a nuclear reactor) and visual scanning requiring rapid shifts in attentional focus (e.g., shooting down enemy aircraft with changing configurations). As noted, research on the efficacy of this type of computer-based treatment has shown mixed results. Anecdotal evidence suggests improved attention for tasks outside the computer room, but the overall findings remain inconclusive.

Memory

In memory rehabilitation, as in improving other areas of cognitive functioning, the major challenge is to develop methods that will prompt the individual with memory impairment to use learned strategies (remembering to remember). The task of identifying situations in which a memory technique should be used is thus an organizational and planning task, which is an executive function.

Improving memory function may involve a strong emphasis on rote, automatic behavior as well as external structures or prompts to activate a strategy. For example, teaching a person to "remember" a daily morning-hygiene routine may require posting a checklist by the bathroom mirror and rehearsing the sequence of getting out of bed, going into the bathroom, and starting the routine by looking at the first item on the list. Similarly, using a memory notebook may require training in the action of writing down specified information (e.g., appointments or the main point of a phone call), and then "building in" the reminder to take out the notebook and use it at certain points during the day, or programming a wristwatch to beep every 30 minutes as a signal to check the notebook (which contains appointments and other reminders).

Memory notebook. This "intervention" consists of a small- to medium-sized notebook with various compartments tailored to compensate for whatever deficits are present. Components may include daily/weekly appointments, sections for writing down events and activities.

The most difficult aspect of training a person to use a memory notebook may be determining how to "remember to remember," i.e., to use it effectively, through tailored prompts and reminders which may be tapping executive functions rather than the memory system.

Mnemonics. Physicians are very familiar with such mnemonic devices as strategies for recalling the optic nerves ("On Old Olympus' Snowy Tops . . . ," etc.). Such techniques have become fairly well known among the general public, owing to a number of books on the topic of improving memory. They are easily taught, but with the schizophrenic population, additional presentation, rehearsal, and prompting may be required. Also, they have been criticized on several points. They are labor-intensive, requiring considerable training and input by the clinician, and are therefore expensive to carry out. They are not necessarily well suited for dealing realistically with problems of day-to-day behavior; they may help in remembering a grocery list or the steps for responding to an emergency, but are less helpful in keeping track of details on an ongoing basis. Relatedly, they have limited generalizability, as they require a fair degree of organization and creativity to generate.

Rehearsal. Research is beginning to show that people with schizophrenia are able to learn information as effectively as those without mental illness, but that they learn more slowly. Thus, they require a greater number of presentations of material, and benefit from using rehearsal strategies. These may include repeating the information out loud, or receiving input through more than one channel, such as reading something while also listening to it being read.

Visuospatial Skills

Training in visuospatial responses consists primarily of cues and prompts to improve visual attention, scanning, and processing. In one-on-one rehabilitation sessions, interventions may range from simple tasks such as counting the number of A's on a page to more ecologically valid tasks such as reading a map or following assembly instructions. At the basic level, the therapist trains the patient to "see," and gives examples of cues in question form (see Table 2).

Executive Function

As mentioned previously, a major question in rehabilitation of executive-function deficits is whether to attempt remediation (teaching a patient how to "think") vs. adaptation (developing and implementing sources of external structure and teaching the patient to utilize and rely on such sources).

Examples of remediation include teaching the patient how to focus on and recognize pertinent information (what is the main idea in this paragraph), how to solve problems (generate ideas, select one, evaluate it, try it out, and review it), and how to make and follow plans (What do you want to do? How can you do that?). In clubhouses and day programs, such tasks are integrated into the program when patients

Table 2 Prompts to Improve Visual Processing

Are you sure you've seen everything on the page? There is more to see.
You haven't found everything yet; can you find it all?
Look over at that part of the page.
What's a way that you can use to keep track of the objects?
Try moving your eyes over here.
Try pointing to each object and saying it out loud. Start here (organizing) and go over here a little bit at a time.

(members) are responsible for planning and preparing meals, organizing outings, and making decisions about events.

Examples of adaptation to executive-function deficits include teaching a patient to use a daily planner or organizer, programming a wristwatch to beep at spaced intervals as a prompt to check one's schedule, setting up a space with storage boxes and cabinets with clear labels and clear definitions of what to put where, etc.

The nature and severity of deficits exhibited by a given patient dictate to a large degree whether one-on-one therapy or group sessions are likely to be more effective. The examples of cognitive exercises shown in Tables 3 and 4 (23), which are provided to give the "flavor" of this kind of therapy, can be conducted either individually or with small groups, depending on the attentional capacities of the patients involved (Tables 3 and 4). As can be deduced from the exercises, thinking about how to think is a considerable challenge, as is training a person to think in a more systematic and/or abstract manner. The issue of remediation vs. adaptation becomes particularly pertinent in this sphere, and is related to "premorbid" functioning as well as the profile of deficits in a given patient. Those whose *overall* intellectual abilities, supported by educational history, are below average are not likely to benefit from this type of approach, and may be better served by receiving training in selected vocational skills. Those with more focal dysfunction and who demonstrate at least average educational and intellectual achievement prior to onset of illness are more likely to be able to develop "thinking skills."

Cognitive-Behavioral Techniques

Cognitive-behavioral therapy (CBT) for psychotic disorders requires the highest degree of insight into illness by the patient compared with other rehabilitation interventions. In CBT, the therapist relabels events or phenomena as being due to pathology. However, when a patient begins to accept the notion that "reality" is mutable and subject to interpretation (due to mental illness), this realization may be a considerable initial blow to self-image and self-esteem ("I can't trust my perceptions because I'm sick"). Thus, while cognitive-behavioral interventions rely primarily on teaching techniques for understanding and countering specific thought processes, several nonspecific factors appear to contribute to successful treatment, especially the development of a therapeutic alliance. The patient must be able to gain insight within the framework of a supportive and empathic relationship with a

Table 3 Rehabilitation of Executive Function

Categories	What could describe a waterfall with the sun shining on it?
	What could describe a marathon runner crossing the finish line?
	What could describe a foreman who has worked two shifts in a row?
	In addition to bread, what can get stale?
	In addition to flashlights, what runs on batteries?
	In addition to glass, what is transparent?
	What are things babies play with?
	What are things that are often stolen?
	What are things that pour slowly?
Name —	An author
	An athlete
	A gangster
Tell me —	Things you talk to that don't talk back
	Things that are expensive but necessary
	Things cooked but eaten cold
	What is a candle made of?
	What is granola made of?
	What is the solar system made of?
Problem solving	Who would you contact if a fallen tree blocked the main road?
	Who would you contact about your health-care benefits?
	Who would you call to complain about air-traffic noise over your home?
Details	What parts does a tree have?
	What parts does a newspaper have?
	What parts does an orchestra have?

Source: Adapted from Ref. 23.

knowledgeable and caring professional. Accordingly, cognitive-behavioral therapists should follow a specific hierarchical sequence, which consists of first engaging the patient to become involved in and agree to the treatment; second, providing understanding of the cognitive process with an accompanying socialization process (i.e., the patient

Table 4 Rehabilitation of Executive Function: Sequencing

Ordering	Put the words in order from smaller to larger: Harp Guitar Violin Marble Eight ball Pea Pie Cookie Pancake
Step-by-step	What steps are involved in: Renting an apartment? Making iced tea? Applying for a loan?
Before and after	Do you swallow pills before or after you take a sip of water? Do you peel an onion before or after you chop it? Do you put oil in an engine before or after it has run out? What occurs before a rainbow? What occurs before a curtain call? What occurs after death?

Source: Adapted from Ref. 23.

accepts that current beliefs or behaviors aren't "working"), and finally, demonstrating and rehearsing specific intervention techniques. The development of such techniques involves three phases of "self-control," as described by Breier and Strauss (24):

1. The patients become aware of the existence of psychotic and prepsychotic symptoms by self-monitoring and identifying target behaviors.
2. Patients recognize the implications of these behaviors and develop a capacity for self-evaluation. At times, they may also rely on others to help in evaluation.
3. Mechanisms of self-control such as self-instruction and specific activities are selected (relaxation or, conversely, "getting busy" as a distraction).

CBT for Delusions

This model focuses on reframing psychosis as distorted thinking, pointing to the (mis)interpretation of experiences (e.g., hallucinations, delusions). Several factors are needed for a successful outcome (see Table 5).

Table 5 Factors in Successful Outcome for CBT for Delusions

The strength of the belief, which may be related to how long the belief has been present (and to some extent the comprehensiveness of the delusional system).
The consequences of relinquishing the belief. Increased social acceptability may be a reason for giving up a belief, but defense of one's self-image may prompt resistance. If one has acted on certain beliefs for a long period of time, "sacrificing" career, family, etc., then the prospect of saying "I was wrong about that" is not going to be very appealing. However, many patients are aware at some level of the "cost" of acknowledging delusions; when asked what it would mean if a (delusional) belief were not true, patients have said "it would mean I was crazy!"
The joint discovery of alternative explanations. This factor relies on the therapist's skill in understanding the beliefs and their antecedents, and the ability to develop pertinent strategies to challenge them in appropriate sequences, as well as persistence to follow them through.
How explanations are presented. Therapists who approach delusional systems with an attitude of modification rather than confrontation tend to have more success.
The therapist–patient relationship. Patients who like and respect their therapists are more likely to accept explanations and tolerate challenges from them.

In developing and implementing a CBT treatment plan to modify beliefs, therapists should follow guidelines that lay out a sequence of "targets." Less strongly held beliefs should be targeted first, because exploration of these beliefs is less likely to generate high anxiety and resistance (as in systematic desensitization). Direct confrontation should be avoided. Instead, the patient should be asked to consider the facts and to entertain possible alternative beliefs. Discussion should be focused not on the belief but on the evidence for it. Finally, the patient should be encouraged to develop and voice arguments against beliefs rather than listening passively as the therapist outlines the illogic of a given delusion. The therapist may gently provide guidance through direct questioning if necessary.

As with other types of CBT, change occurs over a period of weeks and months, and target symptoms may recur during episodes of stress. The clinical axiom that it is useless to argue with a delusional patient may therefore hold true at certain times or in certain situations, but research suggests that CBT can gradually weaken the hold of delusional beliefs, which may in turn reduce the likelihood of acting on a given belief. To say that windmills *are* giants is madness; to say they *might* be giants is progress.

CBT for Hallucinations

For direct intervention (i.e., teaching patients to cope with voices), two diametrically opposite modes have emerged: distraction and focusing (25). However, both are based on a model postulating that the experiencing of hallucinations causes anxiety that interferes with functioning and may therefore perpetuate the phenomenon.

In the *distraction* method, patients are taught to listen to music (e.g., wearing headphones), read, perform mental games, or employ other methods to focus their attention away from internal stimuli. Thus, the hallucinations should be extinguished via a decrease in anxiety and reactivity.

In the *focusing* method, patients follow a desensitization approach to accustom them to the notion that the voices they are experiencing are physiological phenomena over which they can have control. First, they are trained to identify and describe physical characteristics of the hallucinations (number, loudness, gender, accent, location). Tracking the phenomena and articulating the experience serve to demystify the process.

Next, the content of the hallucinations, as well as related thoughts and emotions, are recorded. In reviewing an individual pattern of hallucinations, a patient may begin to realize that they are precipitated by certain stressors, and that they cause considerable anxiety, anger, or despair. Again, recognizing the connection between two such factors reinforces the notion that the voices are not coming from God or the Devil but are due to a surge of dopamine in the limbic system.

Finally, patients are asked to describe what the voices mean to them (belief system—what are the voices, where do they come from?). By sharing their perceptions and the meanings they have assigned to this phenomenon, they become more open to entertaining other explanations, and can then begin to use self-talk to cope with the hallucinations ("I don't have to do what this voice is telling me to do because it's just a surge of dopamine in my limbic system brought on by receiving the gas bill in the mail this morning").

Both approaches appear to be successful to some degree, but individual differences (patient characteristics) are likely to determine effectiveness. Such characteristics include the intensity and quality of the hallucinations and the patient's cultural background, education, capacity for abstraction, and overall defensiveness (25).

Negative Symptoms

Schizophrenics with prominent negative symptoms (flat affect, poverty of speech, decreased initiation, anhedonia, social withdrawal, limited attention) tend to have poor outcome, due in part to limited medication efficacy and perhaps structural brain changes (26,27). Cognitive-behavioral interventions for this syndrome are somewhat similar to those used to improve the lethargy associated with depression, and may include activity scheduling, skills training, and operant conditioning.

Activity scheduling. Initially, patients with marked negative symptoms require a clinician to structure their day for them. They may eventually be able to participate in or take responsibility for developing their own daily routine. The level and variety of activities should be increased incrementally, to avoid overwhelming a patient unaccustomed to a very "stimulating" day. Significantly, this kind of schedule bears a strong resemblance to schedules constructed for brain-injured patients with frontal-lobe deficits. The degree of detail in a patient's "activity chart" is, of course, determined by how much structure is required, and may range from a general guide to a highly specific sequence (see Table 6). For very impaired patients in residential settings, an aide may work with them to provide prompts and positive reinforcement (praise) as they complete each step, until a routine has been developed (28).

An important element of activity scheduling is the presentation of tasks in a graded hierarchy, beginning with suitable and achievable initial targets. The advantages of using an activity-scheduling approach include demonstrating to the patient that change is possible, and helping him to achieve goals that may at first seem difficult or impossible. The skill of the therapist lies to a great extent in helping the patient identify and articulate desired goals and breaking down the sequence of steps to achieve that goal into small, management "units." The structure and guidance provided by the therapist serve to counter the sense of hopelessness and amotivation experienced by many patients with schizophrenia.

Skills training. For patients with marked negative symptoms, skills training should focus on social interaction but may also include developing functional skills such as cooking or job-related activities. The key is to identify and understand the nature of the deficits (e.g., not "lack of motivation"), and break the target skill into small steps that can be taught in a chaining or shaping sequence. Thus, if one is trying to influence the range of affect, one may try to develop a prompt or reminder to "smile!." If one is providing training in how to ride public transportation, one must anticipate the need for a "go" signal without which the patient may never leave the house. Part of the

Table 6 Examples of Activity Schedules for Negative Symptoms

General	7:00	Out of bed
	7:30	Breakfast
	8:00	To day hospital
	4:00	Home from program
	5:30	Supper
	9:00	Take medicine
	10:00	Bed
Specific	7:00	Wake up
		1. Open eyes
		2. Throw back covers
		3. Swing legs to side of bed
		4. Sit up
		5. Stand up
	7:10	Bathroom
		Toilet
		Brush teeth
		Toothpaste on brush
		Brush up and down
		Rinse
		Wash face
		(etc.)

challenge in this type of intervention is developing targets that the patient is interested in achieving (i.e., that have meaning and relevance).

Psychosocial Treatment

The term "psychosocial treatment" often refers to an integrated or comprehensive model of treatment that combines cognitive, cognitive-behavioral, and social-support interventions. Most day-hospital or clubhouse programs characterize themselves as including a psychosocial focus that emphasizes development of "daily living skills" such as social interaction, job skills, and community-living skills.

Social Skills

Several systems or modules are available to improve social skills of persons with chronic mental illness (see, e.g., Ref. 29). Some teach specific skills, while others attempt to address underlying cognitive deficits in the context of social interactions. Outcome studies have not demonstrated any definitive advantage of one model over another; to some extent, funding and staff availability may dictate the feasibility of a given program.

Integrated psychological therapy. Brenner et al. (30) developed integrated psychological therapy (ITP) as a program targeting improvements in social interactions. The model consists of five highly structured subprograms presented in 30–60-minute sessions three times weekly:

Cognitive differentiation
Social perception
Verbal communication
Social skills
Interpersonal problem solving

Spaulding et al. (2) modified the first three subprograms, described as "cognitively targeted." Cognitive differentiation includes activities designed to exercise concept manipulation and related operations. Examples of such activities include having the group sort objects of different size, color, and shape. The social perception subprogram includes activities to exercise the processing of social information, such as a systematic examination and description of individuals involved in social situations. Verbal communication focuses on attention and short-term memory, as represented by sessions in which participants carefully listen to one another's statements, repeating them first verbatim and then in a paraphrased form. Therapists (usually clinical psychologists) should follow a set of interactional rules designed to build rapport and provide effective structure (see Table 7).

Cognitive enhancement therapy. The cognitive enhancement therapy (CET) approach (31) utilizes a model of developmental rehabilitation based on the notion that adult social cognition has not emerged in patients with schizophrenia because of deficits in underlying cognitive processes. The primary goal of CET is to facilitate attainment of social cognitive milestones, such as an effortful and active processing of social content. The program relies heavily on principles of cognitive rehabilitation in brain injury, particular those of Ben-Yishay and Diller (21). It is a holistic approach that seeks to move patients through a process of engagement to an awareness, mastery, and more fluid control of cognitive functions. CET consists of a 24-month sequence of graduated treatments, beginning with computer programs to address deficits in attention, memory, and problem solving, and proceeding to role-play and rehearsal in small groups to improve social functioning.

Table 7 Guidelines for Social-Skills Training

1. Maintain a friendly but matter-of-fact social atmosphere.
2. Never tell patients they're wrong or factually incorrect; instead, elicit group feedback and discussion, and empathetically reflect emotional expressions as they occur.
3. Clarify patients' verbalizations.
4. Encourage participation by all group members.
5. Reflect the affective component of bizarre behavior but otherwise ignore it.
6. Ask patients who exhibit disruptive behavior to leave the group.

Social-skills training. Several manuals are available to facilitate group sessions for training social skills. Teaching those with deficits in social interaction how to act requires focusing on aspects of behavior that most people take for granted. For example, the symptom of flat affect that is associated with schizophrenia is a major barrier to effective social behavior. Thus, the first step in conveying how to be "sociable" may consist of teaching patients verbal and nonverbal behavior, such as body language, how to express interest in posture, how to indicate listening, maintaining an "open" facial expression, and go and no-go signals (is a potential social partner ready to talk?). Next, a module in starting a friendly conversation may be presented by providing patients with a list of possible topics (movies, what was for breakfast, sports, etc.). To sustain the conversation, patients may need to keep in mind what kinds of questions to ask. In this context, discussions may also include such issues as respecting privacy and how to decide about self-disclosure. Patients often need to practice taking turns and to learn to monitor themselves to keep from rambling. Finally, several ways of ending a conversation politely and pleasantly can be rehearsed.

Coping with Schizophrenia

The premise that patients can be taught to manage their illness touches on sociological issues about how the illness is conceptualized and who has the locus of control in the doctor–patient relationship. If schizophrenia is conceptualized as "purely" physiological, then the following cognitive schema are reinforced:

> If I am going to relapse, there's nothing I can do about it.
> I cannot cope with my current symptoms.
> I am powerless to control or influence my illness.

However, a number of studies have shown that targeted interventions can indeed reduce the likelihood of relapse (e.g., Refs. 13, 24, 32,

33), just as outcome studies have identified factors that decrease recidivism, such as "social support" (e.g., Ref. 19). Patients with mental illness who are in steady contact with others—both family members and mental health professionals—are more likely to be able to cope with stress, to take medication as prescribed, and to report exacerbation of symptoms. When dealing with mild to moderate psychotic symptoms, they may be able to rely on others for reality testing and reassurance, rather than acting on beliefs in ways that may have more serious consequences.

As may be apparent, a cognitive-behavioral paradigm is embedded in this model, but the programs tend to focus more on day-to-day problem solving (e.g., "what can I do if I hear voices?"). There are several excellent guidebooks designed to assist practitioners in presenting psychoeducational groups for patients with schizophrenia, which can be provided on both an inpatient and an outpatient basis. Table 8 provides examples of group topics and general content of such a program.

An overarching intention of this type of approach is to demystify and destigmatize the illness. The treatment alliance between staff and patients is given high priority, which allows patients a forum in which to express their fears and concerns and receive validation for their experiences. Improvements in patients' sense of empowerment and self-confidence are considered important outcomes.

Programs of this kind may include modules on teaching information about schizophrenia that provide strategies for symptom management and teach the prodromal symptoms of relapse (see, e.g., Ref. 34). Medication compliance is encouraged, but methods for stress-avoidance and coping strategies for anxiety and tension are also taught, thereby locating an element of responsibility with the patient. Advocacy and self-assertiveness are encouraged through increased awareness of community resources. Patients are guided to set realistic goals that incorporate an understanding of possible limitations.

Job Skills

Often the first step in job training is to teach general expectations and guidelines for the workplace, such as punctuality, dress codes, doing what your boss tells you to do, staying focused on your assignment, and deciding what to disclose about yourself to peers. A young adult chronic patient who has not been able to hold part-time jobs during the prodromal years, and has had several years of bouncing in and out of the hospital due to denial of illness and medication noncompliance, may not have had the opportunity to learn the guidelines that others

Table 8 Coping with Schizophrenia

Definition and diagnosis	Types of schizophrenia
	How the diagnosis is made
	Symptomatology
Course of illness	Age of onset
	Remission
	Exacerbation
Causes of illness	Genetic and diathesis-stress models
	The role of the family, with an emphasis on avoiding blame (i.e., demystification of the "schizogenic mother")
	How family support can improve coping abilities
Treatment approach	Options for treatment
	Mechanisms of medication
Stress factors	Relationship between stress and exacerbation of psychotic symptoms
	Techniques for relaxation and stress avoidance.
Medication management	Dosages
	Side effects
	Advantages of compliance
	Responsibility for following daily medication routine
Relapse prevention	Recognizing possible signals and symptoms of psychosis
	Identifying possible factors (stress, changes, medical factors)
	Taking steps to avoid hospitalization (call your doctor!)
	Need for support system

would consider obvious and that were absorbed without conscious knowledge or training.

Once these general issues have been addressed, vocational assessments that incorporate an understanding of the cognitive and social deficits displayed by many schizophrenics may be useful. Thus, a person with schizophrenia who is interested in being an air-traffic controller might consider other, less stressful options within the aeronautical industry after discussions with a vocational counselor.

Independent Living Skills

As with learning a language, living skills often develop without "lessons." Many of these skills may have been missed by schizophrenics—

younger patients due to the course of illness and resistance to treatment, and older patients due to institutionalization. Further, cognitive deficits as well as psychotic symptoms may interfere with tasks such as renting an apartment, planning a budget, and using public transportation. Therefore, any "transitional living" program that places individuals in group homes or apartments should include support services designed to address skills deficits. Some programs incorporate structured training modules, while others have a learn-by-doing approach. As with the other rehabilitation models described in this chapter, a crucial element in successful outcome is the treatment team's thorough understanding of the nature of the deficits they are trying to remediate.

SUMMARY AND CONCLUSIONS

Schizophrenia is recognized as a devastating mental illness that can profoundly disrupt day-to-day independent functioning as well as potentially prevent the achievement of academic and career goals. The continuing development of antipsychotic medications holds promise for amelioration of the more dramatic symptomatology associated with schizophrenia, including some of the so-called "negative" symptoms. However, even if pharmacological treatment eventually emerges that can successfully treat cognitive and psychosocial impairments, skills deficits are likely to persist. Thus, there is a need for habilitation (if the skill was never developed) or rehabilitation (if the skill was subsumed under the impact of symptom onset).

The role of the clinician in psychiatric rehabilitation includes:

1. Identifying patient deficits
2. Making recommendations about a patient's rehabilitation needs
3. Making referrals to treatment programs based on an evaluation of what a given program offers
4. Monitoring and assessing a patient's rehabilitation progress
5. Applying rehabilitation techniques on an individual basis
6. Participating in rehabilitation programs as a member of the treatment team
7. Designing and/or directing rehabilitation programs

Awareness of treatment efficacy as well as intervention options can help to guide the selection process in finding the best "match" between patient needs and community programs. Types of treatment interventions can be classified into three general categories:

Cognitive/neuropsychological: techniques designed to improve information processing and responses as understood from a neurological model

Cognitive/behavioral: treatment that shapes behavior and teaches patients to cope with symptoms as manifestations of physiological abnormalities

Psychosocial: programs that rely on a skills-deficit model and provide both direct and explicit training in day-to-day-functioning

The majority of rehabilitation programs are based on a psychosocial model, and may have cognitive-behavioral and/or cognitive-neuropsychological elements. Some programs are more specialized, and may be designed specifically for certain types of patients in whom behavioral problems or cognitive impairments present the greatest challenge to independent functioning. The guidelines listed in Table 9 may be useful in determining "goodness of fit."

When talking with patients about coping with schizophrenia, a useful question to ask is: "Do I know everything I need to know about you as a person if I know that you have schizophrenia?" Patients, of course, almost always say (with some healthy indignation) "No!," which provides a lead-in to discussion of accepting realistic limitations but also setting achievable goals. Having something to work toward gives an incentive to stick with the development of needed skills to reach those goals. During discussions of this kind, patients may also bring up their frustrations and disappointments, which are related not only to the onset of schizophrenia but to the stigma of mental illness. A focus on cognitive and psychosocial rehabilitation provides one of the most crucial aspects of successful treatment: hope.

Table 9 Guidelines for Clinicians

Problem	Treatment	Advantages	Disadvantages	Contraindications
Significant cognitive impairment	Computer remediation	Cost-effective; can be practiced at home	Limited efficacy and generalizability	Least effective with executive function deficits
	Individual training	1:1 therapy has shown greatest improvement	Labor-intensive	Limited learning capacity
	Group intervention	Includes social reinforcement	Does not target individual deficits	Limited learning capacity; highly focal deficits
Marked negative symptoms	Activity scheduling	Can be tailored to individual need	May require staff to prompt	Fluctuating daily routine
	Skills training	Functional goals	Limited generalizability	Lack of support system
Persistent hallucinations	Distraction (extinguishing)	Easy to initiate	Outcome dictated by individual differences	Patient's inability to accept model
	Focusing (desensitization)	Recognition of symptom as physiological increases patient empowerment	Labor-intensive	Patient's inability to accept model

Delusions	Cognitive-behavioral	Potential decrease in inappropriate behavior	Requires considerable clinical skill and patience	Extreme defensiveness
Impaired social skills	ITP	Incorporates awareness of cognitive functioning	Labor-intensive	Limited learning capacity
	CET	Incorporates awareness of cognitive functioning	Labor- and time-intensive	Limited learning capacity
	Skills training	Step-by-step process starting with very basic principles	Generalizability may be limited	Limited learning capacity
Deficits in job skills	Skills training	May address non-specific skills	Individual differences may affect outcome	Lack of community resources
Lack of independent living skills	Transitional living programs	Functional goals	Labor-intensive	Lack of community resources

REFERENCES

1. Johnson AB. Out of Bedlam: The Truth About Deinstitutionalization. New York: Basic Books, 1990.
2. Spaulding WD, Fleming S, Reed D, Sullivan M, Storzbach D, Lam M. Cognitive functioning in schizophrenia: implications for psychiatric rehabilitation. Schizophr Bull 1999; 25(2):275–289.
3. Harding C, Brooks G, Ashigaga T, Strauss J, Beier, A. The Vermont longitudinal study of persons with severe mental illness. Am J Psychiatry 1987; 144:727–735.
4. Jaspers K. General Psychopathology. Manchester, England: Manchester University Press, 1963.
5. Berrios G. Delusions as "wrong beliefs": a conceptual history. Br J Psychiatry 1991; 159:6–13.
6. Strauss J, Carpenter W. The prediction of outcome in schizophrenia. I. Characteristics of outcome. Arch Gen Psychiatry 1971; 27:739–746.
7. Strauss J, Carpenter W. The prediction of outcome in schizophrenia. I. Relationship between predictor and outcome variables. Arch Gen Psychiatry 1972; 31:818–831.
8. Bellak A, Gold J, Buchanan R. Cognitive rehabilitation for schizophrenia: Problems, prospects and strategies. Schizophr Bull 1999; 25(2):257–274.
9. Meichenbaum D, Cameron R. Training schizophrenics to talk to themselves: a means of developing attentional controls. Behav Ther 1973; 4:515–534.
10. Mueser K, Bellack A, Douglas M, Wade J. Prediction of social skill acquisition in schizophrenia and major affective disorder patients from memory and symptomatology. Psychiatry Res 1991; 37:281–296.
11. Hawton K, Salkovskis P, Kirk J, Cark D, eds. Cognitive Behaviour Therapy for Psychiatric Problems. Oxford: Oxford University Press, 1989.
12. Kingdon D, Turkington D. Cognitive-Behavioral Therapy of Schizophrenia. New York: Guildford Press, 1994.
13. Falloon IR, Talbot R. Persistent auditory hallucinations: coping mechanisms and implications for management. Psychol Med 1981; 11:329–339.
14. Rutter D. Language in schizophrenia. Br J Psychiatry 1985; 146:399–404.
15. Alford B, Correia C. Cognitive therapy of schizophrenia: theory and empirical status. Behav Ther 1994; 25:17–33.
16. Heydebrand G. The Treatment of Mentally Ill Homeless Clients: The Effect of Client Characteristics and Process Variables on Outcome Factors. Doctoral dissertation, University of Missouri–St. Louis, 1995.
17. Grusky O, Tierney K, Manderscheid R, Grusky D. Social bonding and community adjustment of chronically mentally ill adults. J Health Soc Behav 1985; 26:49–63.
18. Hammer M, Makiesky-Barrow S, Gutwirth L. Social networks and schizophrenia. Schizophr Bull 1978; 4:522–545.
19. Stein L, Test AA. Training in community living: one-year evaluation. Am J Psychiatry 1976; 133: 917–918.

20. Ericsson KA, Hastie R. Contemporary approaches to the study of thinking and problem-solving. In: Sternberg RJ, ed. Thinking and Problem-Solving. San Diego: Academic Press, 1994:37–82.
21. Ben-Yishay Y, Diller L. Rehabilitation of cognitive and perceptual deficits in people with traumatic brain damage. Int J Rehabil Res 1981; 4:208–210.
22. Bracy O. Computer-based cognitive rehabilitation. Cogn Rehabil 1983; 1:7–8.
23. Brubaker S. Workbook for Cognitive Skills. Detroit: Wayne State University Press, 1988.
24. Breier A, Strauss JS. Self control in psychotic disorders. Arch Gen Psychiatry 1983; 40:1141–1145.
25. Haddock G, Bentall R, Slade P. Psychological treatment of auditory hallucinations: focusing or distraction? In: Haddock G, Slade P, eds. Cognitive-Behavioural Interventions with Psychotic Disorders. London: Routledge Press, 1996.
26. Andreasen NC, Olsen S, Dennert J, Smith R. Ventricular enlargement in schizophrenia: relationship to positive and negative symptoms. Am J Psychiatry 1982; 139:297–302.
27. Pogue-Geile M, Harrow M. Negative symptoms in schizophrenia: their longitudinal course and prognostic importance. Schizophr Bull 1985; 11:427–439.
28. Hogg L. Psychological treatment for negative symptoms. In: Haddock G, Slade P, eds. Cognitive-Behavioural Interventions with Psychotic Disorders. London: Routledge Press, 1996.
29. Liberman R. Social and Independent Living Skills. Los Angeles: Clinical Research Center for Schizophrenia and Psychiatric Rehabilitation, 1990.
30. Brenner H, Hodel R, Roder V, Corrigan P. Treatment of cognitive dysfunction and behavioral deficits in schizophrenia: Integrated psychological therapy. Schizophr Bull 1992; 18:21–26.
31. Hogarty G, Flesher S. Practice principles of cognitive enhancement therapy for schizophrenia. Schizophr Bull 1999; 25(4):693–708.
32. Tarrier N. An investigation of residual psychotic symptoms in discharged schizophrenic patients. Br J Clin Psychology 1987; 26:141–143.
33. Carr V. Patients' techniques for coping with schizophrenia: an exploratory study. Br J Med Psychol 1988; 339–352.
34. Ascher-Svanum H, Krause A. Psychoeducational groups for patients with schizophrenia: a guide for practitioners. Gaithersburg, MD: Aspen Publications, 1991.
35. Beck A. Successful outpatient psychotherapy of a chronic schizophrenic with a delusion based on borrowed guilt. Psychiatry 1952; 15:305–312.
36. Haddock G, Slade P, eds. Cognitive-Behavioural Interventions with Psychotic Disorders., London: Routledge Press, 1996.

10

Antipsychotic-Drug Side Effects

Assessment, Treatment, and Prevention

Gary Remington, Shitij Kapur, and Robert Zipursky
University of Toronto
Toronto, Ontario, Canada

INTRODUCTION

Antipsychotic drugs, which became available for clinical use in the 1950s, were the first effective therapy for schizophrenia. They rapidly became the cornerstone of treatment programs and confirmed schizophrenia's biological underpinnings. Indeed, efforts to understand the action of these compounds led to the widely heralded dopamine theory of schizophrenia.

As clinical experience with these drugs mounted, two features became evident. First, they were not a panacea, with approximately 30% of individuals proving refractory to them. Second, this group of medications gained notoriety for their side effects, which may have been at least partially related to inappropriately high doses. In the development of new antipsychotic medications, a more benign side-effect profile has taken on as much importance as improved efficacy, and even among newer agents side effects will be an important dimension to distinguish them.

This chapter focuses on side effects related to antipsychotic use. It is not meant to be an exhaustive overview—that is beyond the scope of a single chapter. Instead, the focus here is on assisting the clinician to better conceptualize a practical approach to antipsychotic-related side effects. To do this, a summary is provided of the evolution of antipsychotics, highlighting the changes these drugs have produced from the standpoint of side effects. The focus then shifts to the development of an approach to antipsychotic-induced side effects that can be applied to clinical practice. Finally, selected groups of side effects, chosen to highlight similarities and differences between antipsychotic groups, are evaluated.

It is important at the outset to clarify the terminology used here. Over the years this class of medications has been termed "major tranquilizers," "neuroleptics," and "antipsychotics." We have chosen to use the term "antipsychotics" for several reasons. Both "neuroleptics" and "major tranquilizers" imply a nonspecific action that may or may not be related to antipsychotic activity. In contrast, "antipsychotic" clearly defines the goal in the development of these compounds and avoids the notion of an agent that tries to be ubiquitous, either pharmacologically or clinically. Paradoxically, this is at odds with the recent trend of developing "pharmacologically rich" compounds, for which the hope is that action at other receptors and systems may not only effect greater antipsychotic activity but also bestow clinical benefits for other symptoms as well, e.g., positively influencing affect, anxiety, and cognition. However, at present there may not be sufficient knowledge to create a "broad-spectrum" antischizophrenia drug. We caution against such an approach as it can obfuscate efforts to delineate specific mechanisms of action that underlie clinical changes. In addition, it places the individual at risk for adverse events linked to pharmacological activity that may not be clinically relevant.

We have also chosen to classify the newer antipsychotics as second-generation antipsychotics (SGAs) rather than "novel" or "atypical." The term "novel" is not really suitable, given clozapine's lengthy history and the fact that even newer antipsychotics reflecting different hypothetical models are likely to be forthcoming. As will be discussed, the term "atypical" is misleading because it implies a dichotomous distinction between the conventional and newer antipsychotics, which is not the case.

The SGAs currently available in North America include clozapine, olanzapine, quetiapine, and risperidone. An application for approval of ziprasidone has been submitted in several countries, including the United States and Canada.

BASIC CONCEPTS

The Introduction of Antipsychotics

Shortly after the discovery of chlorpromazine's antipsychotic properties, the term "neuroleptic" (meaning "seizing the nerves") was coined to describe a class of medications that, over and above antipsychotic properties, displayed a variety of other effects such as extrapyramidal symptoms (EPS). In fact, EPS became a marker for dosing based on the notion that specific features such as those revealed via micrographia reflected the dose that might best be associated with clinical response (1).

The initial finding that these compounds had antipsychotic properties was serendipitous; their synthesis was not premised on any particular pharmacological hypothesis. As well as dopamine D_2–blocking properties, which came to be seen as critical in terms of antipsychotic response (2), these drugs influence a number of other receptors that contributed to their side-effect profile. Postural hypotension and sedation, both autonomic side effects and related to blockade of adrenergic receptors, are two examples characterizing the first antipsychotics.

Dopamine and Psychosis

It was not until the early 1960s that dopamine became linked to psychosis, resulting in: 1) the hyperdopaminergic theory of schizophrenia and 2) efforts to develop more selective dopamine-blocking agents. Subsequent work identifying D_2 receptors in the striatum and correlating antipsychotic affinity at D_2 receptors with clinical potency further refined this model (3). Unfortunately, it was also recognized that D_2 blockade accounted for EPS through the nigrostriatal pathway and elevated prolactin through the tuberoinfundibular system.

Ironically, it was an increasing liability for these side effects related to dopamine blockade that came to characterize the newer, more selective D_2 antagonists such as haloperidol.

Sedative vs. Disinhibiting Compounds: The Potency Story

To classify the antipsychotics, an effort was made to distinguish them along a continuum formed by sedation at one end and disinhibition at the other (3). Low-potency antipsychotics—that is, those with a lower affinity for the D_2 receptor and a broader pharmacological profile (e.g., chlorpromazine)—were identified as sedative neurolepics. In contrast, those with more selective D_2 blockade (e.g., haloperidol) characterized the disinhibiting neuroleptics. In clinical practice, it became apparent that these latter compounds also carried a greater risk of EPS.

Clozapine and "Atypicality"

Despite differences in D_2 affinity, both low- and high-potency conventional antipsychotics block D_2 receptors to a degree that links them clinically with elevated prolactin and EPS. Clozapine, in contrast, has not been associated with either sustained prolactin elevation or a substantial risk of EPS, leading to the notion that the definition of "atypical" should include both these features. As we will see, however, this poses something of a problem since the newer antipsychotics available vary along these dimensions (4,5). This has led to the suggestion that "typical" and "atypical" be viewed not as dichotomous but along a continuum that includes other features (6).

Pharmacological Heterogeneity Revisited

It is somewhat paradoxical that in the development of new antipsychotics we are creating agents that, like the earliest neuroleptics, have a varied receptor profile. At least several factors have contributed to this shift. First, despite the development of relatively selective D_2 antagonists, such as haloperidol, clinical evidence demonstrated that a substantial number of patients remained symptomatic (7). This called into question the notion that schizophrenia and similar illnesses are mediated solely by dopaminergic dysfunction. The synthesis of clozapine in the early 1960s and the clinical evidence indicating unique clinical properties further challenged the unitary dopamine model. Its pharmacological profile demonstrated relatively low D_2 occupancy, leading to the notion that other receptors and neurotransmitters may be responsible for its clinical effect. Other lines of investigation also suggested a role for different systems, such as serotonin (8).

The net result was a new generation of antipsychotics, with clozapine as the prototype. These compounds are not premised on a model of D_2 selectivity, and, while clozapine, olanzapine, quetiapine, risperidone, and ziprasidone all have some degree of D_2 antagonism, they also have in common serotonergic 5-HT_{2A}-blocking properties (6,9,10). Beyond these features, they demonstrate a number of pharmacological differences—whether these contribute to differences in clinical efficacy remains unclear at this time. As will be discussed, though, the different pharmacological profiles clearly have implications from the standpoint of side effects.

ANTIPSYCHOTICS IN THE CLINICAL SETTING

Antipsychotic Use

Figure 1 outlines an approach to antipsychotic use, specifically from the standpoint of side effects. It should go without saying that prevention of side effects is a primary goal in the effective use of antipsychotics. We are dealing with a class of medications whose side effects span a continuum from uncomfortable (e.g., sedation) to acutely distressing (e.g., akathisia) to irreversible (e.g., tardive dyskinesia) to life-threatening (e.g., neuroleptic malignant syndrome). Moreover, one should consider the history of antipsychotic use in the clinical setting. First, over the years their role has extended beyond use as antipsychotics, a practice that has recently come under increased scrutiny. As the term "major tranquilizer" implies, they were utilized for their sedating properties, finding a role in the treatment of behavioral disturbances, agitation, anxiety, and insomnia. In addition, agents were developed that combined an antidepressant and antipsychotic for the treatment of depression with accompanying anxiety and agitation (e.g., Etrafon—perphenazine plus amitriptyline). Thus, it was not uncommon to see antipsychotics used indefinitely for the treatment of conditions other than schizophrenia despite evidence indicating an increased risk of tardive dyskinesia in individuals with a diagnosis other than schizophrenia and the recognition that the risk of tardive dyskinesia increases over time (11). Further problems arose from the evolution of a more-is-better approach, culminating in interventions such as "rapid neuroleptization." Over the past decade, abundant evidence from different lines of investigation, in both clinical and basic science, has challenged the benefit of high-dose antipsychotic therapy and underscored the potential for increased side effects (11–13). Paralleling this has been an increased awareness regarding side effects, and a shift in focus from purely symptomatic improvement to functional recovery.

Guidelines for Clinicians in Selecting Antipsychotic Drugs: Psychopathology

Is the diagnosis correct?

Does the diagnosis warrant antipsychotic therapy?

Has a process been followed to inform the individual as soon as possible of the rationale for antipsychotic use and the possible side effects, including those that can be irreversible or life-threatening?

Does the choice of antipsychotic reflect the individual to be treated? For example, the use of a high-potency conventional

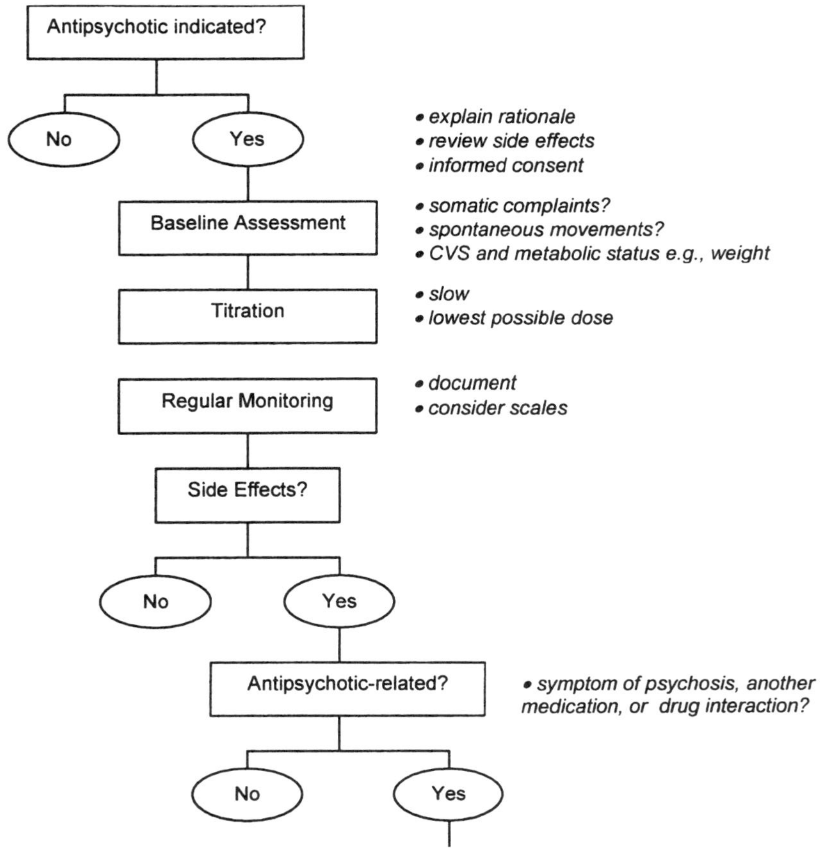
Antipsychotic indicated?
No
Yes
• explain rationale
• review side effects
• informed consent
Baseline Assessment
• somatic complaints?
• spontaneous movements?
• CVS and metabolic status e.g., weight
Titration
• slow
• lowest possible dose
Regular Monitoring
• document
• consider scales
Side Effects?
No
Yes
Antipsychotic-related?
• symptom of psychosis, another medication, or drug interaction?
No
Yes

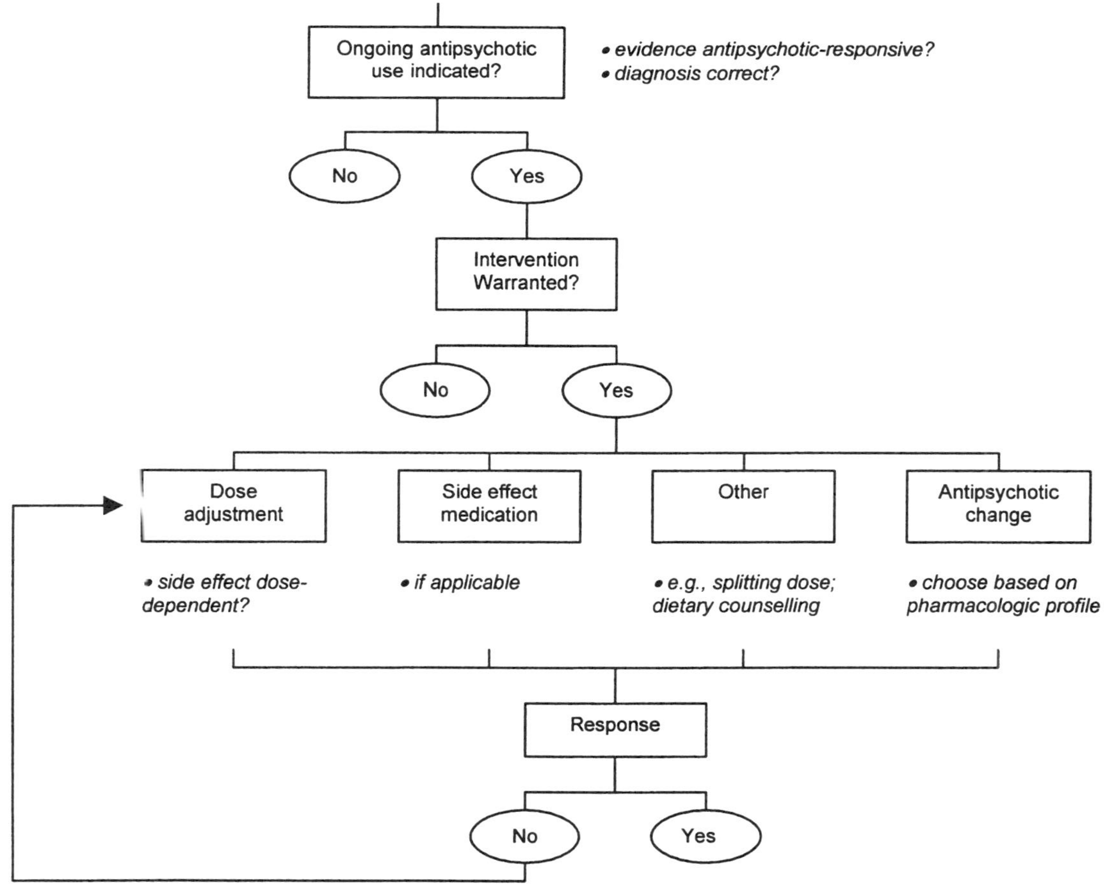

Figure 1 Prevention, assessment, and management of antipsychotic side effects.

antipsychotic in young males carries with it an increased risk of acute dystonic reactions, while antipsychotics with prominent anticholinergic activity carry a greater likelihood of cognitive impairment in the geriatric population.

Are the dose and titration schedule appropriate? There are a lack of data to indicate that doses in excess of 10–12 mg haloperidol equivalents are beneficial (12). Moreover, evidence of response with doses as low as 1–2 mg haloperidol equivalents supports initiating therapy at much lower doses and avoiding rapid titration, which can result in overshooting the optimal clinical dose (14). By treating even acute psychosis with a "low and slow" approach, one can avoid side effects and reduce the need for dose reduction once stabilization has been achieved.

Select populations, e.g., children and geriatric patients, warrant even lower doses and slower titration.

Is a process in place to systematically evaluate clinical symptoms and side effects at regular intervals?

Aim for antipsychotic monotherapy.

Identifying Side Effects

In clinical practice, the identification of side effects can be less than straightforward. Akathisia is often used as an example of this, as it can present in numerous ways other than restlessness (e.g., physical pain, irritability) and can be mistakenly diagnosed as a worsening in the psychosis. Similarly, somatic complaints may have a delusional basis, whereas other physical side effects may go unreported (e.g., sexual dysfunction, constipation).

Guidelines for Clinicians in Selecting an Antipsychotic Drug:
Side Effects

Ask about side effects during each clinical assessment, e.g., restlessness (akathisia), sexual dysfunction.

Look for side effects, e.g., akinesia, tremor, tardive movements.

Pursue their relationship to clinical symptoms, e.g., delusional thinking.

Attempt to link their presence temporally to the onset of the agent in question or to a change in its dose.

Consider the link to other medications (including over-the-counter products), drug interactions, illicit drug and/or alcohol use.

Rule out the possibility of underlying medical conditions. Order appropriate laboratory investigations based on physical findings.

Address clearly identified side effects. In individuals who appear to be responding to treatment, first consider lowering the dose if the side effect is dose-related, e.g., parkinsonism. Adding another medication to treat the side effect is a satisfactory, but second-choice, consideration. If an individual has not shown a clinical response despite a reasonable trial, in terms of both duration and dose, look to switching the antipsychotic.

Categorizing Side Effects

The negative impact of side effects on the individual's well-being and compliance with treatment necessitates a systematic and comprehensive approach to their assessment.

It is a daunting task to try and remember the side effects for each antipsychotic, given the number of drugs available and the list of potential side effects for each. Moreover, many patients are on different medications, making it necessary to consider the side-effect profile of several agents, as well as the possibility of drug interactions. However, this only underscores the importance of having a system in place that allows for a systematic approach to antipsychotic side effects. Various dimensions can be used to categorize side effects, for example, system (cardiovascular, respiratory, gastrointestinal, etc.), severity, and time of onset. Another dimension is pharmacological profile, in that it allows one to link side effects (and therefore treatments) to postulated mechanisms of action. Of course, the relationship between pharmacology and side-effect profile is not absolute, as adverse events are influenced by a number of factors, including individual variability, dosing, previous antipsychotic exposure, concomitant medications, and our limited knowledge regarding relationships between specific receptor binding and resultant side effects. However, this approach does offer general principles that permit the clinician to predict what side effects to look for with a particular compound.

Table 1 outlines our current knowledge regarding the relationship between specific receptor binding and side effects, and Table 2 outlines the more common side effects for the currently available SGAs. Table 3 identifies relative degrees of receptor binding for these same agents, followed by relative risks for the more common and troublesome side effects. Haloperidol has been added here as a conventional antipsychotic comparator, since it remains the most widely prescribed conventional antipsychotic.

As with the assessment of clinical symptoms, the use of scales to evaluate side effects can be particularly useful. Clinicians are often

Table 1. Possible Adverse Effects of Receptor Blockade by Antipsychotics

Receptor / effect
Dopamine D_2 receptors
EPS: dystonia, parkinsonism, akathasia, tardive dyskinesia, rabbit syndrome
Endocrine effects: prolactin elevation (galactorrhea, gynecomastia, menstrual changes, sexual dysfunction in males)
α_1-adrenoceptors
Postural hypotension, dizziness
Reflex tachycardia
Nasal congestion
Histamine H_1 receptors
Sedation
Drowsiness
Weight gain
Muscarinic receptors
Blurred vision
Attack or exacerbation of narrow-angle glaucoma
Dry mouth
Sinus tachycardia
Constipation
Urinary retention
Memory dysfunction
Serotonin 5-HT receptors
? Weight gain
? Sexual dysfunction

Source: Adapted from Ref. 15.

apprehensive about the use of scales, viewing them as burdensome from the standpoint of time. In fact, they may actually streamline the process by providing a framework for a systematic approach and, in doing so, ensuring that the evaluation is complete. As well, they provide clear documentation that such an assessment has been carried out, and done at regular intervals they offer an objective means of reviewing change over time. Table 4 outlines at least some of the side-effect scales available for movement disorders.

Drug Interactions

In evaluating side effects we often deal with individuals who are on multiple medications. These may include several antipsychotics, other psychotropics, and CNS-active agents prescribed for different reasons. Over-the-counter medications may also be used, as well as nonpre-

Table 2 Second-Generation Antipsychotics: Most Common Side Effects Based on Clinical Trial Data (%)

Drug	Side effect
Clozapine	Drowsiness (39)
	Hypersalivation (31)
	Tachycardia (25)
	Dizziness (19)
	Constipation (14)
Olanzapine	Somnolence (26)
	Agitation (23)
	Insomnia (20)
	Headache (17)
	Nervousness (16)
Quetiapine	Headache (20)
	Somnolence (18)
	Dizziness (10)
	Constipation (9)
	Postural hypotension (8)
Risperidone[a]	Insomnia (26)
	Agitation (22)
	EPS (17)
	Headache (14)
	Anxiety (12)
Ziprasidone	Somnolence (14)
	Nausea (10)
	Constipation (9)
	Dyspesia (8)
	Akathisia (8)

Certain side effects may not have been evaluated/reported, e.g., prolactin changes, weight gain.
[a]≤10 mg/day (6–8-week controlled clinical trials).
Source: Adapted from Refs. 16 and 17.

scribed compounds that can interact with antipsychotics or alter the clinical picture, e.g., alcohol, street drugs, nicotine, and caffeine.

Antipsychotics are metabolized through the hepatic system, specifically involving the cytochrome P450 isoenzymes. In the same way that we can better appreciate possible side effects through an understanding of an antipsychotic's receptor-binding profile, we can more fully understand possible drug interactions through knowledge of the isoenzymes involved in the metabolism of a particular antipsychotic

Table 3 Pharmacological and Selected Side-Effect Profile of "Atypical" Antipsychotics

Agent	Haloperidol	Clozapine	Risperidone	Olanzapine	Quetiapine	Ziprasidone[a]
Chemical class	Butyrophenone	Dibenzo-diazepine	Benzisoxazole	Dibenzazepine	Dibenzo-thiazepine	Benzothiazolyl-piperazine
Receptor binding[b]						
D_1	+++	++	—	+++	+	+
D_2	++++	++	+++	+++	++	+++
5-HT_2	+	++++	++++	++++	+++	+++
α_1	++	+++	+++	+++	++++	++
α_2	—	+++	+++	—	+	—
H_1	—	++++	+	++++	++++	+
M_1	—	++++	—	++++	+++	—
Side effects						
EPS	++++	+	+++	++	+	+++
Prolactin	++++	+	+++	+	+	+
Weight gain	+	++++	++	++++	++	—
Abnormal GTT[c]	+	+++	+	+++	?	?
Lipid increase[c]	—	+++	?	+++	++	?

[a]Pending regulatory approval in North America.
[b]D = dopamine; 5-HT = serotonin; α = adrenergic; H = histamine; M = acetylcholine (muscarinic).
[c]Limited published data available.
Source: Adapted from Ref. 18.

Table 4 Clinical Scales to Measure the Presence of Extrapyramidal Side Effects (EPS)

Scale	Measure
Simpson-Angus Neurologic Rating Scale	EPS
Abnormal Involuntary Movement Scale (AIMS)	Tardive dyskinesia
Extrapyramidal Symptoms Rating Scale (ESRS)	Acute EPS, tardive dyskinesia, dystonia
St. Hans Rating Scale for Extrapyramidal Syndromes	Acute EPS, tardive dyskinesia, dystonia
Akathisia Rating Scale	Akathisia
Barnes Rating Scale for Drug-Induced Akathisia	Akathisia
Hillside Akathisia Scale	Akathisia

Source: Data from Refs. 19–24.

and concomitant medications that might be metabolized through similar pathways.

It is beyond the scope of this chapter to identify all such interactions; the reader is referred to more recent reviews that address this topic in greater detail (25–27). Table 5 identifies the major isoenzymes involved in the metabolism of different SGAs.

TREATING SIDE EFFECTS: INTEGRATING THEORY AND CLINICAL PRACTICE

Once again, it is impossible to review here all antipsychotic-related side effects; accordingly, certain groups of side effects have been chosen. These include side effects related to D_2 antagonism (e.g., EPS, hyperprolactinemia), as well as sedation, postural hypotension, and anticholinergic side effects (e.g., dry mouth, blurred vision, and constipation). Weight gain and diabetes are selected for discussion because of their increased prevalence with at least some of the SGAs. The induction of obsessive-compulsive symptoms warrants comment as this is a feature that has been reported uniquely with SGAs. Neuroleptic malignant syndrome is addressed briefly because of the mortality risk. Finally, a cluster of other side effects are reviewed because of their association with particular SGAs and the implications for additional testing: hematological, hepatic, cardiac, and ocular.

Table 5 Cytochrome P450 Isoenzymes Involved in Metabolism of Second-Generation Antipsychotics

Clozapine	1A2,[a] 2D6, 3A4
Olanzapine	1A2,[a] 2D6
Quetiapine	3A4
Risperidone	2D6
Ziprasidone	3A4

[a]Linked to more prominent role.

Extrapyramidal Side Effects

Acute/Chronic Effects

The triad of acute EPS consists of dystonia, akathisia, and parkinsonism (Figure 2) (28). D_2 blockade at the level of the nigrostriatal pathway has been implicated, and more recent work involving positron emission tomography (PET) has indicated that the risk is associated with D_2 blockade exceeding 80%. This threshold is an important one, because there is also evidence to indicate that D_2 occupancy in the range of 65–70% is necessary to optimize the chance of clinical response. Thus, there is a relatively narrow "window" of efficacy before the threshold for EPS is reached (14,29–31).

Guidelines for Clinicians for Treatment of EPS

Acute laryngeal/pharyngeal dystonia, presenting as respiratory distress, is a medical emergency, requiring immediate treatment, e.g., i.m. or i.v. benztropine.

Certain risk factors are associated with acute dystonic reactions: conventional antipsychotic (especially high-potency) drugs; high dose; being young, male, and/or antipsychotic-naïve; and previous history of antipsychotic-induced dystonia. In individuals with some combination of these factors who are being started on conventional antipsychotics, prophylactic antiparkinsonian medication is warranted. Reassess with the goal of discontinuation within 4–7 days; more than 90% of acute dytonic reactions occur during this period (32).

Akathisia may or may not respond to anticholinergics. Options include benzodiazepines, e.g., lorazepam 1–6 mg daily, or β-blockers, e.g., propanolol 20–160 mg daily; their efficacy suggests a role for other etiological mechanisms in akathisia, e.g., noradrenaline, γ-aminobutyric acid (GABA) (32).

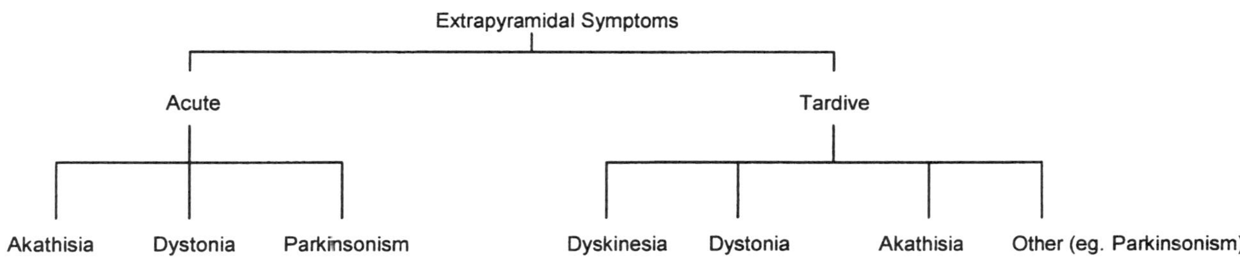

Figure 2 Neuroleptic-induced movements. (Adapted from Ref. 28.)

Based on rates of D_2 occupancy of the SGAs available, risperidone and olanzapine have the greatest risk of dose-related EPS (5,33,34). However, clinically olanzapine appears to have a comparatively lower risk of EPS, possibly related to its muscarinic properties. Data on ziprasidone are still pending, while quetiapne and clozapine have a low risk.

Tardive Effects

Tardive (late-onset) side effects are not confined to dyskinesia (TD); tardive dystonia, akathisia, parkinsonism, and others have also been described (Figure 2). By definition, such movements are described as tardive if their onset occurs after at least 12 weeks of antipsychotic exposure (1 month in the case of individuals age 60 years or over) (35). Many risk factors (Table 6) and treatments (Table 7) for TD have been investigated. The number of treatments evaluated reflects the limited efficacy of any one agent, and speaks to our lack of clear understanding regarding the pathophysiology of these unwanted movement disorders.

With conventional antipsychotics, the reported risk of TD is in the range of 5% per year initially, with a lifetime risk of approximately 60%. In the geriatric population this risk increases considerably (e.g., up to 25% within 1 year's exposure) (11,36). Differences in the risk of TD between low- and high-potency antipsychotics have not been clearly demonstrated, perhaps because the use of high doses of such drugs has historically created a "ceiling effect" that masked differences.

Guidelines for Clinicians: Identifying and Treating Tardive Side Efects

As many as 20–25% of individuals with schizophrenia may have spontaneous movements before antipsychotic exposure (37); thus, it is imperative that patients be assessed at baseline.

Patients must be informed of the risk of tardive side effects as soon as possible, with documentation. Re-evaluations should be done on a regular basis (i.e., every 6–12 months) and documented.

Tardive dyskinesia and tardive dystonia may be mediated, at least in part, by different pathophysiological mechanisms, and different treatments may be warranted.

Tardive movements are not necessarily irreversible, nor do they always increase across time with ongoing antipsychotic exposure. In fact, they can fluctuate within and between days.

Table 6 Tardive Dyskinesia: Postulated Risk Factors

Age	Race	*Obstetric complications*
Gender	Familial	*Soft neurological signs*
EPS	Dose	*Neurocognitive impairment*
Antiparkinsonian drugs	Potency	*Handedness*
Duration	Formulation	*Smoking*
Diabetes	Drug-free intervals	*Alcohol*
Diagnosis	Organicity	*Substance abuse*

Italics indicate factors that may be related to organicity.

There is evidence of diminished TD risk for clozapine, making it a first choice in this respect. Other SGAs (risperidone, olanzapine, and quetiapine) may share this advantage (38,39), making them reasonable alternatives to clozapine and preferable to conventional antipsychotics. Clozapine, olanzapine, and risperidone also have been reported to decrease existing tardive movements (38). One would expect quetiapine and ziprasidone to confer this same benefit, but data are lacking as of yet. There are not yet enough comparative data to establish the comparative risk of TD between the different SGAs.

A syndrome of acute self-induced water intoxication has been reported in a subgroup of patients with schizophrenia, and one hypothesis suggests that this may be a tardive variant, associated with cold intolerance and possibly linked to dopaminergic supersensitivity at the level of the hypothalamus (41). There are reports that the SGAs improve the polydipsia in some individuals (41–43).

There is no proven treatment for TD. Switching to an SGA if the individual is not on one and requires ongoing antipsychotic treatment should be a first step. The evidence regarding vitamin E, in doses up to 1600 IU daily, is less compelling. Tetrabenazine, a reserpine-like compound, has proven useful in some cases at doses of 25–75 mg/day but is not without its own side effects (e.g., hypotension, sedation, possible depressinogenic properties) (44).

For tardive dystonia (e.g., tardive torticolis), localized botulinuum toxin injections have proven useful, although response may be time-limited (i.e., several months), with reinjections required (44).

Table 7 Treatment of Tardive Dyskinesia

Dopamine	**γ-Aminobutyric acid**
Depleting agents	Agonists
α-methyl-tyrosine	Baclofen
Reserpine[a]	Muscimol
Tetrabenazine[a]	4,5,6,7-tetrahydroisoxazolo-(5, 4-c)pyridine-3-ol (THIP)
Calcium-channel blockers	Transaminase inhibitors
Diltiazem	γ-Vinyl GABA
Nifedipine	Sodium valproate
Verapamil	Receptor enhancers
Agonists	Benzodiazepines
Amantadine	Clonazepam
Apomorphine	Diazepam
Bromocriptine	**Norepinephrine**
Levodopa	Depleting agents
Antagonists	Reserpine[a]
Buspirone	Tetrabenazine[a]
Acetylcholine	Agonists
Synthesis enhancing agents	Clonidine
Choline	Antagonists
Deanol	Isororbide
Lecithin	β-blockers
Acetylcholinesterase inhibitors	Propranolol
Physostigmine	**Opioid**
Tacrine	Antagonists
Serotonin	Naloxone
Depleting agents	**Other**
Reserpine[a]	Electroconvulsive therapy
Tetrabenazine[a]	Dihydrogenated ergot alkaloids
Agonists	Essential fatty acids, e.g., dihomo-μ-linolenic acid
Buspirone	Lithium
Antagonists	Vitamin E
Clozapine[b]	
Olanzapine[b]	
Risperidone[b]	
Cyproheptadine	

[a]Effects on dopamine, norepinephrine, and serotonin.
[b]Antidyskinetic properties may be influenced via influence on serotonin.
Source: Adapted from Ref. 28.

Hyperprolactinemia

Hyperprolactinemia has been linked to D_2 blockade in the tuberinfundibular pathway. The relationship between D_2 occupancy and prolactin elevation is less clear than for EPS, but appears to be in the range of 50–75% (14,45).

Since all antipsychotics have some degree of D_2 binding, all are capable of producing hyperprolactinemia. Certainly all conventional antipsychotics can produce sustained hyperprolactinemia and, therefore, the related clinical sequelae. Initial PET data have suggested that clozapine and quetiapine have relatively low D_2 binding at therapeutic doses, i.e., less than 50% (14,46). However, more recent work has indicated that these agents show transient D_2 occupancy. Antipsychotics such as haloperidol result in D_2 occupancy that is sustained for days following a single dose. In contrast, after a rapid rise in D_2 occupancy, clozapine, quetiapine, and similar drugs come off the receptor quickly and by 12–24 hours measured D_2 blockade is quite low (46-48). This pattern of receptor occupancy may have important implications for diminished risk of EPS as well as transient increases in prolactin. While olanzapine's transience at the D_2 receptor is less rapid, it is also not associated with prolonged hyperprolactinemia (49). In contrast, risperidone's risk of prolactin elevation is at least in keeping with conventional antipsychotics such as haloperidol (50–52), perhaps reflecting more sustained occupancy of the D_2 receptor, an active metabolite (9-hydroxy-risperidone), and poor permeability at the level of the blood–brain barrier (BBB). Because the anterior pituitary is positioned outside the BBB, the net result is one of substantial and prolonged D_2 occupancy. Limited data are available regarding ziprasidone, but one report suggests less prolactin elevation compared with haloperidol (53).

Guidelines for Clinicians:
Identifying and Treating Hyperprolactinemia

- All conventional antipsychotics produce sustained hyperprolactinemia.
- Not all SGAs are devoid of this side effect. They may be characterized by transient prolactin elevation, with the exception of risperidone, with which the risk of hyperprolactinemia is comparable to that with conventional antipsychotics.
- Inquire about side effects linked to sustained hyperprolactinemia (e.g., amenorrhea, breast engorgement, decreased libido).

- While ameliorative treatments are available (e.g., bromocriptine), SGAs that spare sustained prolactin elevation should be preferred.
- In evaluating prolactin, the possibility of an organic etiology (e.g., prolactin-secreting tumors) should not be overlooked.

Anticholinergic Side Effects

Cholinergic (or muscarinic) receptors have been classified into four subtypes pharmacologically and five genetically (M_3 and M_5 receptors are expressed to a lesser extent in the brain). The newer antipsychotics differ in their pattern of subtype binding, as well as their muscarinic activity in general (clozapine, olanzapine > risperidone, quetiapine, and ziprasidone) (9,54). As a class, low-potency conventional antipsychotics tend to have greater anticholinergic activity than high-potency drugs.

Guidelines for Clinicians: Identifying and Treating Anticholinergic Side Effects

- Geriatric patients are especially susceptible to these side effects, with increased concern regarding cognitive impairment.
- Caution should be used when combining compounds with anticholinergic activity (e.g., most antiparkinsonians) and antipsychotics that also have substantial anticholinergic effects.
- Patients should be regularly re-evaluated for the need for ongoing antiparkinsonian medications.
- Cholinergic "rebound" (e.g., influenza-like symptoms, insomnia, agitation, confusion, diaphoresis) can occur following abrupt discontinuation of compounds with anticholinergic activity. Gradual tapering is indicated when discontinuing such drugs. This syndrome may also occur when switching from an antipsychotic with high anticholinergic activity (e.g., clozapine) to one with little or no such activity (e.g., risperidone).
- While in vitro work indicates that olanzapine has potent anticholinergic activity, related side effects have not been as evident clinically.

Obsessive-Compulsive Symptoms

Obsessions and compulsions are not new to the list of symptoms and signs that can be seen in the context of schizophrenia. Of note, though, are recent reports of obsessive-compulsive symptoms (OCS) seen more recently in conjunction with the use of SGAs (55–57); one hypothesis suggests a link to the 5-HT antagonism that is a common feature of each.

Guidelines for Clinicians: Identifying and Treating OCS

- They have been reported within days following treatment initiation, and seen both *de nouveau* and in individuals with preexisting OCS.
- OCS may be dose-related, and have been reported with several SGAs in the same individual.
- Use of agents to treat OCD, e.g., selective serotonin-reuptake inhibitors (SSRIs), may be useful in some cases.
- OCS may abate with discontinuation of the SGA.
- Paradoxically, there are also reports documenting the efficacy of SGAs in individuals with refractory obsessive-compulsive disorder and related illnesses (58–60).

Neuroleptic Malignant Syndrome

Neuroleptic malignant syndrome (NMS) is rare, with an incidence of ≤1% for patients treated with conventional antipsychotics; however, it is associated with a relatively high mortality rate. Cases of NMS have recently been reported with the newer antipsychotics. The onset of NMS is generally rapid, and includes pyrexia, rigidity, and autonomic dysregulation. Other features include agitation, fluctuating levels of consciousness, and abnormal laboratory findings (e.g., leukocytosis and elevated ESR, liver transaminases, and creatinine phosphokinase). NMS shares features in common with malignant hyperthermia, lethal catatonia, and heatstroke. A relationship to D_2 blockade has been implicated but not proven (61–64).

Guidelines for Clinicians: Identifying and Treating NMS

- NMS has been reported with all SGAs available for clinical use in North America. The relative risk of NMS in patients treated with SGAs vs. conventional antipsychotics is not clear. NMS may have been overdiagnosed in the past, and the degree of clinical experience with at least some of the newer antipsychotics is too limited to establish specific risk figures.
- Data on NMS risk factors are not well established. However, high antipsychotic doses, rapid titration, and concomitant lithium use should be avoided. Patient factors that seem to increase risk include extreme agitation, dehydration, organic cerebral

disease, a previous episode of NMS, and a diagnosis of affective disorder.

Suggested treatments for NMS include dopamine agonists, dantrolene sodium, benzodiazepines, β-adrenergic antagonists, calcium-channel blockers, and ECT. None has proven to be categorically effective. Regardless of whether these treatments are employed, two interventions are fundamental: antipsychotic discontinuation and supportive care (e.g., hydration).

Antipsychotic rechallenge can occur, but is associated with a diminished risk of NMS recurrence if delayed for a period of several weeks.

Weight Gain and Diabetes

With the exception of molindone, all conventional antipsychotics have been associated with weight gain. While the SGAs have made significant gains from the standpoint of EPS and hyperprolactinemia, they may have no advantages in terms of weight gain. Indeed, olanzapine and clozapine appear to carry a high risk of weight gain (65–67). The risk for risperidone and quetiapine may be more in keeping with conventional antipsychotics, although few data are available on the latter drug (65–68). Ziprasidone may be "weight-neutral" (16,65); however, this drug has not yet been released for widespread clinical use to confirm or refute this claim.

The problem of weight gain with use of SGAs is really just beginning to receive attention, and there is considerable need for further study. Some experts have suggested that it may become the EPS of the SGAs. In addition, reports of type II diabetes are emerging with these agents (69), which may not be confined to patients with weight gain, and elevated triglycerides (70–72), both risk factors for cardiovascular disease. Such side effects are even more troublesome considering that schizophrenia is an illness frequently characterized by a sedentary lifestyle, financial constraints that restrict environmental changes, and smoking rates as high as 90%. Taken together, these risk factors emphasize the need to pay more attention to cardiovascular morbidity and mortality in this population.

Different mechanisms have been implicated in the increased weight gain seen with the newer antipsychotics. Particular attention has been paid to the possible role of antihistamine activity, a feature characterizing both clozapine and olanzapine, but other mechanisms have also been postulated (e.g., dopaminergic, serotonergic, opioid, peptide) (67,73,74).

Guidelines for Clinicians:
Identifying and Treating Weight Gain

Clozapine and olanzapine have been associated with the greatest risk of weight gain. A clear relationship between weight gain and antipsychotic dose has not been demonstrated (75–77).

Increase in weight tends to occur soon after treatment, with most of the weight gain occurring in the first months (76,77).

Factors predicting weight gain are not entirely clear. In the case of olanzapine, weight gain has been associated with lower baseline body-mass index (BMI), males, younger age, and better clinical outcome (78). Studies with clozapine suggest that patients with lower baseline weight may be at increased risk of weight gain (77).

Patients prescribed antipsychotics should be monitored for cardiovascular risk factors. Attention should be paid to baseline weight, blood pressure, diet, alcohol and smoking history, family history, and selected laboratory measures (e.g., ECG, fasting blood glucose, triglycerides). The evaluation of risk factors should be guided by clinical history and evidence of weight change. However, changes in blood glucose may not be simply a function of weight gain, and routine monitoring may be required at regular intervals, e.g., every 3–6 months.

Efforts should be made to educate the individual and to assist in making lifestyle changes that can lead to weight loss.

It is unclear yet whether weight gain can be reversed by switching from one SGA to another.

Treatments are currently being evaluated for treatment of weight gain, including topiramate, orlistat, and buproprion.

Hematological Effects

Only clozapine requires routine hematological monitoring because of its association with a risk of agranulocytosis (<1%). The mechanisms underlying this side effect remain unclear, so regular monitoring must continue for the duration of treatment. There is a network in place, the Clozaril Support and Assistance Network (CSAN), to coordinate this process. CBC and differential should be monitored weekly for the first 26 weeks and then biweekly thereafter. CSAN guidelines allow for three possibilities based on reported results: green (allowing for ongoing treatment), yellow (repeat blood testing before the next scheduled date), and red (clozapine should be discontinued).

Guidelines for Clinicians: Clozapine-Induced Agranulocytosis

The risk of granulocytopenia and agranulocytosis is not dose-related (79).

The period of maximum risk occurs within 18 weeks after clozapine initiation; approximately 80% of cases occur within the first 26 weeks (80).

An increased risk exists in individuals over the age of 50, and in those who have demonstrated a hematopoietic reaction to other medications (17).

There is no clear evidence that other agents that can cause agranulocytosis, such as carbamazepine, increase the risk in a synergistic fashion (81). However, it is common to avoid such combinations in favor of alternatives (e.g., sodium valproate).

Hepatic Effects

Antipsychotics are metabolized through the liver, so it is not surprising that altered liver-function tests (LFTs) have been reported. Although scattered reports of hepatitis and jaundice have occurred with the conventional antipsychotics, such events are not frequent, and it is not common to see clinicians routinely monitoring LFT. It is of note, though, that two of the SGAs—olanzapine and quetiapine—have been associated with elevated transaminases (82,83).

Guidelines for Clinicians: Hepatic Toxicity

ALT (SGPT) elevation is the most common side effect in this category.

The risk appears to be in the range of about 5–10%, and the elevations are often transient, resolving within 6–8 weeks in 70–80% of cases.

Baseline and regular monitoring of LFT is advocated for those with a history of previous hepatic dysfunction, exposure to hepatotoxic drugs (which would include alcohol abuse), or clinical evidence of hepatic disease (17).

In cases of moderate increases—e.g., ALT/AST (SGPT/SGOT) >1.5 times the upper limit of normal (ULN)—repeat monitoring should be carried out within the following week. The antipsychotic should be immediately discontinued with increases >3 times ULN. Consultation with experts may be warranted to guide future treatment decisions.

Cardiac Effects

Various ECG changes and cardiac arrhythmias were reported with chlorpromazine, the first antipsychotic available clinically. Caution has also been raised with pimozide, a high-potency conventional antipsychotic, following reports of increased risk of sudden death at doses ≥20 mg daily. However, the frequency and severity of these events with conventional antipsychotics have not warranted baseline and routine monitoring of all patients.

At present, patients treated with SGAs are not routinely monitored, although certain events have raised the visibility of potential cardiac complications, particularly QT prolongation. This conduction change has been associated with various ventricular arrhythmias, syncope, and sudden death, especially when the Qtc interval exceeds 440 milliseconds (84). QTc prolongation has also been proposed as the factor accounting for pimozide's risk of sudden death at higher doses, and for this reason it is contraindicated in individuals with a history of cardiac disease.

Clozapine has been associated with QTc prolongation, which appears to be dose-related, in a small number of cases (85). Risperidone and quetiapine have also been linked to QTc prolongation, but in these cases the data have not indicated increases in clinical risk compared to control samples (86,87). Sertindole, a SGA also characterized by greater activity of 5-HT_2 vs. D_2, was released briefly but subsequently withdrawn because of scattered deaths thought to be related to cardiac disturbances, specifically QTc prolongation. Finally, application for approval of ziprasidone, also known to cause QTc prolongation, has been delayed in the United States (88). Its clinical approval is being held pending collection and review of additional ECG data.

On July 31, 2000, Novartis notified clinicians that thioridazine, an older conventional antipsychotic, has also been linked to conduction abnormalities through QTc prolongation.

Guidelines for Clinicians: Cardiac Toxicity

At present, all individuals being started on antipsychotics do not require baseline and routine cardiac monitoring.

However, clinicians should ensure that an adequate history and clinical examination related to cardiac risk factors is carried out. ECG monitoring, and even expert consultation, is indicated in individuals with a cardiac history or current disease.

Clinicians should remain aware of potential drug interactions involving concomitant use of agents that induce conduction abnormalities, including agents that increase plasma antipsychotic levels through competition at the level of the cytochrome P450 isoenzymes.

Further recommendations for cardiac monitoring are likely in the future, based on evidence related to increased weight gain, diabetes, and elevated triglycerides in association with the SGAs.

Ocular Effects

Ocular side effects related to antipsychotic use are not uncommon, and were identified years ago in conjunction with phenothiazine use. Lenticular changes were reported with chlorpromazine use, while pigmentary retinopathy was noted in conjunction with thioridazine (>800 mg daily). Moreover, blurred vision is a common side effect in antipsychotics with anticholinergic activity.

Quetiapine is the only SGA currently available that requires specific monitoring for such side effects. Animal work with dogs noted the development of cataracts following high doses of quetiapine, leading to the clinical recommendation that eye examinations (including slit-lamp) be carried out shortly after initiation of quetiapine treatment and at subsequent 6-month intervals (17,89). Discontinuation of quetiapine should be considered with any evidence of lens changes.

Guidelines for Clinicians: Ocular Toxicity

Many individuals still being treated with conventional antipsychotics should be monitored for ocular changes.

Guidelines for ophthalmological monitoring in quetiapine-treated patients should be followed. However, data from 300,000 individuals treated short-term with quetiapine indicate an incidence of 0.005% for lens opacities, less than the analogous risk in the general population (90).

Recent data from a survey of individuals with schizophrenia in a community setting suggest a much higher incidence of cataracts than in the general population (91), a further reminder that this population should receive careful and complete medical evaluations on a regular basis.

SUMMARY

By the strict definition of "atypicality" (i.e., decreased EPS, lack of prolactin elevation), SGAs represent a significant advance over the conventional antipsychotics. However, there are differences on these measures among the newer agents, in some cases as a function of dose. This supports the notion that a typical-atypical distinction is best viewed along a continuum, rather than as dichotomous.

Clinicians are using the SGAs with increasing frequency, and so these newer agents will gradually replace their conventional counterparts. However, it is important to recognize that improvements in D_2-related side effects represent only part of the side-effect story. With the increased use of SGAs, we are faced with different, and perhaps new, side effects. For example, some of these agents have more anticholinergic activity (e.g., clozapine). While the precise mechanisms underlying weight gain are not clear, this side effect appears to be more of a problem with the SGAs. A growing number of reports identifying diabetes and elevated triglycerides is alarming given that SGAs are used in a population already at risk for cardiovascular disease. Other side effects highlighted with one or more of these newer agents (e.g., hepatic, cardiac, ocular) will be better understood with more widespread clinical use. NMS, a rare but potentially fatal side effect, has not been eliminated with the SGAs.

From our clinical experience with conventional antipsychotics, we have learned that more is not better. To minimze side effects, antipsychotic monotherapy is preferred at the lowest possible dose. The use of excessively high doses has not been associated with improved clinical outcome but has been linked to a greater likelihood of side effects. For example, higher clozapine doses increase the risk of seizures, and the risk of EPS rises with higher doses of risperidone and olanzapine. Combining antipsychotics, including two SGAs, can negate the D_2-related benefits (i.e., decreased EPS, lack of prolactin elevation) that may be seen with each individually. Additive side effects can also be seen (e.g., sedation), and unexpected side effects that cannot be predicted based on the profiles of the individual agents may also emerge.

Clinicians should aim to prevent side effects. Judicious use of antipsychotics can optimize this happening, but in actual practice we will encounter some side effects in many, if not most, individuals, even with the newer antipsychotics. Therefore, detection and treatment become as important as prevention, and clinicians must ensure that a systematic and comprehensive approach to side-effect monitoring is in place.

REFERENCES

1. Bitter I, Volavka J, Scheurer J. The concept of the neuroleptic threshold: an update. J Clin Psychopharmacol 1991; 11:28–33.
2. Seeman P. Dopamine receptor sequences: therapeutic levels of neuroleptics occupy D_2 receptors, clozapine occupies D4. Neuropsychopharmacology 1992; 7:261–284.
3. Deniker P. The neuroleptics: a historical survey. Acta Psychiatr Scand 1990; 82(suppl 358):83–87.
4. Remington G, Kapur S. Atypical antipsychotics: are some more atypical than others? Psychopharmacology (Berlin) 2000; 148:3–15.
5. Kapur S, Zipursky RB, Remington G. Clinical and theoretical implications of 5-HT_2 and D_2 receptor occupancy of clozapine, risperidone, and olanzapine in schizophrenia. Am J Psychiatry 1999; 156:286–293.
6. Waddington JL, Scully PJ, O'Callaghan E. The new antipsychotics, and their potential for early intervention in schizophrenia. Schizophr Res 1997; 28:207–222.
7. Brown WA, Herz LR. Response to neuroleptic drugs as a device for classifying schizophrenia. Schizophr Bull 1989; 15:123–129.
8. Baldessarini RJ, Frankenburg FR. Clozapine: a novel antipsychotic agent [comments]. N Engl J Med 1991; 324:746–754.
9. Gerlach J, Peacock L. New antipsychotics: the present status. Int Clin Psychopharmacol 1995; 10(suppl 3):39–48.
10. Meltzer HY, Matsubara S, Lee JC. Classification of typical and atypical antipsychotic drugs on the basis of dopamine D-1, D-2 and $serotonin_2$ pKi values. J Pharmacol Exp Ther 1989; 251:238–246.
11. Jeste DV, Caligiuri MP. Tardive dyskinesia. Schizophr Bull 1993; 19:303–315.
12. Baldessarini RJ, Cohen BM, Teicher MH. Significance of neuroleptic dose and plasma level in the pharmacological treatment of psychoses. Arch Gen Psychiatry 1988; 45:79–91.
13. Bollini P, Pampallona S, Orza MJ, Adams ME, Chalmers TC. Antipsychotic drugs: is more worse? A meta-analysis of the published randomized control trials. Psychol Med 1994; 24:307–316.
14. Kapur S, Zipursky R, Jones C, Remington G, Houle S. Relationship between dopamine D_2 occupancy, clinical response, and side effects: a double-blind PET study of first-episode schizophrenia. Am J Psychiatry 2000; 157:514–520.
15. Richelson E. Receptor pharmacology of neuroleptics: relation to clinical effects. J Clin Psychiatry 1999; 60:5–14.

16. Tandon R, Harrigan E, Zorn SH. Ziprasidone: a novel antipsychotic with unique pharmacology and therapeutic potential. J Serotonin Res 1998; 4:159–177.
17. Welbanks L, ed. Compendium of Pharmaceuticals and Specialists (CPS). 25th ed. Toronto: Webcom, 2000.
18. Kapur S, Remington G. Atypical antipsychotics: new opportunities and new challenges in the treatment of schizophrenia. In: Coggins C, ed. Annual Review of Medicine. Vol 52. Palo Alto: Annual Reviews, 2001:503–517.
19. Simpson GM, Angus JWS. A rating scale for extrapyramidal side effects. Acta Psychiatr Scand 1970; 212:11–19.
20. Guy W, ed. Assessment Manual for Psychopharmacology. DHEW publication (ADM) 76–338. Rockville, MD: National Institute of Mental Health, 1976.
21. Chouinard G, Ross-Chouinard A, Annable L, Jones BD. Extrapyramidal Symptom Rating Scale (ESRS). Can J Neurol Sci 1980; 7:233–243.
22. Brown KW, Glen SE, White T. Low serum iron status and akathisia. Lancet 1987; i:1234–1236.
23. Barnes TR. A rating scale for drug-induced akathisia. Br J Psychiatry 1989; 154:672–676.
24. Gerlach J, Korsgaard S, Clemmesen P, Lauersen AM, Magelund G, Noring U, Povlsen UJ, Bech P, Casey DE. The St. Hans Rating Scale for extrapyramidal syndromes: reliability and validity. Acta Psychiatr Scand 1993; 87:244–252.
25. Goff DC, Baldessarini RJ. Drug interactions with antipsychotic agents. J Clin Psychopharmacol 1993; 13:57–67.
26. DeVane CL. Drug interactions and antipsychotic therapy. Pharmacotherapy 1996; 16:15–20.
27. Flockhart DA, Oesterheld JR. Cytochrome P450-mediated drug interactions. Child Adolesc Psychiatr Clin North Am 2000; 9:43–76.
28. Remington G, Kapur S. Neuroleptic-induced extrapyramidal symptoms and the role of combined serotonin/dopamine antagonism. J Clin Psychiatry Monograph 1996; 14:14–24.
29. Farde L, Nordstrom AL, Wiesel FA, Pauli S, Halldin C, Sedvall G. Positron emission tomographic analysis of central D_1 and D_2 dopamine receptor occupancy in patients treated with classical neuroleptics and clozapine: relation to extrapyramidal side effects. Arch Gen Psychiatry 1992; 49:538–544.
30. Nordstrom AL, Farde L, Wiesel FA, Forslund K, Pauli S, Halldin C, Uppseldt G. Central D_2-dopamine receptor occupancy in relation to antipsychotic drug effects: a double-blind PET study of schizophrenic patients. Biol Psychiatry 1993; 33:227–235.
31. Remington G, Kapur S. D_2 and 5-HT_2 receptor effects of antipsychotics: bridging basic and clinical findings using PET. J Clin Psychiatry 1999; 60(suppl 10):15–19.

32. Remington G, Bezchlibnyk-Butler K. Management of acute antipsychotic-induced extrapyramidal syndromes. CNS Drugs 1996; 5(suppl 1):21–35.
33. Kapur S, Remington G, Zipursky RB, Wilson AA, Houle S. The D_2 dopamine receptor occupancy of risperidone and its relationship to extrapyramidal symptoms: a PET study. Life Sci 1995; 57:103–107.
34. Kapur S, Zipursky RB, Remington G, Jones C, DaSilva J, Wilson AA, Houle S. 5-HT_2 and D_2 receptor occupancy of olanzapine in schizophrenia: a PET investigation. Am J Psychiatry 1998; 155:921–928.
35. American Psychiatric Association. Diagnostic and Statistical Manual of Mental Disorders. 4th ed. Washington, DC: American Psychiatric Press, 1994.
36. Jeste DV. Tardive dyskinesia in older patients. J Clin Psychiatry 2000; 61:27–32.
37. Fenton WS, Wyatt RJ, McGlashan TH. Risk factors for spontaneous dyskinesia in schizophrenia. Arch Gen Psychiatry 1994; 51:643–650.
38. Glazer WM. Expected incidence of tardive dyskinesia associated with atypical antipsychotics. J Clin Psychiatry 2000; 61(suppl 4):21–26.
39. Glazer WM, Morgenstern H, Pultz JA, Yeung PP, Rak IW. Incidence of tardive dyskinesia may be lower with quetiapine treatment than previously reported with typical antipsychotics in patients with psychoses. 38th Annual Meeting of the American College of Neuropsychopharmacology, Acapulco, Mexico, Dec 12–16, 1999.
40. Koczapski AB, Ashby YT, Ibraheem S, Pareded J, Jones BD. "Afternoon radiator-sitting syndrome": hypothermia and early diagnosis of self-induced water intoxication [letter]. Br J Pschiatry 1987; 151:133–134.
41. Kern RS, Marshall BD, Kuehnel TG, Mintz J, Hayden JL, Robertson MJ, Green MF. Effects of risperidone on polydipsia in chronic schizophrenia patients [letter]. J Clin Psychopharmacol 1997; 17:432–435.
42. Fuller MA, Jurjus G, Kwon K, Konicki PE, Jaskiw GE. Clozapine reduces water-drinking behavior in schizophrenic patients with polydipsia. J Clin Psychopharmacol 1996; 16:329–332.
43. Littrell KH, Johnson CG, Littrell SH, Peabody CD. Effects of olanzapine on polydipsia and intermittent hyponatremia [letter]. J Clin Psychiatry 1997; 58:549.
44. Egan MF, Apud J, Wyatt RJ. Treatment of tardive dyskinesia. Schizophr Bull 1997; 23:583–609.
45. Nordstrom AL, Farde L. Plasma prolactin and central D_2 receptor occupancy in antipsychotic drug-treated patients. J Clin Psychopharmacol 1998; 18:305–310.
46. Kapur S, Zipursky R, Jones C, Shammi CS, Remington G, Seeman P. A positron emission tomography study of quetiapine in schizophrenia: a preliminary finding of an antipsychotic effect with only transiently high dopamine D_2 receptor occupancy. Arch Gen Psychiatry 2000; 57:553–559.
47. Kapur S, Seeman P. Antipsychotic agents differ in how fast they come off the dopamine D_2 receptors: implications for atypical antipsychotic action. J Psychiatry Neurosci 2000; 25:161–166.

48. Seeman P, Tallerico T. Rapid release of antipsychotic drugs from dopamine D_2 receptors: an explanation for low receptor occupancy and early clinical relapse upon withdrawal of clozapine or quetiapine. Am J Psychiatry 1999; 156:876–884.
49. Tran PV, Hamilton SH, Kuntz AJ, Potvin JH, Andersen SW, Beasley C Jr, Tollefson GD. Double-blind comparison of olanzapine versus risperidone in the treatment of schizophrenia and other psychotic disorders. J Clin Psychopharmacol 1997; 17:407–418.
50. Chung Y-C, Eun H-B. Hyperprolactinaemia induced by risperidone [letter]. Int J Neuropsychopharmacol 1998; 1:93–94.
51. Schreiber S, Segman RH. Risperidone-induced galactorrhea [letter]. Psychopharmacology (Berlin) 1997; 13:300–301.
52. Dickson RA, Dalby JT, Williams R, Edwards AL. Risperidone-induced prolactin elevations in premenopausal women with schizophrenia [letter]. Am J Psychiatry 1995; 152:1102–1103.
53. Goff DC, Posever T, Herz L, Simmons J, Kletti N, Lapierre K, Wilner KD, Law CG, Ko GW. An exploratory haloperidol-controlled dose-finding study of ziprasidone in hospitalized patients with schizophrenia or schizoaffective disorder. J Clin Psychopharmacol 1998; 18:296–304.
54. Reus VI. Olanzapine: a novel atypical neuroleptic agent. Lancet 1997; 349:1264–1265.
55. Baker RW, Chengappa KNR, Baird JW, Steingard S, Christ MAG, Schooler NR. Emergence of obsessive compulsive symptoms during treatment with clozapine. J Clin Psychiatry 1992; 53:439–442.
56. Remington G, Adams M. Risperidone and obsessive-compulsive symptoms [letter]. J Clin Psychopharmacol 1994; 14:358–359.
57. Morrison D, Clark D, Goldfarb E, McCoy L. Worsening of obsessive-compulsive symptoms following treatment with olanzapine [letter]. Am J Psychiatry 1998; 155:855.
58. Young CR, Bostic JQ, McDanald CL. Clozapine and refractory obsessive-compulsive disorder: a case report [letter]. J Clin Psychopharmacol 1994; 14:209–210.
59. Stein DJ, Bouwer C, Hawkridge S, Emsley RA. Risperidone augmentation of serotonin reuptake inhibitors in obsessive-compulsive and related disorders. J Clin Psychiatry 1997; 58:119–122.
60. Koran LM, Ringold AL, Elliot MA. Olanzapine augmentation for treatment-resistant obsessive-compulsive disorder. J Clin Psychiatry 2000; 61:514–517.
61. Buckley P. Neuroleptic malignant syndrome. J Neurol Neurosurg Psychiatry 1995; 58:271–273.
62. Sternberg DE. Neuroleptic malignant syndrome: the pendulum swings. Am J Psychiatry 1986; 143:1273–1275.
63. Kornhuber J, Weller M. Neuroleptic malignant syndrome. Curr Opin Neurol 1994; 7:353–357.
64. Bristow MF, Kohen D. How malignant is the neuroleptic malignant syndrome? Br Med J 1993; 307:1223–1224.

65. Allison DB, Fontaine KR, Heo M, Mentore JL, Capelleri JC, Chandler LP, Weiden PJ, Cheskin LJ. The distribution of body mass index among individuals with and without schizophrenia. J Clin Psychiatry 1999; 60:215–220.
66. Ganguli R. Weight gain associated with antipsychotic drugs. J Clin Psychiatry 1999; 60:20–24.
67. Wirshing DA, Wirshing WC, Kysar L, Beresford MA, Goldstein D, Pashdag J, Mintz J, Marder SR. Novel antipsychotics: comparison of weight gain liabilities. J Clin Psychiatry 1999; 60:358–363.
68. Jones AM, Rak IW, Raniwalla J, Phung D, Melvin K. Weight changes in patients treated with Seroquel (quetiapine). 38th Annual Meeting of the American College of Neuropsychopharmacology, Acapulco, Mexico, Dec 12–16, 1999.
69. Wirshing DA, Spellberg BJ, Erhart SM, Marder SR, Wirshing WC. Novel antipsychotics and new onset diabetes. Biol Psychiatry 1998; 44:778–783.
70. Dursun SM, Szemis A, Andrews H, Reveley MA. The effects of clozapine on levels of total cholesterol and related lipids in serum of patients with schizophrenia: a prospective study. J Psychiatry Neurosci 1999; 24:453–455.
71. Gaulin BD, Markowitz JS, Caley CF, Nesbitt LA, Dufresne RL. Clozapine-associated elevation in serum triglycerides. Am J Psychiatry 1999; 156:1270–1272.
72. Sheitman BB, Bird PM, Binz W, Akinli L, Sanchez C. Olanzapine-induced elevation of plasma triglyceride levels [letter]. Am J Psychiatry 1999; 156:1471–1472.
73. Stanton JM. Weight gain associated with neuroleptic medication: a review. Schizophr Bull 1995; 21:463–472.
74. Baptista T. Body weight gain induced by antipsychotic drugs: mechanisms and management. Acta Psychiatr Scand 1999; 100:3–16.
75. Kinon BJ, Basson B, Szymanski K, Tollefson GD. Predictors of weight gain during olanzapine treatment. XXIst Collegium Internationale Neuro-psychopharmacologicum (CINP) Congress, Glasgow, July 12–16, 1998.
76. Kinon BJ, Basson BR, Gilmore JA, Tollefson GD. Effect of long-term olanzapine treatment on weight change in schizophrenia. XXIInd Collegium Internationale Neuro-psychopharmacologicum (CINP), Brussels, July 9–13, 2000.
77. Hummer M, Kemmler G, Kurz M, Kurzthaler I, Oberbauer H, Fleischhacker WW. Weight gain induced by clozapine. Eur Neuropsychopharmacol 1995; 5:437–440.
78. Kinon BJ, Basson BR, Szymanski K, Tollefson GD. Predictors of weight gain during olanzapine treatment. XXIst Collegium Internationale Neuropsychopharmacologicum (CINP), Glasgow, July 12–16, 1998.
79. Alvir JM, Lieberman JA, Safferman AZ, Schwimmer JL, Schaaf JA. Clozapine-induced agranulocytosis: incidence and risk factors in the United States. N Engl J Med 1993; 329:162–167.
80. Krupp P, Barnes P. Leponex-associated granulocytopenia: a review of the situation. Psychopharmacology (Berlin) 1989; 99:S118–121.

81. Chong SA, Remington G. Clozapine augmentation: safety and efficacy. Schizophr Bull 2000; 26:421–440.
82. Fulton B, Goa KL. ICI-204,636: an initial appraisal of its pharmacological properties and clinical potential in the treatment of schizophrenia. CNS Drugs 1995; 4:68–78.
83. Fulton B, Goa KL. Olanzapine: a review of its pharmacological properties and therapeutic efficacy in the management of schizophrenia and related psychoses. Drugs 1997; 53:281–298.
84. Welch R, Chue P. Antipsychotic agents and QT changes. J Psychiatry Neurosci 2000; 25:154–160.
85. Kang UG, Kwon JS, Ahn YM, Chung SJ, Ha JH, Koo YJ, Kim YS. Electrocardiographic abnormalities in patients treated with clozapine. J Clin Psychiatry 2000; 61:441–446.
86. Brecher M, Lemmens P, Baelen BV. Tolerability and cardiovascular safety of risperidone. 35th Annual Meeting of the American College of Neuropsychopharmacology, San Juan, Puerto Rico, Dec 9–13, 1996.
87. Borison RL, Arvanitis LA, Miller BG, and the US Seroquel Study Group. ICI 204,636, an atypical antipsychotic: efficacy and safety in a multicenter, placebo-controlled trial in patients with schizophrenia. J Clin Psychopharmacol 1996; 16:158–169.
88. Daniel DG, Copeland LF. Ziprasidone: comprehensive overview and clinical use of a novel antipsychotic. Exp Opin Invest Drugs 2000; 9:819–828.
89. Abramowicz M, ed. Quetiapine for Schizophrenia. Vol 39:1016. New Rochelle, NY: Medical Letter, 1997.
90. Nasrallah HA, Dev V, Rak I, Raniwalla J. Safety update with quetiapine and lenticular examinations: experience with 300,000 patients. 38th Annual Meeting of the American College of Neuropsychopharmacology, Acapulco, Mexico, Dec 12–16, 1999.
91. Smith D, Pantelis C, McGrath J, Tangas C, Copolov D. Ocular abnormalities in chronic schizophrenia: clinical implications. Aust N Z J Psychiatry 1997; 31:252–256.

11

Violence and Forensic Issues in Schizophrenia

John Rabun
St. Louis Psychiatric Rehabilitation Center
St. Louis, Missouri

Susan K. Boyer
Washington University School of Medicine
and St. Louis Psychiatric Rehabilitation Center
St. Louis, Missouri

One concept addressed in forensic psychiatry is the assessment of violence. Violence is often a sleeping volcano. A volcano manifests a calm demeanor and occasionally rumbles over months and even years, then suddenly turns into a cataclysmic event. Scientists over time have outlined the evolving behavior of a quiescent volcano becoming active. They have learned through painstaking research what circumstances are vital for determining the risk of an eruption. And we all, especially those living near volcanoes, are greatly indebted to them.

Just as most volcanoes remain quiescent, most people with schizophrenia are not violent. While assessment of potential violence in those with schizophrenia is feasible, actual prediction is difficult. Monahan (1) has noted that predictions of violent behavior among the mentally ill are accurate only one-third of the time. Why is this? Well-trained psychiatrists face the same problem when attempting to screen for any infrequent event, such as suicide or homicide—relatively small errors in sensitivity and specificity become huge errors in predicting outcomes. It turns out that psychiatrists overpredict violence by 40 to 90% (2).

Therefore, determining a rare event—e.g., when a person with schizophrenia will act violently—is a keen professional challenge. The literature enriches our knowledge but increases the complexity of our decision making by demonstrating the ambivalent views of our colleagues. This is because some studies support the relationship between violence and schizophrenia, while others do not. Why is that?

The target we are aiming at—the relationship between schizophrenia and violence—appears to be a moving one. Researchers' definitions of violence include or exclude such things as violence toward an object, physical violence toward another person or oneself, use of weapons, and/or verbal threats. Researchers also gather information from various sources, e.g., police records, family, and observations in the hospital. They study violence retrospectively or prospectively. Ultimately, many methods of studying violence have been used in the absence of a real "gold standard," which illustrates the difficulty of addressing violence as it pertains to schizophrenia and demonstrates how these different approaches can have conflicting outcomes.

Does this mean no attempt should be made to assess violence potential in our patients? Thanks to the Tarasoff case, we have been forced to practice forensic psychiatry to some degree, and are required to assess violence potential. As we recall, Tatiana Tarasoff was a college student who was murdered by a classmate named Poddar in 1969. Two months prior to her death, Poddar discussed his homicidal thoughts with his therapist, who did not warn Tarasoff. After two separate court proceedings, the well-known Tarasoff rule evolved to its current standard: if "a therapist determines, or according to the standard of his profession, should determine that his patient presents a serious danger of violence to another, he incurs an obligation to use reasonable care to protect the intended victim from danger" (3). It may call for us to warn the intended victim or notify the police, to increase medications, or to involuntarily hospitalize the patient—essentially, to take whatever steps are reasonable to protect the third party. Ultimately, the therapist is required to protect third parties from harm, regardless of the difficulty in assessing potential violence.

However, the question remains whether we as clinicians should assess violence potential in our patients. Clearly, as the literature points out, psychiatrists have no special ability to predict future violence. Moreover, psychiatrists should not place themselves in the precarious situation of predicting that a particular patient will act violently given the inherent difficulty in forecasting an infrequent event. In fact, making a prediction in a court of law that a specific patient will act violently could be construed as a misrepresentation of one's expertise. Despite these admonitions, psychiatrists have been thrust into the role of barometers of violence potential of their patients. Courts across the Unites States allow, and in many instances expect, psychiatrists to give opinions on the issue of violence potential in civil commitment proceedings. Further, psychiatrists are now allowed to opine as to the likelihood of future sexual violence in a select population of prisoners facing commitment in the states that adopted the Kansas vs. Hendricks model (4).

What should psychiatrists do when faced with questions about "future dangerousness"? Obviously, given the current legal climate, psychiatrists cannot ignore such questions. On the other hand, psychiatrists should not overreach their knowledge base and actually predict that a particular patient will act violently. Instead, prudent psychiatrists should offer a risk assessment based on a known group of factors that are associated with potential violence. Psychiatrists should familiarize themselves with the accepted risk factors and use these factors as an anchor for clinical judgment when they interview patients. Even though psychiatrists have not demonstrated the ability to make accurate predictions of long-term dangerousness, they can predict imminent dangerous behavior (2).

The process of risk assessment should be similar to assessing risk for suicide potential: eliciting known risk factors and then adjusting the level of risk based on information unique to the patient. For example, the literature on suicide suggests that a middle-aged white male, divorced and living alone, with a weapon, and having trouble with alcohol and depression is similar to a population of individuals who have completed suicide. Therefore, a psychiatrist, even merely listening to such a case as presented by a primary care physician, would immediately consider the patient at an increased risk for suicide. The psychiatrist might contemplate voluntary or involuntary hospitalization while listening to the case presentation. Subsequently, the psychiatrist might conduct an interview and learn that this individual abhors suicide for religious and familial reasons. Suddenly, the increased risk for suicide is converted to an acceptable risk for suicide, allowing the psychiatrist to comfortably treat this individual on an outpatient basis.

The process of assessing violence potential should be approached in a like manner. During an evaluation, the psychiatrist asks about known risk factors and at the same time considers information distinct to this patient. Such a process calls for psychiatrists not only to remain abreast of the current literature in this area but also to continually assess their patients for violence potential. In other words, the process is grounded in static guides and then repeatedly honed by gathering dynamic features.

This means that every time each of us sees a patient in his office, or even speaks to a patient on the phone, we are in effect assessing dangerousness. Keep in mind that clinicians are more easily faulted in malpractice litigation for failure to collect relevant data than for making an incorrect assessment of violence. Also, a clinical determination that a patient is at an increased risk does not necessarily indicate that the patient is going to commit a violent act. Rather, such a determination represents a judgment that the patient poses an unacceptable risk of causing harm.

IS THERE AN ASSOCIATION BETWEEN SCHIZOPHRENIA AND VIOLENCE?

Determining whether there is an association between schizophenia and violence is the ultimate question. We believe that in certain circumstances there has indeed been a link between acute schizophrenic symptoms and violence. Although studies may differ regarding violence toward others, it has been clearly documented that people with schizophrenia are at an increased risk of violence toward themselves. Roughly 10% of people with schizophrenia will die by suicide (5). It is not difficult to fathom that in this group already predisposed to such desperate acts as suicide, given the right circumstances, desperate and violent acts could be inflicted on others.

Multiple studies have concluded there is a relationship between schizophrenia and violence. For example, the Epidemiological Catchment Area (ECA) study revealed that 12% of those with schizophrenia admitted to being violent in the previous year, as opposed to only 2% of the non–mentally ill (6). In addition, the ECA study showed that even though most mentally ill people do not commit assaultive acts, serious mental disorder by itself is quite significantly associated with violence, as shown by odds ratios in the range of 2.4 to 3.6 (7). Also, the Northwick Park study evaluating first episodes of schizophrenia found that, of the 253 first-episode patients, over one-third had behaved violently in the month before they were admitted to the hospital (6). Given the practical knowledge we have as clinicians, and the numerous studies that point to a relationship between schizophrenia and violence, it would be foolish to ignore a sleeping volcano. Even though authors have used different methods and definitions of violence, useful information can be garnered to provide a template to guide clinical decisions.

In conclusion, there is a weak relationship between schizophrenia and violence. The argument appears to be over how strong the association is.

Let us turn to the risk factors for potential violence in the general population and the factors unique to schizophrenia.

RISK FACTORS IN THE GENERAL POPULATION

Certain general factors hold true for assessing potential violence whether or not someone has a mental illness. These factors need to be looked at in all patients, including those with schizophrenia, because the combination of factors is likely to have a synergistic effect.

Demographics

Violence typically peaks between the ages of 15 and 24 (8). In the nonpsychiatric population, violence peaks at about age 18. In psychiatric patients it occurs around the mid-20s (9,10). Males are more likely to commit violent acts in nonpsychiatric populations (11). However, among people with mental disorders, males and females do not significantly differ (8). Violence is three times more likely to occur in the lowest socioeconomic class than in the highest (8). The lower the IQ, the greater the likelihood of violence (12). According to Resnick (2), violence increases with the use of substances, lower levels of education, unemployment, and unstable living circumstances. Homeless mentally ill individuals commit 35 times more crimes than those in a stable living situation (13).

Personality Traits

Certain personality traits are associated with violence. According to Reid and Balis (14), these traits include impulsivity, low frustration tolerance, reckless driving, inability to tolerate criticism, repetitive antisocial acts, entitlement, and a tendency to have superficial relationships and to dehumanize others. The mental-status examination may show glibness and a tendency to project internal difficulties on the environment. According to Widiger and Trull (15), violent behavior is the defining feature for two personality disorders: borderline and antisocial.

The violence committed by those with antisocial personality disorder typically has revenge as the motive, or has occurred during a period of heavy drinking. The violence lacks the emotionality common among nonpsychopaths (16). Lack of empathy, failure to accept responsibility for one's actions, shallow affect, lack of remorse, poor behavior controls, and impulsivity are psychopathic traits that contribute to aggression (15).

Childhood Factors

If a child is brutalized by a parent, he is more likely to become violent (17). Boys typically become aggressive, whereas girls seem to replicate their victimization (18). Other factors associated with violence are truancy, school failures, and lower IQs (2). Finally, childhood hyperactivity or serious inattention (19), arrest for prior assault (20), first psychiatric hospitalization before age 18 (21), and the triad of enuresis, fire setting, and cruelty to animals (22,23) are all associated with higher violence potential.

Drug and Alcohol Use

The ECA study in 1990 surveyed thousands of people in the community regarding self-reported violence in the last year. Twenty-five percent of those who met criteria for alcohol abuse or dependence were reportedly violent within the past year; 35% of those who met criteria for other drug abuse or dependence were also violent within the past year (10). It was noted that the combination of substance abuse with other major psychopathology was more volatile than either alone. According to Swanson (7), substance abuse alone and comorbidity were about five times more prevalent among those who reported violence than among those who did not; the ECA data revealed that mental illness alone caused less violence than substance abuse, being about twice as prevalent in the subgroups identified as violent. He went on to say that mentally disordered individuals with substance abuse comorbidity were significantly more likely to be violent than those with mental disorder alone, with odds ratios ranging from 3.1 to 4.3.

Situational Factors

The likelihood of violence increases if someone has ready access to weapons, if the victim is easily accessible, and if the perpetrator is homeless, unemployed, and noncompliant with medication.

However, *the strongest indicator for future violent behavior is past violent behavior* (21). If someone has previously been violent, it is important to access the situation to look for a pattern of behavior and triggers for the previous violence.

RISK FACTORS IN SCHIZOPHRENIA

Particular Subtype

Does a specific subtype of schizophrenia pose an increased risk for violence? Clinical experience suggests that an individual suffering from structured delusions would be more likely to act on those beliefs than the person with disorganized delusions. Moreover, it is reasonable to assume that the person afflicted by organized paranoid delusions may be at a distinct risk for violence. In fact, the literature suggests that a person who has been diagnosed with paranoid schizophrenia is at a higher risk for violence outside of a structured setting than those in other diagnostic groups (24).

Further, based on anecdotal experience, we have also found that a patient with paranoid schizophrenia is at greater risk for acting on his delusions than other mentally ill individuals. The finding in the literature is consistent with clinical acumen. Clearly, the patient who firmly believes that his family is involved in a plot to harm him is of more concern to the psychiatrist than the patient who believes that he has communicated with aliens. Moreover, because the person with paranoid schizophrenia has relatively preserved cognitive functioning, he is more likely to be able to formulate a plan of action, in contrast to the individual with disorganized schizophrenia who shows disintegration in cognitive capacity.

Particular Delusions

Are there particular delusions that place an individual at higher risk for violence? As previously noted, the literature suggests that the patient with paranoid schizophrenia is more likely to act violently in the community than are other mentally ill individuals. If we accept this finding, then the next question is: what causes the patient with paranoid schizophrenia to become more likely to act violently? Is it paranoid schizophrenia per se, or is it a set of delusions that increase the potential for violence? It appears, based on the literature and anecdotal experience, that specific types of delusions create the threat of violence.

According to the literature, individuals with psychosis are more likely to act on persecutory delusions than any other category of delusion (24–27). Other studies suggest that patients are more likely to act, possibly violently, on persecutory delusions when they are frightened, anxious, or saddened by their delusions (28–30). Further, in one study conducted at a forensic hospital, the frequency of committing murder was highest in the paranoid psychotic group (31). We have also found, in our own experience in the forensic setting, that the person with a paranoid psychosis is more likely to formulate a plan and act in a seriously aggressive manner, especially if he senses that his life is in danger. To understand why the individual with persecutory delusions is more likely to respond violently, it is important to accept for a moment that the delusions are real. With this in mind, it becomes intuitively obvious that if a person believes that a specific individual is plotting to harm him and that his life is in imminent peril, then he may devise a plan and act accordingly.

For example, one of the authors evaluated an individual who held the persecutory delusion that his father was harassing him, plotting against him, and having him followed by various people. Subsequently, he purchased a firearm and shot and killed his father. Prior to the shooting, he had perceived that he could not hide from or evade the people pursuing him. In addition, he had never divulged his homicidal intentions or his plan. This example not only highlights that paranoid delusions can fuel violent behavior but emphasizes another finding noted in the literature, that among paranoid individuals the resulting violence is frequently planned, potentially life-threatening, and consistent with the delusion (24). Similar findings were reported in a study that focused on violence in geriatric patients who were afflicted by late-onset paraphrenia (32). In addition, the example demonstrates that the paranoid psychotic patient is more likely to target a known individual and to hide his intentions from others (33).

Another type of delusional system associated with increased risk for violence is in misidentification syndrome. The most common misidentification sydrome is the Capgras delusion, sometimes referred to as the delusion of doubles (34). The patient with Capgras delusion believes that the physical appearance of an individual remains the same while the psychological identity is completely different (35). Individuals suffering from misidentification delusions often exhibit paranoid ideas and hostility toward the perceived psychological stranger (34). Moreover, these patients are at increased risk for planning and executing a violent act directed at the psychological stranger. The literature suggests that the risk for violence is significantly greater in the patient with a delusional misidentification syndrome (34,36).

We have also been involved in forensic cases in which the resulting violent act flowed directly from a misidentification delusion. The violence driven by a misidentification delusion is understandable when the belief system is recognized as a reality. If a patient starts to believe that a previously familiar person is now a clever imposter who has assumed that person's appearance, then he will naturally develop paranoid ideas about the perceived stranger. Such a combination of paranoia and misidentification may facilitate aggression, especially since the patient is no longer emotionally attached to the perceived stranger.

For example, one of the authors evaluated an individual who shot and killed two family members after developing Capgras delusions and concluding that, although both family members retained their original physical appearance, they were no longer themselves. This individual was of the opinion that evil entities had not only taken the form of these two people but in fact had murdered them. She asserted that, because the evil impostors planned to kill her next, a pre-emptive homicidal act was necessary and appropriate. This example demonstrates how a patient with a misidentification syndrome no longer feels emotionally connected to the perceived stranger, making it much easier to act in an aggressive manner.

Research on psychosis and violence has also targeted a set of delusions termed "threat/control-override" that may increase a patient's risk for aggression (37). The term threat/control-override defines a specific set of delusions that cause the afflicted individual to lose internal psychological control, enhancing the probability that violence will emerge. Such delusions are characterized by thought insertion, thought control, and the fear of personal harm. Since persecutory delusions have already been addressed, the following discussion focuses on thought insertion and control.

In an early study, researchers found that people who were former and current patients of mental health professionals showed an increased rate of police contacts and violence when compared with never-treated community residents (38). The differences in rates of violence and illegal acts were accounted for by the presence of psychotic symptoms in the patient groups. In a subsequent study, researchers discovered that a specific group of psychotic symptoms explained the noted difference: designated as threat/control-override delusions (37). The association between violence and threat/control-override delusions was confirmed in a later study (26). The later study enunciated the principle that if either of the threat or control-override delusions was experienced as real, it would lead to real behaviors and result in an increased risk for violence.

The results of these earlier studies have been challenged by new data that suggest that threat/control-override delusions are not associated with higher rates of violence in patients recently discharged from psychiatric hospitals (39). Despite new data, clinicians were cautioned in this study to avoid the conclusion that delusions never lead to violence. This study noted that professional experience and earlier studies suggested that delusions could spark an aggressive act. Further, this study pointed out that the new data did not refute the tenet frequently voiced by experts that if a patient has a past history of delusion-driven violence he might behave similarly in the future. We agree with the latter admonitions and concur with the maxim established by clinical wisdom that recognizes that acute delusions of a threat/control-override nature accepted as reality can lead to an increased risk for violence.

What appears to be important in assessing these types of delusions is whether the patient has surrendered to the psychotic belief and now holds it as genuine (30,37). At that point, any violent act that springs from the delusion could be viewed as an understandable or rational reaction to an irrational stimulus (25,37). Stated differently, the violent act is seen as a natural corollary of the threat/control-override delusion. Therefore, the psychiatrist should not only ask about the presence of such delusions but also inquire as to their content and test the resolve with which they are held.

For example, one of the authors reviewed the medical records of a person accused of killing both parents. The individual had had multiple psychiatric hospitalizations prior to the incident and had expressed delusions of paranoia and thought control, and stated the belief that one parent was responsible for the perceived mind and body control. Unfortunately, the link between this individual's threat/control-override delusion and the homicides cannot be firmly established because only a chart review was conducted. It is significant, however, that one of the victims was the focus of the threat/control-override delusion. In addition, the chart review suggested that this individual unquestionably adopted his delusional constructs.

In summary, persecutory delusions are more likely to be acted on than any other type of delusion. Violence is more likely to occur if individuals feel they are losing control, e.g., if they believe that their minds are being dominated by other forces, that thoughts are being put into their head, or that they are being followed. Of note, psychotic symptoms not associated with increased aggression include feeling dead and that one's thoughts are being broadcast. Remember that violence is more likely if delusions are persecutory and systematized and have been acted on before. Importantly, on the rare occasions when individuals with schizophrenia do act out violently, it is usually during the acute phase of their illness and their victims are rarely strangers.

Particular Hallucinations

Just as certain delusions are associated with violence, there appear to be particular hallucinations that place an individual at higher risk for violence. Auditory hallucinations that produce negative emotions, i.e., anger, anxiety, and sadness, are more likely to generate violent behavior in patients with schizophrenia than positive emotions are (40). For instance, one of the authors evaluated an individual with paranoid schizophrenia who had been arrested for reckless endangerment after a multistate police chase while driving a truck. He was driving fast and erratically, causing several cars to seek shelter on the shoulder of the highway. After his arrest, he said he had heard several voices talking to each other and to him. The voices made statements about wanting to kill him, his family, and the President of the United States. He could not figure out whether the voices were coming from the truck radio or the air. Eventually, the voices began saying there was a bomb in the cab of his truck and that if he did not reach a particular city within three hours it would detonate. He therefore drove at a fast pace, frightened that he would not make the "deadline," and ultimately drove his truck into a large body of water in an attempt to defuse the "bomb." This example illustrates how negative emotions, i.e., fear and anxiety, produced by auditory hallucinations can lead to violent behavior.

Also, the risk of violence is increased when hallucinations are related to delusions (41). For instance, one of the authors was involved in a case in which an individual was evaluated after allegedly hijacking an interstate bus and stabbing one of the passengers. The attacker described a pattern of symptoms consistent with paranoid schizophrenia. According to this individual, while riding the bus, he heard a woman yelling "let me out" and "you are going to kill me." At first he believed that the woman had been trapped in the baggage compartment by accident. After several hours, he concluded that the bus driver and several passengers were involved in a plot to kill him and others. He contended that the woman in the baggage compartment had been the first victim of this perceived plot. Eventually, he no longer heard the voice and surmised that the woman had died from exhaust fumes. Subsequently, the individual, thinking he heard two passengers talking about killing everyone on the bus, assaulted one of them with a knife and hijacked the bus. The incident ended when he stopped the bus and requested help. This example demonstrates how the content of a hallucination can further fuel a delusion and consequently enhance violence potential.

Furthermore, studies have revealed a relationship between hallucinations' giving commands and subsequent compliance with the commands (41). For instance, Junginger (42) conducted a study in which 52 of 93 subjects, the majority of whom carried a diagnosis of schizophrenia, reported at least partial compliance with their most recent command hallucination; 40 of 93 reported full compliance. In this study, Junginger also found that the level of compliance was higher for harmless commands and if the subject could identify the hallucinated voice. Also, violent commands toward others are less frequently obeyed than harmless commands and commands to harm oneself (43). We have treated psychotic individuals who have attempted suicide because of command hallucinations, e.g., a patient with schizophrenia who jumped off a bridge and sustained bilateral ankle fractures in response to command hallucinations telling him to kill himself to gain "salvation."

In addition, studies based on quantitative clinical ratings of patients with psychosis have shown a significant positive relationship between hallucinations and violent behavior, particularly in the presence of other positive psychotic symptoms such as thinking disturbance and conceptual disorganization (44). For instance, one of the authors performed a risk assessment on a person with paranoid schizophrenia who was charged with robbery, menacing, criminal mischief, and harassment. He smashed windows at a church, threatened one onlooker and struck another with an umbrella, and waved a pair of scissors near someone's throat. At the time, the individual exhibited incoherence in his speech with a disorganized flow of thought. He did say that he was chased out of his house by a voice that told him to go to the church to get money to escape (to where he did not know). This example illustrates how the combination of auditory hallucinations and thinking disturbance can lead to violent behavior.

ANECDOTAL FACTORS

Our experiences in forensic psychiatry have led to additional insights regarding risk factors for violence and psychosis, albeit anecdotal but in some instances supported by the literature. We are of the opinion that individuals with schizophrenia are at higher risk for acting on delusions than in response to hallucinations. The literature addressing psychotic motivation for offending suggests findings similar to our experiences (45,46). Moreover, in one study on pretrial prisoners, researchers noted that males with schizophrenia were more likely to have engaged in serious violence if their illness was characterized by an almost exclusive delusional course (47).

Along the same lines, we have observed that individuals with schizophrenia who categorically believe in their delusions are at an increased risk for acting on those beliefs. Our observations are supported by research that has studied the link between delusions and violence (30,37). Further, we have found that persons with schizophrenia who committed a violent crime usually showed an earlier onset of disease. One study, which looked in part at the course of paranoid schizophrenia, has confirmed our conclusion that violent behavior is more likely in patients with an earlier onset of symptoms (48).

We have also noted that, among those who had been previously diagnosed with schizophrenia, repeated hospitalizations and noncompliance defined the illness before the index offense. Finally, based on several cases, we believe that when a persecutory delusion shares a synergistic relationship with either delusional grandiosity or jealousy, the patient's potential for violence is significantly enhanced. The possibility of aggression flowing from a mixture of delusional persecution and jealousy is supported by one study (49). A stark example of how delusions of persecution and grandiosity can promote aggression was encountered by one of the authors. A patient suffering from schizophrenia was evaluated to address issues related to conditional release. The patient had been adjudicated not guilty by reason of insanity after murdering an acquaintance. He elaborated grandiose and persecutory delusions about the victim, which were intertwined and served to aggravate one another. Contending that he had the power to control certain events and that the victim was plotting to harm him to obtain his powers, he decided to act first and killed the victim. Thus, the patient's belief that the victim meant to harm him was wedded to the grandiosity, and both were buttressed by the delusion that the victim was jealous of his powers. This example signifies how grandiose and persecutory delusions can increase the risk for violence.

USE OF THE RISK FACTORS: THE ARGUMENT FOR GUIDED JUDGMENT

It has recently been demonstrated that specific actuarial instruments are useful in assessing the risk of sexual recidivism (50). The actuarial instruments are based on research that has identified specific items correlated with an increased risk for recidivism in a select population of offenders (51). These instruments are advantageous because the technique employed forces the clinician to consider scales associated with an increased rate of recidivism (50) and hence serve as a guide or anchor for the risk assessment. The instruments are then balanced by an interview that addresses information unique to the individual. The final risk calculus is an appraisal of both actuarial data and distinct information gleaned from the interview.

We believe that the assessment of violence potential in a patient with schizophrenia should follow a similar course. When psychiatrists are presented with a potentially violent patient, they should first consider the general risk factors and then explore the items unique to schizophrenia. By following this procedure, psychiatrists will allow their judgment to be guided by the literature and not "gut" instinct. Only then should they offer their opinion as to a patient's risk for violence. Further, the opinion should be presented as a risk assessment, not as a prediction that a particular patient will act violently. A statement such as the following is acceptable: "this patient's acute symptoms and demographics are similar to a set of known factors associated with an increased risk for violence." Psychiatrists should eschew the inherent and often expected conclusion that a patient will actually commit violence.

In summary, we contend that the factors listed below should be used as guidelines in risk assessment. A detailed vignette is included afterward to illustrate many of the identified factors.

General Factors Associated with an Increased Risk for Violence

Gender: male
Age: late teens and early 20s
Substance use: current abuse of alcohol or drugs
Weapons: ownership or access to weapons
Training: military, paramilitary, or police experience
Personality: cluster B features, nosology from DSM-IV-TR (5)
Employment: unemployed or unstable employment
Education: high school or less
Current family dynamics: estranged from or lack of family support
Housing: homeless or living alone
Marital: single
Legal: criminal record, particularly of violent acts
Intelligence: below-average IQ, particularly borderline or less
Organic status: history of head injuries and/or present cognitive deficits
Childhood: history of conduct disorder or attention deficit/hyperactivity disorder
Abuse: history of sexual or physical abuse as a child
Family history: unstable parenting and/or poor role models

Thoughts: documented history of homicidal ideas, from statements or records

Factors in Schizophrenia Associated with an Increased Risk for Violence

Diagnostic subtype: paranoid schizophrenia
Onset: early age of onset
Present state of illness: acute psychosis
Particular delusions: persecutory, threat/control-override, and misidentification
Combined delusions: persecutory delusions linked to delusional grandiosity or jealousy
Delusional structure: systematized
Delusional target: risk-enhancing delusions that target a specific person
Delusional resolve: risk-enhancing delusions that are unquestionably adopted
Delusional course: illness defined by an almost exclusive delusional course
Delusional action: a history of acting on risk-enhancing delusions
Affect and delusions: delusions causing sadness, fright, or anxiety
Course of illness: repeated hospitalizations
Insight: lack of insight and noncompliance with treatment
Combined psychotic symptoms: hallucinations that accentuate risk-enhancing delusions
Hallucinations: auditory commands to engage in a violent act; auditory hallucinations that produce negative emotions
Type of hallucination: familiar voice
Hallucinations and action: a history of acting on risk-enhancing hallucinations
Hallucinations and resolve: risk-enhancing hallucinations that are firmly believed

CASE STUDY

One of the authors was retained to evaluate an individual charged with murder. The man, in his mid-30s, had allegedly stabbed a neighbor to death. The individual told the police that he believed that the victim had been involved in a plot to kill him. He indicated that other neighbors were involved in the plot, including the victim's adult child. He explained that he had targeted the victim as the principal actor in the plot. The individual also informed the police that he felt that the victim and others were trying to control him and were listening to his conversations. He admitted to the recent use of marijuana, and a urine drug screen revealed cannabis metabolites.

The man's personal history revealed some important factors. There was axis I pathology in two close family members, one of whom suffered from a paranoid disorder. He was raised by a grandparent even before his parents' divorce. He was described by a family member as being "hyper" as a child although no formal evaluation had ever been performed. He quit high school and ran away from home. He joined the military but was discharged for medical reasons during basic training. He was arrested several times as an adult for nonviolent offenses and was twice incarcerated in prison. While in prison, he developed a paranoid psychotic illness and was treated with antipsychotic medication. His prison records revealed that the treating psychiatrist suspected the possibility of paranoid schizophrenia. Prior to the charged offense, he was sporadically attending an outpatient psychiatric center where he was diagnosed with paranoid schizophrenia. The records from the outpatient provider noted that he was noncompliant with treatment and lacked insight into his mental illness. Further, he was unemployed and living alone around the time of the alleged offense. In addition, he was estranged from his family because of his paranoia and maintained an isolated existence in the vicinity of the incident. He had abused cocaine and methamphetamine in the past, but was smoking marijuana daily around the time of the index offense.

The evaluation found that the individual was suffering from acute persecutory delusions involving the victim, believing that the victim and others were plotting to harm him. He was convinced of the reality of his beliefs and almost terminated the interview when his delusions were challenged. He appeared to be frightened by his persecutory delusions. In addition, he described auditory hallucinations related to his persecutory delusions in that he thought that he heard the victim and others talking about him and mocking him through the walls. Moreover, he expressed ideas that suggested he was homicidal and suicidal.

The individual was diagnosed with paranoid schizophrenia and cannabis abuse. The final opinion was that the behavior flowed from his acute psychotic state. After a report was generated, a second opinion was sought. The second opinion resulted in similar conclusions.

REFERENCES

1. Monahan J. The prediction of violent behavior: toward a second generation of theory and policy. Am J Psychiatry 1984; 141(1):10–15.
2. Resnick P. Violence risk assessment. American Academy of Psychiatry and the Law Conference, New Orleans: Oct 19, 1998.
3. Tarasoff vs. Regents of the University of California, 551 P.2d 334 (1976).
4. Kansas vs. Hendricks, 117 S. Ct. 2072 (1997).
5. American Psychiatric Association. The Diagnostic and Statistical Manual of Mental Disorders. 4th ed, text revision. Washington, DC: American Psychiatric Press, 2000.
6. Wessely S. The epidemiology of crime, violence, and schizophrenia. Br J Psychiatry 1997; 170(32):8–11.
7. Swanson J. Mental disorder, substance abuse, and community violence: an epidemiological approach. In: Monahan J, Steadman HJ, eds. Violence and Mental Disorder: Developments in Risk Assessment. Chicago: University of Chicago Press, 1994:101–136.
8. Borum R, Swartz M, Swanson J. Assessing and managing violence risk in clinical practice. J Pract Psychiatry Behav Health 1996; 2(4):205–215.
9. Pearson M, Wilmot E, Padi M. A study of violent behaviour among inpatients in psychiatric hospitals. Br J Psychiatry 1986; 149:232–235.
10. Swanson JW, Holzer CE, Ganju, VK, Jono RT. Violence and psychiatric disorder in the community: evidence from the Epidemiologic Catchment Area surveys. Hosp Commun Psychiatry 1990; 41:761–770.
11. Tardiff K, Sweillam A. Assault, suicide, and mental illness. Arch Gen Psychiatry 1980; 37:164–169.
12. Quinsey V, MacGuire A. Maximum security psychiatric patients: actuarial and clinical prediction of dangerousness. J Interpersonal Violence 1986; 1:143–171.
13. Martell, DA, Rosner R, Harman RB. Base-rate estimates of criminal behavior by homeless mentally ill persons in New York City. Psychiatr Serv 1995; 46(6):596–601.
14. Reid WH, Balis GU.Evaluation of the violent patient. In: Hales RE, Frances AJ, eds. American Psychiatric Association Annual Review 1987:491–509.
15. Widiger TA, Trull TJ. Personality disorders and violence. In: Monahan J, Steadman HJ, eds. Violence and Mental Disorder: Developments in Risk Assessment. Chicago: University of Chicago Press, 1994:203–226.
16. Williamson S, Hare RD, Wong S. Violence: criminal psychopaths and their victims. Can J Behav Sci 1987; 19:454–462.
17. Yesavage JA, Brizer DA. Clinical and historical correlates of dangerous inpatient behavior. In: Brizer DA, Crowner M, eds. Current Approaches to the Prediction of Violence. Washington, DC: American Psychiatric Press, 1989.

18. Carmen EH, Reiker PP, Mills T. Victims of violence and psychiatric illness. Am J Psychiatry 1984; 141:378–379.
19. Manuzza S, Klein RG, Konig PH, Giampino TL. Hyperactive boys almost grown up. IV. Criminality and its relationship to psychiatric status. Arch Gen Psychiatry 1989; 46:1073–1079.
20. Convit A, Jaeger J, Lin, SP, Meisner M, Volavka J. Predicting assaultiveness in psychiatric inpatients: a pilot study. Hosp Commun Psychiatry 1988; 39:429–434.
21. Klassen D, O'Connor WA. A prospective study of predictors of violence in adult male mental health admissions. Law Hum Behav 1988; 12:143–158.
22. Hellman D, Blackman N. Enuresis, firesetting, and cruelty to animals: a triad predictive of adult crime. Am J Psychiatry 1966; 122:1431–1435.
23. Felthous AR, Kellert SR. Childhood cruelty to animals and later aggression against people: a review. Am J Psychiatry 1987; 144:710–717.
24. Krawkowski M, Volavaka J, Brizer D. Psyopathology and violence: a review of literature. Compr Psychiatry 1986; 27(2):131–148.
25. Junginger J. Psychosis and violence: the case for a content analysis of psychotic experience. Schizophr Bull 1996; 22(1):91–103.
26. Link BG, Stueve A, Phelan J. Psychotic symptoms and violent behaviors: probing the components of "threat/control-override" symptoms. Soc Psychiatry Psychiatr Epidemiol 1998; 33:S55–S60.
27. Wessely S, Buchanan A, Reed A, Cutting J, Everitt B, Garety P, Taylor PJ. Acting on delusions. I. Prevalence. Br J Psychiatry 1993; 163:69–76.
28. Appelbaum PS, Robbins PC, Roth LH. Dimensional approach to delusions: comparison across types and diagnoses. Am J Psychiatry 1999:156(12); 1938–1943.
29. Buchanan A, Reed A, Wessely S, Garety P, Taylor PJ, Grubin D, Graham D. Acting on delusions. II. The phenomenological correlates of acting on delusions. Br J Psychiatry 1993; 163:77–81.
30. Taylor PJ, Garety P, Buchanan A, Reed A, Wessely S, Ray K, Dunn G, Grubin D. Delusions and violence. In: Monahan J, Steadman HJ, eds. Violence and Mental Disorder: Developments in Risk Assessment. Chicago: University of Chicago Press, 1994:161–182.
31. Benezech M, Bourgeois M, Yesavage J. Violence in the mentally ill: a study of 547 patients at a French hospital for the criminally insane. J Nerv Ment Dis 1980; 168:698–700.
32. Petrie WM, Lawson EC, Hollender MH. Violence in geriatric patients. JAMA 1982; 248:443–444.
33. Addad M, Benezech M, Bourgeois M, Yesavage J. Criminal acts among schizophrenics in French mental hospitals. J Nerv Ment Dis 1981; 169:289–293.
34. Silva JA, Leong GB, Weinstock R. The dangerousness of persons with misidentification syndromes. Bull Am Acad Psychiatry Law 1992; 20(1):77–86.

35. Silva JA, Leong GB, Shaner AL. A classification system for misidentification syndromes. Psychopathology 1990; 23:27–32.
36. Nestor PG, Haycock J, Doiron S, Kelly J, Kelly D. Lethal violence and psychosis. a clinical profile. Bull Am Acad Psychiatry Law 1995; 23(3):331–341.
37. Link BG, Stueve A. Psychotic symptoms and the violent/illegal behavior of mental patients compared to community controls. In: Monahan J, Steadman HJ, eds. Violence and Mental Disorder: Developments in Risk Assessment. Chicago: University of Chicago Press, 1994:137–159.
38. Link BG, Andrews HA, Cullen FT. The violent and illegal behavior of mental patients reconsidered. Am Sociol Rev 1992; 57:275–292.
39. Appelbaum PS, Robbins PC, Monahan J. Violence and delusions. data from the MacArthur Violence Risk Assessment Study. Am J Psychiatry 2000; 157(4):566–572.
40. Cheung P, Schweitzer I, Crowley K, Tuckwell V. Violence in schizophrenia: role of hallucinations and delusions. Schizophr Res 1997; 26:181–190.
41. Junginger J. Predicting compliance with command hallucinations. Am J Psychiatry 1990; 147:245–247.
42. Junginger J. Command hallucinations and the prediction of dangerousness. Psychiatr Serv 1995; 46(9):911–914.
43. Kasper ME, Rogers R, Adams PA. Dangerousness and command hallucinations: an investigation of psychotic inpatients. Bull Am Acad Psychiatry Law 1996; 24:219–224.
44. McNiel D. Hallucinations and violence. In: Monahan J, Steadman HJ, eds. Violence and Mental Disorder: Developments in Risk Assessment. Chicago: University of Chicago Press, 1994:183–202.
45. Taylor PJ. Motives for offending among violent and psychotic men. Br J Psychiatry 1985; 147:491–498.
46. Martell DA, Dietz PE. Mentally disordered offenders who push or attempt to push victims onto subway tracks in New York City. Arch Gen Psychiatry 1992; 49:472–475.
47. Robertson G, Taylor PJ. The presence of delusions and violence among remanded male prisoners with schizophrenia. In: Gunn J, Taylor P, eds. Forensic Psychiatry: Clinical, Ethical and Legal Issues. Oxford: Heinemann-Butterworth, 1993:338–339.
48. Calcedo-Barba AL, Calcedo-Ordonez A. Violence and paranoid schizophrenia. Int J Law Psychiatry 1994; 17(3):253–263.
49. Silva JA, Ferrari M, Leong GB, Penny G. The dangerousness of persons with delusional jealousy. J Am Acad Psychiatry Law 1998; 26(4):607–623.
50. Hanson RK, Thornton D. Improving risk assessments for sex offenders: a comparison of three actuarial scales. Law Hum Behav 2000; 24(1):57–66.
51. Hanson RK, Bussiere MT. Predicting relapse: a meta-analysis of sexual offender recidivism studies. J Consult Clin Psychol 1998; 66(2):348–362.

12

Impact of Substance Abuse and Dependence on Patients with Schizophrenia

Collins E. Lewis
Washington University School of Medicine
St. Louis, Missouri

INTRODUCTION

Schizophrenia is a chronic, severe mental disorder that occurs in about 1% of the population and has equal prevalence in men and women. The etiology of the disorder has not been clearly elucidated; however, genetic factors and early brain injury from prenatal and obstetric complications have been implicated. Hypotheses have been formulated involving dysfunction of the dopamine and glutamate neurotransmitter systems (1).

Onset is usually occurs between the late teens and the mid-30s. The illness is characterized by symptoms such as delusions, hallucinations, disorganized speech, disorganized behavior, and negative symptoms (e.g., affective flattening, alogia, and avolition). This symptom picture is accompanied by psychosocial deterioration with marked impairment in employment, interpersonal relations, and self-care. Ideally, the disorder should be diagnosed in the absence of major mood disorders, pervasive developmental disorders, and major contributions from substance use and medical disorders (2).

The onset of schizophrenia may be either abrupt or insidious with gradual social withdrawal, loss of interest in school or work, deterioration in hygiene, unusual behavior, and emotional outbursts. More pronounced positive symptoms may subsequently appear and co-occur with negative symptoms and cognitive impairment. The course of the disease is variable; there may be either a slow, gradual deterioration or a series of exacerbations and remissions leading to progressively more compromised interepisode functioning.

Schizophrenia alone has a dramatic impact on psychosocial functioning. Failure to complete school, hold employment, initiate a family or hold one together, as well as multiple psychiatric hospitalizations and loss of independent living, are all too common. The disorder also confers an increased mortality through increased rates of suicide, violent death, and cardiovascular disorders. Finally, schizophrenia exerts an additional impact on the patient in that it dramatically increases the risk of substance use disorder. This added morbidity not only makes schizophrenia itself more difficult to treat but also markedly accelerates the psychosocial decline. Substance use disorders increase rates of noncompliance, psychotic exacerbation, refractoriness to antipsychotic treatment, hospitalization, tardive dyskinesia, violence, suicide, and homelessness (3).

This chapter explores the relationship between schizophrenia and substance use disorders and addresses comorbid, neurobiological, diagnostic, psychotherapeutic, and pharmacotherapeutic issues.

COMORBIDITY

The lifetime risk of comorbidity of substance use disorder in patients with schizophrenia is approximately 50% (1). Estimates of the lifetime prevalence of substance use disorders in schizophrenia have ranged from 10% to over 65%; however, most studies were carried out in treatment populations, which can have artificially higher rates of substance use disorders. The most compeling evidence of the association of substance abuse and schizophrenia comes from the Epidemiologic Catchment Area (ECA) study, which reported a 16.7% prevalence of substance use disorder in the general population and a 47.0% prevalence in schizophrenics. An odds ratio of 4.6 indicated that people with schizophrenia were at least four times more likely than the general population to have substance use disorder (3).

Studies have characterized substance-abusing schizophrenics as young males with a low educational level, an early age of first hospitalization, poor treatment compliance, a high relapse rate, and high risk of suicide.

The etiology of substance abuse in schizophrenia appears to involve both peer-group availability and genetics (4). Family studies have shown that substance-abusing schizophrenics have a higher prevalence of substance abuse and affective disorder in their families than non-substance-abusing schizophrenics. Twin studies have indicated that individuals who have both alcoholism and schizophrenia have a genetic predisposition for both disorders.

In addition to genetic vulnerability, negative symptoms, peer group, and medication effects also contribute to the risk of chemical dependence in the schizophrenic.

An important component of substance abuse among schizophrenics may be self-medication; however, the literature has been varied and contradictory (5,6). Some studies have reported a decrease in psychotic symptoms with alcohol use; others have reported an increase. Cannabis has been reported to cause both pleasant and unpleasant effects. Some schizophrenics report that drinking decreases anxiety, insomnia, depression, and energy, and increases calm and trust.

Noordsy and coworkers (5) studied outpatient schizophrenics and schizoaffectives, 50.7% of whom had a lifetime alcohol use disorder. Over 50% of the subjects stated that alcohol relieved social anxiety, tension, dysphoria, apathy, anhedonia, and insomnia. In contrast, no more than 15% reported relief of any specific psychotic symptom. For those who reported relief of the positive symptomatology, alcohol appeared to relieve the dysphoria related to the psychosis and not the psychosis itself. As one subject said, "Drinking doesn't make the voices go away, but they don't bother me as much."

Addington and Duchak (6) also studied the self-reported reasons for substance abuse in schizophrenics and found that over 50% reported that the reasons for alcohol use were to: relax, increase pleasure, "get high," reduce depression, become more talkative, and belong to the group. Figures for cannabis use were similar. Hence, these authors concluded that there was some support for the self-medication hypothesis, although the reasons for substance use were not so much to reduce psychotic symptoms as to relieve nonpsychotic symptoms (dysphoria, tension, apathy, anhedonia, insomnia, etc.) and social isolation.

Finally, medications used for treatment may present a biological risk for substance abuse in schizophrenics (4). Some studies have shown that chronic neuroleptic administration enhances the reinforcing effects of stimulants. Psychotic patients have reported substantial euphoria from modest doses of cocaine even while continuing their neuroleptics. Haloperidol has also been shown to increase the reinforcing effects of cocaine in rodents, perhaps due to up-regulation of the postsynaptic dopamine receptors in response to chronic blockade. In addition, schizophrenics who abuse stimulants and marijuana have reported amelioration of the dysphoric effects of the neuroleptics (4,7).

COMORBID NEUROBIOLOGY

The neurobiological and neuroanatomical abnormalities of schizophrenics may make them even more vulnerable to the neurotoxic effects of alcohol and illicit substances. Further, substance use disorder may exacerbate the cognitive deficits already present in the schizophrenic patient. Cortical atrophy and ventricular enlargement have been observed in a subset of schizophrenic patients, and the additional sulcal widening and ventricular dilation due to pathological drinking would appear to exacerbate the already present neuropathology (1).

In a 6-month follow-up study of schizophrenics and affective psychotics, Kovasznay and coworkers (8) reported that schizophrenics appeared to be more vulnerable to the effects of substance abuse than affective psychotics. Their results indicated that in schizophrenics the clinical deterioration related to substance abuse lasted well beyond the course of active use. This suggested that exposure to substance abuse may cause lasting neuropathological damage.

Although it would appear logical that schizophrenics with substance abuse or dependence have significantly more neuropathology than schizophrenics without, this has been difficult to show objectively. Sullivan and coworkers (9) studied the distinguishing neuropathological features of alcoholics and schizophrenics with MRI. They reported that the "schizophrenic group had tissue volume deficits selective to cortical gray matter, whereas the alcoholic group had tissue volume deficits in gray matter and white matter," and concluded that "distinct pathophysiological processes [were] underlying the structural abnormalities seen in alcoholism and schizophrenia." In accordance with this, Scheller-Gilkey and coworkers (10) hypothesized that schizophrenics with substance use disorder have more structural brain pathology than schizophrenics without; however, their investigation found no significant differences in MRI scans between substance-abusing (61.2% had abused alcohol) and non-substance-abusing schizophrenics.

Mathalon and coworkers (11) studied MRI scans of schizophrenics only, alcoholics only, and people with both disorders. The three groups differed significantly with respect to cortical gray-matter volume in six regions of interest. The schizophrenic group had greater volume deficits than the alcoholics, and the comorbid group was intermediate. Group-by-region interaction showed that the three groups differed significantly in their gray-matter-deficit profile, and the schizophrenics had more frontal and temporal deficits than the alcoholics. The comorbid group's gray-matter-deficit profile did not differ from that of the schizophrenics but did differ from the alcoholics'.

These studies do not point to a simple additive model in which alcoholic schizophrenics automatically show more neuropathological deficits than alcoholics or schizophrenics alone. One simple explanation is that not all schizophrenics have similar levels of cognitive and neuropathological deficit at the outset and that it is the ones with the lesser degrees of impairment who later develop substance abuse. However, a multitude of additional factors may explain these results, and more research is required for better understanding.

DIAGNOSTIC ISSUES

Schizophrenic patients with substance use disorder fall under the general heading of "dual diagnosis"; however, as Kathleen Sciacca (12) has pointed out, this term is an ambiguous one. In 1986, the New York State Commission on Quality of Care for the Mentally Disabled introduced the terms *mentally ill chemical abusers and addicted* (MICAA) and *chemical-abusing mentally ill* (CAMI) to better clarify the interface between psychiatric illness and chemical dependency. The term MICAA denotes individuals with severe, persistent mental illness, accompanied by chemical abuse and/or addiction (Table 1), and CAMI denotes individuals with severe alcohol and/or drug addiction with associated symptoms of mental illness but who are not severly mentally ill (Table 2).

Thus, in evaluating a patient who presents with an active psychosis and active substance abuse, it is critical to determine whether the psychiatric symptomatology is dependent on or independent of the substance abuse. This question must be answered to make an accurate diagnosis and to properly treat the patient. In this discussion, the differential diagnosis is between schizophrenia and substance-induced psychosis.

Rosenthal and Miner (13) pointed out that the most difficult task is the differential diagnosis of psychotic patients who present for treatment. Is the psychosis due only to the abuse of substances in a patient without schizophrenia, to the exacerbation of schizophrenia with minimal input from the substance abused, to an exacerbation caused primarily by the abused substance and not by the disease itself, or to both the substance abuse and schizophrenia?

Although primary and substance-induced psychoses may appear similar, they have different prognostic and therapeutic implications. The

Table 1 Characteristics of the Mentally Ill Chemical Abusers and Addicted (MICAA)

1. Severe mental illness exists independently of substance abuse; persons would meet the diagnostic criteria of a major mental illness even if a substance abuse problem were not present.
2. MICAA persons have a DSM axis I diagnosis of a major psychiatric disorder, such as schizophrenia or major affective disorder.
3. MICAA persons usually require medication to control their psychiatric illness; if medication is stopped, specific symptoms are likely to emerge or worsen.
4. Substance abuse may exacerbate acute psychiatric symptoms, but these symptoms generally persist beyond withdrawal of the precipitating substances.
5. MICAA persons, even when in remission, frequently display the residual effects of major psychiatric disorders (for example, schizophrenia), such as marked social isolation or withdrawal, blunted or inapproprate affect, and marked lack of initiative, interest, or energy. Evidence of these residual effects often differentiates MICAA persons from substance abusers who are not severely mentally ill.

Table 2 Characteristics of the Chemical Abusing Mentally Ill (CAMI)

1. CAMI patients have severe substance dependence (alcoholism, heroin, cocaine, amphetamine, or other addictions), and frequently have multiple substance abuse and/or polysubstance abuse or addiction.
2. CAMI persons usually require treatment in alcohol or drug treatment programs.
3. CAMI persons often have coexistent personality or character disorders (DSM axis II).
4. CAMI patients may appear in the mental health system because of "toxic" or "substance-induced" acute psychotic symptoms that resemble the acute symptoms of a major psychiatric disorder. In this instance, the acute symptoms are always precipitated by substance abuse, and the patient does not have a primary axis I major psychiatric disorder.
5. CAMI patients' acute symptoms remit completely after a period of abstinence or detoxification. This period is usually a few days or weeks, but may be months.
6. CAMI patients do not exhibit the residual effects of a major mental illness when acute (substance abuse) symptoms are in remission.

current default is to assume that the psychosis is exogenously induced until demonstrated otherwise; this strategy reduces the harm of untreated withdrawal as well as of unnecessary exposure to neuroleptics.

The DSM-IV (2) criteria for the diagnosis of substance-induced psychotic disorder can assist the psychiatrist in differentiating psychosis due to exogenous substances from that due to endogenous psychiatric disorders. The criteria are shown in Table 3.

In summary, substance-induced psychotic disorders should be diagnosed only when the psychotic symptoms are:

1. Judged in excess of those usually associated with intoxication or withdrawal
2. Sufficiently severe to warrant independent attention

Table 3 DSM-IV Diagnostic Criteria for Substance-Induced Psychotic Disorder

A. Prominent hallucinations or delusions. Note: Do not include hallucinations if the person has insight that they are substance-induced.
B. There is evidence from the history, physical examination, or laboratory findings of either (1) or (2):
   1. The symptoms in criterion A developed during, or within a month of, substance intoxication or withdrawal
   2. Medication use is etiologically related to the disturbance
C. The disturbance is not better accounted for by a psychotic disorder that is not substance-induced. Evidence that the symptoms are better accounted for by a psychotic disorder that is not substance-induced might include the following: the symptoms precede the onset of the substance use (or medication use); the symptoms persist for a substantial period of time (e.g., about a month) after the cessation of acute withdrawal or severe intoxication, or are substantially in excess of what would be expected given the type or amount of the substance used or the duration of use; or there is other evidence that suggests the existence of an independent non-substance-induced psychotic disorder (e. g., a history of recurrent non-substance-related episodes).
D. The disturbance does not occur exclusively during the course of a delirium.

Note: This diagnosis should be made instead of a diagnosis of substance intoxication or substance withdrawal only when the symptoms are in excess of those usually associated with the intoxication or withdrawal syndrome and when the symptoms are sufficiently severe to warrant independent clinical attention.

Source: Adapted from Ref. 2

3. Not recognized to be substance-induced by the patient
4. Not associated with delirium
5. Not accounted for by a psychotic disorder that is not substance-induced

Substance-induced psychotic disorders can occur in association with intoxication with: alcohol, amphetamine and related substances, cannabis, cocaine, hallucinogens, inhalants, opiods (meperidine), phencyclidine and related substances, sedatives, hypnotics, anxiolytics, and other or unknown substances.

Substance-induced psychotic disorders can also occur in association with withdrawal from: alcohol, sedatives, hypnotics, anxiolytics, and other or unknown substances.

Medications reported (those most frequently used are italicized) to evoke psychotic symptoms include anesthetics and analgesics, anticholinergic agents, anticonvulsants, antihistamines, antihypertensive and cardiovascular medications, antimicrobial medications, antiparkinsonian medications, chemotherapeutic agents (e.g., cyclosporine and procarbazine), *corticosteroids*, gastrointestinal medications, muscle relaxants, nonsteroidal anti-inflammatory medications other than over-the-counter medications (e.g., phenylephrine, *pseudoephedrine*), antidepressant medication, and disulfram. Toxins reported to induce psychotic symptoms include anticholinesterase, organophosphate insecticides, nerve gases, carbon monoxide, and volatile substances such as fuel or paint.

The differential diagnosis of acutely psychotic patients can be difficult and challenging. The following steps should be taken in their evaluation (14). The physician should obtain a history from the patient and collateral informants, review all obtainable medical and psychiatric records and accompanying laboratory reports, and conduct a complete physical examination and laboratory assessment.

The co-occurrence of psychological and substance abuse problems is more likely to bring a patient into a clinical setting than having either one alone. However, substance-abusing patients often minimize their use and try to keep their problems hidden from the physician. For these reasons, information from collateral sources is important, and past medical and psychiatric histories should be reviewed. In addition, a physical examination and the appropriate laboratory tests, including CBC, liver-function tests, and toxicology screen, should be performed.

The psychiatrist's task is to make a diagnosis and treat the syndrome. Of course, substance abuse makes this task more challenging because alcohol and drugs can cause signs and symptoms that mimic most psychiatric disorders.

Determining the timeline of substance abuse and psychiatric symptoms can be essential in the determination of the independence of the two disorders. The age at which the patient developed problems and fulfilled criteria for substance abuse should be noted. Psychiatric symptomatology should also be reviewed in the course of the substance abuse history to determine parallels and correlations between the two. Framing symptomatology with anchor points such as graduations, wedding dates, deaths, and military discharge dates can help the patient remember critical periods. It is also important to probe for periods of abstinence of three or more months and to determine their relationship to psychiatric symptoms.

If major psychiatric symptoms occurred before the onset of substance abuse or during periods of *prolonged* abstinence, then the individual most likely suffers from two independent disorders. If no major syndrome can be demonstrated either before or in the *prolonged* absence of substance abuse, the psychiatric syndrome is probably secondary to the substance abuse.

TREATMENT

Programmatic Treatment

Until the last decade, addictive disorders and psychiatric disorders were treated separately (15,16). In psychiatric settings addictive disorders tended to be underdiagnosed, and in addiction settings psychiatric disorders tended to be underdiagnosed. Psychiatric treatment has traditionally emphasized nurturance. However, additional therapeutic strategies are needed to effectively rehabilitate substance abusers. Many addiction programs have emphasized self-control and personal responsibility and have used direct confrontation as a therapeutic strategy. However, these approaches may not be suited to schizophrenics who have difficulties in understanding the relationship between psychiatric symptoms and behavior, who have cognitive deficits, and who have an increased vulnerability to interpersonal stress.

The factors that facilitate abstinence are high levels of motivation and the ability to exert self-control in the face of temptation. Unfortunately, many schizophrenics have limitations in these very areas and suffer from low levels of motivation, poor self-control, residual symptoms, cognitive impairment, and social isolation. Many see no reason for abstinence. With no employment, no family support, and no positive relationships, they have nothing, and they have nothing to lose.

Thus, the traditional psychiatric and substance abuse treatment programs often do not have sufficient expertise to treat the dually diagnosed (MICAA) patient, so psychiatric patients with addictive disorders often do not receive comprehensive care.

In order to address the problems of comorbidity, both psychiatric and addiction settings have had to make alterations. Many addiction treatment programs have added trained psychiatric staff and established special tracks for the dual patient. In addition, the use of medication to treat comorbid psychiatric disorders has gained increasing acceptance in the addiction treatment community.

Models for the treatment of comorbity in psychiatric settings have included the serial, parallel, and integrated treatment models.

The serial model encompasses initial psychiatric stabilization at one site and addiction treatment at a separate, independent site. Since neither the psychiatric nor the addictive staff participates in combined treatment, the psychiatric and addictive approaches often remain apart and in conflict. Neither staff is knowledgeable about the approach of the other, and treatment may be fragmented and antagonistic.

The parallel model also encompasses psychiatric and addictive treatment by different staff members at separate sites, but concurrently. The limitations of this model are similar to those of the serial model, and treatment may be further complicated by the patient's being concurrently involved in two systems with different and potentially conflicting approaches.

The integrated model has one staff that simultaneously provides psychiatric and addictive therapeutic modalities. The staff members are trained in both disciplines, the patient receives treatment from a unified system, and the needs of both disorders are met at the same time. The integrated model is indicated for the MICAA patients who can benefit from a less confrontational and more supportive approach.

A major limitation of the integrated model is that it may lead to undertreatment of addictive disorders and overdiagnosis and overtreatment of psychiatric disorders in patients with only an addictive disorder. For severely addicted CAMI patients who come to treatment for the psychiatric consequences of their addiction (e.g., suicidal or homicidal ideation, psychosis, severe anxiety, or depression), the integrated model may not provide the required level of intensity of addiction treatment.

Integrated Treatment

Dually diagnosed patients need a program that integrates both psychiatric and substance abuse treatment. They also require careful assessment since patients may differ widely in their ability to actively participate in the program, assume responsibility for their behavior, and resist temptation. Treatment for substance abuse in schizophrenia needs to be integrated with broad-based psychosocial rehabilitation because there is no clear demarkation between substance abuse problems and the psychosocial problems characteristic of the illness.

Minkoff (16) has described a model for conceptualizing comorbid psychiatric and addictive disorders in which both are considered primary, chronic, and requiring specific and intensive treatment. Recovery is subdivided into four phases:

1. Acute stabilization
2. Engagement
3. Prolonged stabilization
4. Rehabilitation/recovery

The engagement and last two treatment phases have been further subdivided into engagement, persuasion (education), active treatment, and relapse prevention. Each phase requires specific intervention strategies.

In Minkoff's model, general principles have been developed for treating addictions in psychiatric populations.

1. Treatment of addictions should be the same as in nonpsychiatric populations, with elements of intervention, education, empathic confrontation of denial, relapse prevention, and intensive, ongoing recovery in self-help and professionally led groups. Pharmacotherapy should be adjunctive and not a primary method of intervention.
2. Standard addiction treatment should be modified before it is applied to psychiatric patients. Modifications include special preparation for 12-Step programs, simplifications of traditional step assignments to accommodate cognitive limitations, modification of group or step work to include dual-diagnosis questions, and special social-skills training. Dual diagnosis AA meetings in which individuals may speak more comfortably about their psychiatric symptoms and medications are important.

In addition, intensive case management with assertive outreach should be part of the program (17). Case managers should actively moniter progress, provide crisis intervention, educate patients about both substance abuse and mental health, reiterate treatment recommendations, and coordinate planning across community services.

Drake and Mueser (18) conducted a comprehensive review of the psychosocial approaches to dual diagnosis. Although there are few outcome studies of dual-diagnosis programs, investigation is under way to determine the efficacy of this integrated treatment approach (19).

Pharmacotherapy

From the literature, there appear to be at least three major risk factors for the intiation and continuation of substance abuse in the schizophrenic patient that are amenable to pharmacotherapeutic intervention: nonpsychotic symptoms, neuroleptic side effects, and alcohol craving.

Krystal and coworkers (7) have reviewed the pharmacotherapy of comorbid substance abuse in schizophrenics and have developed guidelines for the treatment of substance abuse risk factors, including EPS, positive and negative symptoms, emotional distress, cognitive dysfunction, and residual withdrawal symptoms. They have advocated the use of atypical antipsychotics as one important strategy for reducing negative symptoms, emotional stess, and cognitive dysfunction.

Nonpsychotic dysphoric states have been associated with substance use and abuse (5,6). Thus, it is important for the physician to treat low mood, tension, anhedonia, insomnia, and the negative symptoms of schizophrenia as aggressively as the psychotic symptoms. The use of atypical antipsychotics, buspirone, antidepressants, and benzodiazepines are clearly indicated to ameliorate this symptomatology. Also, newer atypical antipsychotics have clear advantages over the older typical ones in that they are effective in treating the negative symptoms and also offer additional anxiolytic and antidepressant effects.

The efficacy of clozapine in reducing substance abuse in schizophrenics has been reported. Several case reports (20,21) have revealed that clozapine decreases both psychosis and concurrent substance abuse in previously refractory patients. Recently Zimmet and coworkers (22) reported that over 85% of their schizophrenic and schizoaffective patients with active substance abuse decreased their use after the initiation of clozapine in the Clozapine Clinic at the Massachusetts Mental Health Center. Drake and coworkers (23) reported that alcohol-abusing schizophrenic and schizoaffective patients in a dual-diagnosis program showed significant reductions in drinking days and alcohol abuse and significant improvement in treatment progress when they were taking clozapine. However, the reason for the decrease in substance use was not clear in either study, and Zimmet and coworkers pointed out that it may have been related to the effect of clozapine on psychiatric symptoms or to its benign extrapyramidal profile rather than to a distinct effect of clozapine on comorbid substance abuse. In addition, weekly visits required for the monitoring of clozapine patients may also be beneficial.

Krystal and colleagues (7) stated, "Extrapyramidal symptoms are an important source of neuroleptic-induced dysphoria." Addington and Duchak (6) found that 24% of their schizophrenic/schizoaffective subjects reported that they used alcohol, and 38% used cannabis to decrease the "slowed-down" feeling caused by prescribed medication. Hence, the psychiatrist should strive to minimize neuroleptic-induced side effects by lowering the dose of neuroleptic medication, optimizing adjuvant medications, or switching to an antipsychotic with a lower side-effect profile.

Alcoholism research has been stimulated by the appearance of three new products—naltrexone, acamprosate, and nalmefene—that have been demonstrated to reduce drinking, craving, and relapse rates, and so may hold new hope for the dually diagnosed patient (24–27). Naltrexone and nalmefene are opiate-receptor antagonists, and acamprosate is an amino acid derivative (calcium acetylhomotaurinate) that affects γ-aminobutyric acid (GABA) and glutamate neurotransmission.

Naltrexone, which is currently available in the United States, has been shown in multiple studies to significantly reduce relapse rates in alcohol-abusing and -dependent patients. It has also been shown to be safe and tolerable when given to schizophrenic patients taking neuroleptics (28).

Acamprosate has been used in Europe but has not been approved for use in the United States. European studies suggest that it can significantly improve retention in treatment, increase time to first alcohol consumption, and increase abstinent days. Nalmefene has also been shown to decrease alcohol relapse rates (29,30). However, more research needs to be carried out.

SUMMARY

It is important for the psychiatrist to realize that about half of patients with schizophrenia also have a substance use disorder (see Table 4). Because patients may not give a complete history of their chemical

Table 4 Summary of Main Points

1. About half of schizophrenic patients have substance use disorder.
2. Nonpsychotic symptoms, neuroleptic side effects, and social isolation appear to be important treatable risk factors for substance abuse.
3. It is important to differentiate the patient with a psychosis independent of substance abuse from the patient with a psychosis dependent on substance abuse. The DSM-IV criteria for substance-induced psychotic disorder will aid in this differentiation.
4. The schizophrenic with substance abuse or dependence requires an integrated program that will simultaneously address both the mental illness and chemical dependency.
5. Atypical antipsychotics address negative symptomatology and also have fewer side effects. This may decrease the risk of the initiation of substance abuse or of its continuance. Recent data indicate that clozapine decreases substance abuse in schizophrenic patients.
6. Naltrexone may become an important part of the pharmacological treatment of the schizophrenic alcoholic. It has been shown to be efficacious in preventing relapse in nonschizophrenic alcoholics, and one study indicates that it is well tolerated in schizophrenic patients taking neuroleptics. Acamprosate and nalmefene may also prove effective when available in the United States.

abuse, information from collateral sources should be obtained. It is important to differentiate psychosis related to exogenous factors from that related to an endogenous illness. This can be facilitated by using the DSM-IV criteria for substance-induced psychotic disorder and by taking a thorough and careful history. Nonpsychotic symptoms, neuroleptic side effects, and social isolation in patients with schizophrenia should be treated aggressively because studies have found them to be risk factors for substance abuse.

For psychosocial treatment of the schizophrenic substance abuser, dual-diagnosis programs and support groups should be encouraged and assertive case management applied (see Table 5). For the pharmacological treatment, atypical antipsychotics show much promise because of their efficacy with negative symptoms and their low side-effect profile. Clozapine has been shown to reduce substance abuse in schizophrenic patients in individual case reports and in recent studies. Naltrexone also appears to be a valuable addition to the pharmacological armamentarium because of it efficacy in preventing alcohol relapse.

Table 5 Guidelines for Physicians

1. In evaluating and treating patients with schizophrenia physicians should actively look for the signs and symptoms of substance abuse. Patient history should be verified with collateral informants, medical records, and laboratory tests.
2. Patients who do have a substance use disorder should be directed to dual-diagnosis programs or support groups if they are available. Assertive case management is important in the follow-up of the dual-diagnosis patient.
3. Nonpsychotic symptoms, neuroleptic side effects, and social isolation should be aggressively treated because they are reversible risk factors for substance abuse.

REFERENCES

1. Newcomer JW. Schizophrenia and delusional disorders. In: Guze SB, ed. Washington University Adult Psychiatry. St. Louis: Mosby, 1997:211–240.
2. American Psychiatric Association. Diagnostic and Statistical Manual of Mental Disorders. 4th ed. Washington, DC: American Psychiatric Press, 1994.
3. Mueser KT, Bellack AS, Blanchard JJ. Comorbidity of schizophrenia and substance abuse: implications for treatment. J Consult Clin Psychol 1992; 60(6):845–856.
4. Kosten TR, Ziedonis DM. Substance abuse and schizophrenia. Schizophr Bull 1997; 23(2):181–186.
5. Noordsy DL, Drake RE, Teague GB, Osher FC, Hurlbut SC, Beaudett MS, Paskus TS. Subjective experiences related to alcohol use among schizophrenics. J Nerv Ment Dis 1991; 179(7):410–414.
6. Addington J, Duchak V. Reasons for substance use in schizophrenia. Acta Psychiatr Scand 1997; 96:329–333.
7. Krystal JH, D'Souza DC, Madonick S, Petrakis IL. Toward a rational pharmacotherapy of comorbid substance abuse in schizophrenic patients. Schizophr Res 1999; 35:S35–S49.
8. Kovasznay B, Fleischer J, Tanenberg-Karant M, Jandorf L, Miller AD, Bromet E. Substance use disorder and the early course of illness in schizophrenia and affective psychosis. Schizophr Bull 1997; 23(2):195–201.
9. Sullivan EV, Mathalon DH, Lim KO, Marsh L, Pfefferbaum A. Patterns of regional cortical dysmorphology distinguishing schizophrenia and chronic alcoholism. Biol Psychiatry 1998; 43:118–131.
10. Scheller-Gilkey G, Lewine RR Caudle J, Brown FW. Schizophrenia, substance use, and brain morphology. Schizophr Res 1999; 35:113–120.
11. Mathalon DH, Sullivan EV, Lim KO, Pfefferbaum A. Gray matter deficits in schizophrenia-alcoholism comorbidity. Biol Psychiatry 1995; 37:629.

12. Sciacca K. An integrated treatment approach for severely mentally ill individuals with substance disorders. In: Minkoff K, Drake RE, eds. Dual Diagnosis of Major Mental Illness and Substance Disorder. San Francisco: Jossey-Bass, 1991:69–84.
13. Rosenthal RN, Miner CR. Differential diagnosis of substance-induced psychosis and schizophrenia in patients with substance use disorders. Schizophr Bull 1997; 23(2):187–193.
14. Anthenelli RM. The initial evaluation of the dual diagnosis patient. Psychiatr Ann 1994; 24(8):407–411.
15. Minkoff K. Program components of a comprehensive integrated care system for serious mentally ill patients with substance disorders. In: Minkoff K, Drake RE, eds. Dual Diagnosis of Major Mental Illness and Substance Disorder. San Francisco: Jossey-Bass, 1991:13–27.
16. Minkoff K. Models for addiction treatment in psychiatric populations. Psychiatr Ann 1994; 24(8):412–417.
17. Drake RE, Osher FC, Wallach MA. Homelessness and dual diagnosis. Am Psychologist 1991; 46(11):1149–1158.
18. Drake RE, Mueser KT. Psychosocial approaches to dual diagnosis. Schizophr Bull 2000; 26(1):105–118.
19. Ho AP, Tsuang JW, Liberman RP, Wang R, Wilkins JN, Eckman TA, Shaner AL. Achieving effective treatment of patients with chronic psychotic illness and comorbid substance dependence. Am J Psychiatry 1999; 156(11):1765–1770.
20. Albanese MJ, Khantzian EJ, Murphy SL, Green AI. Decreased substance use in chronically psychotic patient treated with clozapine. Am J Psychiatry 1994; 151(5):780–1781.
21. Tsuang JW, Eckman TA, Shaner AL, Marder SR. Clozapine for substance-abusing schizophrenic patients. Am J Psychiatry 1999; 156(7):1119–1120.
22. Zimmet SV, Strous RD, Burgess ES, Kohnstamm S, Green AI. Effects of clozapine on substance use in patients with schizophrenia and schizoaffective disorder: a retrospective survey. J Clin Psychopharmacol 2000; 20(1):94–98.
23. Drake RE, Xie H, McHugo GJ, Green AI. The effects of clozapine on alcohol and drug use disorders among patients with schizophrenia. Schizophr Bull 2000; 26(2):441–449.
24. Anton RF. New directions in the pharmacotherapy of alcoholism. Psychiatr Ann 1995; 25(6):353–362.
25. Litten RZ, Allen JP. Advances in development of medications for alcoholism treatment. Psychopharmacology 1998; 139:20–33.
26. Kranzler HR, Amin H, Modesto-Lowe V, Oncken C. Pharmacologic treatments for drug and alcohol dependence. Psychiatr Clin North Am 1999; 22(2):401–423.
27. Garbutt JC, West SL, Carey TS, Lohr KN, Crews FT. Pharmacological treatment of alcohol dependence: a review of the evidence. JAMA 1999; 281(14):1318–1325.

28. Sernyak MJ, Glazer WM, Heninger GR, Charney DS, Woods SW, Petrakis IL, Krystal JH, Price LH. Naltrexone augmentation of neuroleptics in schizophrenia. J Clin Psychopharmacol 1998; 18(3):248–251.
29. Mason BJ, Ritvo EC, Morgan RO, Salvato FR, Goldberg G, Welch B, Mantero-Atienza E. A double-blind, placebo-controlled pilot study to evaluate the efficacy and safety of oral nalmefene HCL for alcohol dependence. Alcoholism: Clin Exp Res 1994; 18:1162–1167.
30. Mason BJ, Salvato FR, Williams LD, Ritvo EC, Cutler RB. A double-blind, placebo-controlled study of oral nalmefene for alcohol dependence. Arch Gen Psychiatry 1999; 56:719–724.

13

Family Education

A Guide for Developing a Program

Mary Will
Metropolitan St. Louis Psychiatric Center
St. Louis, Missouri

INTRODUCTION

Family education is now considered an essential component of any comprehensive treatment program for patients with schizophrenia. This chapter describes how one hospital, Metropolitan St. Louis Psychiatric Center (MSLPC), developed a family education program, its reasons for doing so, and the results that were obtained. It is my hope that by following the suggestions in this chapter you will easily be able to develop an education program for your setting.

MSLPC considers families a vital resource in the treatment and rehabilitation of severely mentally ill persons. Families are often the only support system available to the ill person. The stress and burden of caring for a mentally ill relative can be enormous and have devastating effects on families. It is extremely difficult—sometimes impossible—to meet the many needs and demands of the ill person. It adds to the stress when family members have little or no understanding of mental illness, or believe they may have contributed to their relative's developing the illness.

As noted, families may feel guilt and blame themselves for having a mentally ill relative. To manage the situation, families need to muster all the skills and knowledge currently available. Many families new to the system have no idea how to access information about mental illness and so are unable to adequately develop a knowledge base or gain skills to cope with schizophrenia. Even those who have a relative with a chronic mental illness do not always have the knowledge and necessary skills to support the patient.

Why then are there so few formal family education programs? Before we developed such a program at MSPLC our physicians were more than willing to meet with families and did so; however, physicians alone could not meet all the needs of families for information and education. Conflicts in work schedules and time constraints made it difficult for physicians and families to meet. Without a formal family education program that met on a regular bases, family contact was on a catch-as-catch-can basis even though all parties concerned were willing to meet.

There are many reasons why education to families has been overlooked or neglected in the past. Some families work during hours when staff are available. Clients may not give permission for family involvement. In some hospitals, rapid turnover of clients in an acute care setting is a disincentive to family involvement and staff may be occupied in other responsibilities when families do visit. However, no matter how legitimate these reasons are for not providing systematic education to families, a formal program that addresses family needs in a logical, organized fashion is now considered essential.

Prior to developing a formal program, it is wise to seek advice from other nearby hospitals or centers that already have a family education program. In our case, we contacted all state facilities and private hospitals in the St. Louis area. To our surprise, no facility had a formally organized program. Most professionals were rather pessimistic in discussing the development of a program, saying, "Nobody will come . . . we tried it and it didn't work . . . people aren't interested." Despite such daunting input, we forged ahead. A literature search was conducted to evaluate the approaches for our education program. While no one "best" approach was identified, we did discover a range of different approaches to dealing with family education (1–4). Books were selected based on this literature review to develop an educational approach for the program. These materials provided a systematic, organized process that could easily be adapted to a range of settings, including an acute care hospital, long-term residential care, and an outpatient setting. It is best to take a concrete, realistic approach to developing an educational program. In our case, we needed a short-term (4-week) program that would meet the requested needs of families.

GETTING STARTED

The time and effort expended in getting started are extremely important and—except for some action-oriented people—difficult to muster. Although beginning is a slow process, perseverance is essential. Designing the curricula, arranging the schedule, and selecting presenters all entail research, decision making, and patience. The time spent in preparation is worthwhile because, once this work is completed, presenting the program is relatively easy.

Prior to planning, it is essential to identify who will be responsible for developing and implementing the program. One person, rather than a committee or a taskforce, with the input and assistance of other staff, should be responsible for this task. The person selected should have a strong investment in family education and be committed to developing a quality program. In 1998, the Social Work Department and the Patient/Family Education Team at MSLPC were charged with developing our family education program. As the director of the Social Work Department and team leader of the Education Team, I was ultimately responsible for developing and implementing the program.

Agnes Hatfield, in *Family Education in Mental Illness*, defined preplanning as follows: "The essence of planning programs for education is to direct attention to three basic questions: what do we want to accomplish, how can we accomplish it and how well did we accomplish it?" (5).

There are four crucial steps to follow prior to starting a program. First and foremost, one must get the support of hospital or clinic administration. Although it might seem logical that such support would be automatic, don't assume this is the case. MSLPC was fortunate in that members of our administration served on the board of the local chapter of the National Alliance for the Mentally Ill (NAMI) and so were committed to our efforts. The hospital CEO volunteered to provide an introduction to the program at the first session of each monthly cycle of meetings.

The second step in developing the program might also seem obvious, but it is sometimes not even considered: ask the families in your community what they want. Don't just give them what you, the professionals, think they want or need. At MSLPC our Social Work Department developed a simple survey for families to complete, asking if they wanted a program and, if so, what they wanted to obtain from it.

Third, conduct a literature search to gather as much information as possible related to family education, always keeping in mind your own goals and objectives for the program. You might ask members of your local chapter of NAMI and other mental health support groups for advice. Such groups are extremely helpful, supportive, and enthusiastic about developing such programs and usually also agree to be participants in one or more sessions.

The fourth step in developing a family education program is to consider the setting of the program and the community to which it will be presented. Our hospital is a state-funded acute care psychiatric hospital with a short to moderate average length of stay. It is located in an urban area serving the economically deprived and those not having the access to private care. Since our hospital has a rapid turnover, we needed to reach as many families as possible in a limited time, preferably while their family members were still hospitalized. One of our goals was to build collaborative relationships with families so that they would receive education to assist them in managing the acute as well as long-term needs of their ill relatives. Because of the short length of stay, we wanted to engage families as quickly as possible and encourage them to complete the program even if their relative was discharged from the hospital.

THE SURVEY

We developed a simple survey form and asked families to indicate their interests, the hours and days preferred, and the topics and preferred methods of instruction. The families of our patients did indicate an interest in a program and expressed their preferences for topics and instructional methods. Most responses indicated that the greatest interest was in learning about serious mental illness and how the medications would help. Our families were also interested in how to obtain support in the community and other local resources. The survey asked about barriers to attendance, such as transportation and possible childcare problems, but such barriers were not always acknowledged as problems. Our families' preferred instruction methods were lectures with handouts, pamphlets, and video presentations. However, our survey was not especially helpful in determining a day or time for the program—because the responses reflected no consensus, we selected a time when all presenters would be available. The disciplines represented in the program were psychiatry, pharmacy, nursing, psychology, and social work. Our program was held on four consecutive Tuesdays with two presentations during each weekly session.

THE LITERATURE SEARCH

Because our hospital had had no previous formal family education program, thorough research in the field of family education was needed. After extensive review of the literature, we selected two books by designers of such programs. The first book selected was *Family Education in Mental Illness*, by Agnes B. Hatfield, Ph.D. (4). This book is invaluable for professionals working in the field of mental illness and providing family education, and ought to be on the required reading list for all professionals preparing for work with families who have a mentally ill relative. At our hospital, each member of the social work staff who would serve as group facilitators for the program was given his or her own copy and required to read it and discuss it in department meetings. This and many other books have been written by Dr. Hatfield in her dual role as mother of a mentally ill son and one of the founders of the Maryland Alliance for the Mentally Ill.

The second book selected was *Educating Patients and Families about Mental Illness*, by Cynthia Carson Bisbee, Ph.D. (5). This is a manual that breaks down the development of a family education program into simple steps. It presents a how-to approach with course content, outlines, handouts, forms, and anything else one might need for such a program. This manual can be strongly recommended to anyone because it may be adapted to any type of program, including those needed for acute care hospitals, long-term residential care facilities, and outpatient clinics. Dr. Bisbee's book addresses patient education as well as education for the family. It presents a wealth of information, much of it invaluable for designing a family education program. For our purposes, Dr. Hatfield's book and Dr. Bisbee's manual, our principal resources, best met our needs and approach to family education.

POPULATION AND SETTING

At MSLPC the families we serve are mainly from an economically disadvantaged population in an urban area. We also serve clients from surrounding rural counties, who also generally are economically disadvantaged. Because MSLPC is a state-funded acute care psychiatric hospital we typically serve persons without insurance or whose insurance has expired. Many of our families are employed but they must care for a mentally ill relative and sometimes for aging parents as well. Such families typically have many constraints on their time, and have little time or desire to devote to outside activities. For this reason, we designed a short, 4-week program to meet the needs of our families. However, our local chapter of NAMI has a 9-week family education course to which we can refer families after completion of our program.

CONTENT OF THE PROGRAM

The content of the program was based on our review of the literature, our survey results, and staff experiences in working with families. Most families wanted in-depth information about serious mental illness and how the medications could help. In addition, many families wanted to know what to do when prescribed medicine didn't work. They were interested in finding help in the community and knowing what resources were available for their ill relatives. Because caring for an ill relative can be very stressful, stress-reduction techniques and problem-solving methods were included in the program. Sometimes four videos relating to families and their experiences with mentally ill relatives would be shown in lieu of stress-reduction techniques or problem solving. The videos chosen were the three "Bonnie Tapes," which discuss mental illness from the points of view of a family, a patient, and the patient's sister. The fourth video, "Families Coping with Mental Illness," shows 10 persons discussing coping with a relative with schizophrenia or bipolar disorder. The length of the program was based on the amount of time needed for the above presentations and the perceived attention span of the audience. Our initial prediction was that family members would not attend for more than 4 weeks, and this prediction was borne out by our attendance records.

PROGRAM MATERIALS

A flyer describing the MSLPC family education program was framed and placed in our emergency room, in our lobby, and at the entrance to each treatment unit. Brochures were also placed in the lobby and emergency room, and were sent to several agencies that provide outpatient services to discharged clients. We solicited public service announcements and advertisements in several local newspapers. Our hospital wanted families in the community to understand that the program was accessible even to those whose relatives used private hospitals or outpatient services.

Social workers on the treatment units were selected to personally invite family members to the program because they had the most consistent contact with families. An invitation letter and a brief description of the program were sent to families by the unit social worker. Handouts relating to each week's topics were either developed or obtained from other sources. Sign-in and evaluation forms to be used weekly were created. This way attendance could be tracked and each presentation could be individually evaluated. (The manual written by Dr. Bisbee (5) was very helpful in developing forms, although they would probably need to be customized for a particular program and locale.)

Brochures were obtained from other agencies that provided services to the mentally ill, such as vocational rehabilitation agencies, day programs, and consumer groups. Folders to hold each week's handouts were distributed at the first session each month. Additional handouts, matched to the particular presentations, were distributed each week. These folders were to be kept by family members attending the program. New information regarding mental illness and treatment that we discovered during the course of the 4 weeks was also distributed to the participants. Some of our speakers developed overhead presentations for such topics as psychiatric medications, community resources, stress management, and problem-solving methods.

PRESENTATIONS AND PRESENTERS

Family education should be interdisciplinary. Presenters in the various disciplines should provide education according to their particular expertise. With the support of your administration, you should be able to obtain volunteers from different disciplines. At our hospital, social work staff was chosen to facilitate the program each month and also present at the fourth session on community resources. Our medical director, who reviewed basic information on the psychiatric diagnosis, presented the first session of the program. Presenters from pharmacy, nursing, and psychology also lent their expertise to the program.

Finally, in the last session, the associate director of our local chapter of NAMI gave one of our most important presentations. This presentation added credibility to the program because the speaker was the mother of a mentally ill son and a tireless worker with NAMI (Table 1). Frequently family members who have "been through the mill" discuss a particularly difficult decision or problem. Having a presenter who also has a mentally ill relative and who has "been there and done that" is invaluable.

We selected the hours of 6–8 P.M. for the program, giving families ample time to visit their hospitalized relatives (visiting hours at our

Table 1 Weekly Topics

Week 1	Symptoms and causes of mental illness
Week 2	Medications
	Noncompliance, civil commitment, guardianship
Week 3	Problem-solving methods
	Stress reduction
	Family videos and discussion
Week 4	Community resources
	Family support

hospital last until 9 P.M.). The program was held on four consecutive Tuesday evenings each month. One presentation was held on the first evening and two presentations were held on each of the next three. No session was held on a fifth Tuesday in a month unless there was a special request for coverage of a specific topic.

The sequence of the presentations was as follows. The first week's presentation was on the symptoms and causes of serious mental illness. Schizophrenia and mood disorders were featured as these are the predominant diagnoses in our hospital. On the second Tuesday, a pharmacist and nurse presented on psychiatric medications, another popular topic, and a member of the social work stafff provided information on noncompliance, civil commitment, and guardianship. The third week's session opened with a presentation by a psychologist on approaches to problem solving. In the second hour, a family video was shown, followed by open discussion. Following the second week's presentations, families were given the option to request particular topics for the third week, but rarely was anything requested other than the planned presentations.

The fourth week's presentation provided information on community resources and family support groups. The facilitating social worker presented the information on community resources and how to access them. During the second hour of this presentation, information on NAMI and family support was provided. The presenter for this hour was the associate director of the St. Louis chapter of NAMI, also the mother of a mentally ill son. The family members appreciated that the presenter was "one of them" and understood the problems that families face.

RECRUITMENT OF FAMILY MEMBERS

The key to successful recruitment is personal contact and follow-up. As mentioned earlier, the unit social workers at MSLPC personally invite families to the program, although any staff member could also do so. The only criterion for selection is that the family member have a relative with a serious mental illness. After being personally invited, families receive an invitation letter with the referring social worker's name and phone number in case more information is needed. Finally, the social worker makes follow-up calls on the evening prior to each Tuesday meeting to remind families of the program. In addition to the families of our patients, families were sometimes referred to attend the program from the community or from friends who had attended previously.

One may ask why so much effort needs to be expended in recruitment. There are several reasons. Feedback we had received from other institutions who had tried to establish a family education program was pessimistic about recruiting families to attend. Further, our own prior experience in trying to arrange meetings with families was that cancelations were frequent. Because of work schedules, conflicting responsibilities, or lack of transportation, family members are not always able to accept additional commitments.

It's important to remember to act like a successful salesperson when recruiting families. Believe in your product. Be enthusiastic and upbeat about your product, which, after all, is education. Without follow-up, it is doubtful that many families will attend the program. Thus, recruitment must be an ongoing process, not merely to start the program. When participating staff become tired of recruiting, they should be reminded of its importance. When attendance dwindles, a reminder memo to staff from the program director can increase attendance. Another incentive to increase the attendance of family members is refreshments. It is easy and effective to serve cookies, coffee, tea, and lemonade.

TRAINING STAFF

Members of our social work staff served as group facilitators for our program. Assigned on a monthly-rotation schedule, it was their responsibility to keep the sessions running smoothly and to redirect any attendees who tended to dominate the sessions or dwell overly long on their own issues. Some staff expressed concern about being able to facilitate such groups. *Material from Family Education in Mental Illness* (4) was helpful in training group presenters.

Participating staff thoroughly reviewed their own material as well as general material from Dr. Hatfield's book prior to their presentations. This brought some measure of relief to those unsure of their ability to facilitate or present, and gave them guidelines regarding situations likely to be encountered. Successful presenters are flexible and adaptable and can gauge the needs of the audience. Even though selected topics were scheduled for each week, we were not rigid in our approach. If it was observed that the audience wanted to veer from a topic, the facilitator adapted to this need.

It is important for the success of any program to address the concerns of participating staff when they voice anxiety and to take time and effort to assist them. This consideration also decreases resistance to adding yet another assignment to an already heavy workload. Social workers, and other presenters, became more at ease with the Family Education Program and came to consider it one of their more rewarding assignments.

OVERHEAD PRESENTATIONS AND VIDEOS

All visual materials, such as slides and overheads, were designed to be simple and to the point, and to highlight the salient features of various presentations. Videos related to family education can be ordered and should be reviewed prior to selection for the program. As noted earlier, for our program we selected "The Bonnie Tapes" and "Families Coping with Mental Illness." In the "Bonnie Tapes" series there are three videos: one from the family's perspective, one from the patient's, and one from that of the patient's "well" sister. The sister's video, which represents a perspective not often heard, is particularly moving. "Families Coping with Mental Illness," also an excellent video, shows 10 family members discussing having a relative with mental illness. A positive feature of this video is the diversity of the participating family members.

It is also important to carefully consider the room where you plan to hold your program. If you do not have a choice of rooms, make the one you have as presentable as possible. Besides an overhead projector and television monitor, it helps to have comfortable chairs. If you are fortunate in having more than one available room, choose the one that is more conducive to interaction between families. Our experience suggests that long tables arranged in the shape of a U may be better than round tables, as this facilitates more interaction between presenters and those attending. Don't forget to ensure that the room temperature remains stable—if the room is under- or overheated there are likely to be complaints. Although these issues may seem minor, comfortable surroundings are needed to allow people to concentrate and focus on the presentation.

ATTENDANCE AND EVALUATION

Once all the above steps have been completed and the program is underway, it is time to check the evaluation forms. Examples of forms can be obtained from Dr. Bisbee's manual (5) and are easily adapted for a particular program. One should make the forms as short and simple as possible without sacrificing essential information. During the first months of our program, the evaluation forms were revised several times as we attempted to increase the response rate. The family members appeared to dislike filling out evaluation forms—even a one-page form was rarely fully completed, and this is still often the case.

It is common to find that satisfaction with the program is consistently reported at the 98 to 100% rate. Therefore, it is important to state at the beginning of each session that you want family members to say what they don't like as well as what they do like. Stress that suggestions for improvement will not hurt the feelings of the organizers, who want to improve the program and need the feedback of the participants to do so. These families are usually so appreciative of an opportunity to learn about mental illness that their gratitude outweighs negative aspects they may encounter. However, their hunger for knowledge should not imply that they would accept a program of poor quality. Shoddy presentations are easily recognized as such.

At our hospital, since August 1998, 914 people have attended our family education program—approximately 41 persons per month, 10 for each weekly session. Of the 914 participants, 557 completed evaluation forms and 548 indicated that they were highly satisfied.

Although the number of persons attending each month averaged 41, attendance varied widely on a weekly basis—there might be 20–25 one week and 5 the next. On occasion, there was only one participant. No matter what the attendance, the program proceeded. In fact, when attendance was low, the program was adapted according to the participants' requests. Although low attendance can be discouraging, it is essential to persevere and continue the program. Whatever the number of persons attending, those present state that they find it worthwhile. When only one or two attend, they seem to enjoy the extra attention.

When attendance levels are low, it is important to remember that they will usually improve. Increasing recruitment efforts may help, but such efforts do not always result in higher attendance.

SUMMARY

Two years after implementing a formal family education program, I believe that this type of program is the most efficient and successful way to approach education of family members and the community at large. Program evaluations and remarks from families support this conclusion. However, any program should be an evolving one. The participants in our program are continually asking if there is something more we can offer. We recently added a presentation on the coexistence of mental illness and substance use/abuse. At times facilitators may need to adapt a presentation to the family members attending, especially when their needs are greater than the planned program. Facilitators and presenters must be adaptable and flexible, and still be able to direct the presentation. Being adaptive requires a high degree of skill and experience on the part of the facilitators and presenters, which emphasizes the need to train staff prior to implementation of the program.

Understanding the needs of the audience to which you are directing the program is perhaps one of the most crucial element of a successful program. You are likely to have different levels of need within the same audience, which can be challenging as you tailor the presentations. With training and experience, the skills to tailor each presentation to specific audiences can be acquired by all participants.

It is also important to keep up with new and different approaches to educational programming. This is important because new material is always becoming available for use. For our program, we continually update the material and its content. If presenters feel the need to include new information, this is encouraged. If family members request something different, we try to follow their lead. The bottom line is to be flexible and adaptable and to offer many options.

According to Hatfield (4), "We need to learn how to keep new ways of doing things continually changing and evolving." She stresses the importance of recognizing obstacles to change. In this regard, J. W. Gardner's book *Self Renewal: The Individual and the Innovative Society* (6) may also be helpful. He contends that most obstacles to change exist in people's minds rather than in reality. It is easy to become complacent with a successful program and to feel that you have found the right way to do it. Actually, the "right" way is the one that works best for families and addresses the needs they present. As the experience and treatment of mental illnesses continue to change, these needs must also change.

According to Gardner (6), vested interests can, and often do, develop in new programs. It can become "my program," "my way of doing things," "my success," and this kind of thinking may not lend itself to change or innovation. Of course, we have all had these feelings and had to struggle to overcome them. Institutions can also have a vested interest in the status quo and be unwilling to change or consider new ideas. However, if the person in charge of the program is aware of and alert to this kind of limited perspective, it can be overcome. It is wise to schedule regular discussions about the program to solicit new ideas for improvement.

Developing an educational approach does not mean that being individually supportive to families should be neglected. Families still need and want much individual support. Indeed, the best presenters and facilitators are excellent at providing both support and encouragement to individual families. Also, families should be strongly encouraged to join NAMI and participate in its support groups as well as other available activities.

Eventually, the effectiveness of the program should be formally evaluated. MSLPC has not done this because of other considerations, but is open to this in the future. Participants may be asked to complete pre- and post-tests for this purpose.

This chapter was written to assist with developing your own program. The key points for success we identified are listed in Table 2. At times you may think, "This is too much work," and we sometimes felt this way. However, after two years, most staff members feel that providing education to families has been one of the more rewarding experiences in their careers. We learn much from these families—perhaps more than they learn from us.

Table 2 Helpful Hints for a Successful Program

Assign responsibility for the program
Administrative support
Preplanning
Survey families
Conduct literature search
Determine goals
Consider population and setting
Determine length of program
Select content and topics
Recruit presenters
Select program materials
Design family education brochure
Advertise
Select program facilitators
Train facilitators
Recruitment of families
Start program
Evaluate (ongoing)
Be flexible and adaptable
Update information
Be open to change

REFERENCES

1. Bernheim KF, Lehman AF. Working with Families of the Mentally Ill. New York: Norton, 1985.
2. McFarlane WR, ed. Family Therapy in Schizophrenia. New York: Guilford Press, 1983.
3. Torrey EF. Surviving Schizophrenia: A Family Manual. New York: Harper & Row, 1983.
4. Hatfield AB. Family Education in Mental Illness. New York: The Guilford Press, 1990.
5. Bisbee CB. Educating Patients and Families About Mental Illness. Birmingham, AL: Partnership for Recovery, 1995.
6. Gardner JW. Self Renewal: The Individual and the Innovative Society. New York: Harper & Row, 1965.

BIBLIOGRAPHY

Goldstein MJ. New Developments in Interventions with Families of Schizophrenics. San Francisco: Jossey-Bass, 1981.

Lamb HR. Treating the Long-Term Mentally Ill. San Francisco: Jossey-Bass, 1982.

Lamb HR, Oliphant. Schizophrenia through the eyes of the family. Hosp Commun 1978; 29:803-806.

Wasow M. Coping with Schizophrenia: A Survival Manual. Palo Alto, CA: Science and Behavior, 1982.

14

Schizophrenia from the Life-Cycle Perspective

John Lauriello, William P. Horan,* and Juan Bustillo
University of New Mexico
Albuquerque, New Mexico

Schizophrenia is a chronic mental illness that has a severe impact on patients and those who are close to them. Kraepelin's classic description of schizophrenia ("dementia praecox") as a unitary degenerative disease that inevitably results in a grossly deteriorated end state has been refuted on empirical grounds, with contemporary research supporting a more optimistic prognostic picture. However, schizophrenia is a disorder that persists across the lifespan at varying degrees of severity and requires a multifaceted, long-term treatment approach as the needs of patients change over time. To optimally treat patients with schizophrenia, the unique issues that emerge during each patient's progression through the different stages of life must be addressed.

Several factors about schizophrenia must be acknowledged at the outset in describing phases of illness and their accompanying implications for treatment. First, schizophrenia is a heterogeneous clinical syndrome with a course that is characterized by considerable inter- and intraindividual variability. Second, data regarding the natural history of schizophrenia are scarce and rarely prospective, which considerably

*_Current affiliation:_ Western Psychiatric Institute and Clinic, University of Pittsburgh School of Medicine, Pittsburgh, Pennsylvania.

limits attempts to link clinical features of the illness at different time points with underlying pathophysiological processes (see Refs. 1 and 2 for reviews). Third, patients with schizophrenia very often present with a variety of comorbid psychiatric and medical conditions that influence course and treatment. Fourth, the course of schizophrenia is determined by the interplay of the unique biological, environmental, and protective factors that affect individuals with this disorder. Thus, attempts to identify sharp divisions between different phases of schizophrenia can be oversimplifications and probably do not directly correspond to underlying pathophysiological processes.

Nonetheless, delineation of phases of illness on the basis of available evidence and their accompanying treatment issues may provide a useful framework for treating patients who suffer from this complex disorder, which is ideally accomplished through an approach that integrates pharmacological, psychosocial, and rehabilitative interventions. In this chapter, four broad phases of schizophrenia are delineated: the premorbid/prodromal, early, middle, and late phases. For each phase, the major clinical characteristics are described in terms of positive and negative symptoms, mood symptoms, and cognitive functioning, and prognostic implications are discussed. We then describe treatment issues that accompany each phase and discuss strategies to address the treatment goals of ameliorating symptoms, reducing relapse risks, and improving psychosocial functioning.

THE PREMORBID/PRODROMAL PHASE

Clinical Characteristics

The premorbid phase of schizophrenia refers to the period from birth to the onset of identifiable acute or positive schizophrenic symptomatology. The first episode of schizophrenia symptoms typically occurs during late adolescence or early adulthood, with a somewhat earlier age of onset found for males (17–27 years) than females (17–37 years). Research has increasingly focused on the premorbid phase in light of a growing body of evidence that supports the conceptualization of schizophrenia as at least in part a neurodevelopmental disorder. A number of subtle behavioral and socioemotional abnormalities, presumed to reflect the underlying pathophysiology of schizophrenia, have been identified in preschizophrenics that appear to be relevant for long-term prognosis. Immediately preceding the onset of acute psychotic symptoms an initial prodromal period is usually identifiable, although a clearly defined prodromal period is not pathognomonic for the illness.

Whereas characteristic traits of abnormal premorbid adjustment are regarded as habitual and enduring for the preschizophrenic individual, prodromal symptoms refer to a marked change (i.e., "ego-dystonic") from habitual adaptive functioning and cognitive experiences.

Premorbid Adjustment

Considerable variability in timing, course, and severity of symptoms is found in the premorbid period. A range of behavioral abnormalities has been found to differentiate many, but not all, preschizophrenics from normals (3). Psychosocial abnormalities identified among preschizophrenic individuals include increased social isolation, delayed social-sexual development, diminished social drive, and reduced emotional responsivity. Poor scholastic adjustment, disruptive behaviors, and impulsivity have also been identified. Neurocognitive abnormalities, such as attentional impairment, and poor motor and sensorimotor coordination, may also be present. Disturbances in some social behaviors, such as diminished emotional responsiveness and expression, have been detected as early as in infancy (4).

Prodromal Period

The duration of prodromal symptoms typically ranges from several weeks up to approximately one year, but may be prolonged and last up to several years. Prodromal symptoms, which are detectable in the majority of schizophrenia patients, are characterized by positive or negative symptoms in attenuated form. Examples of prodromal symptoms, as described in DSM-III-R (5), include marked social isolation and withdrawal; marked impairment in role functioning; markedly peculiar behavior; marked impairment in personal hygiene and grooming; blunted or inappropriate affect; digressive, vague, overelaborate, or circumstantial speech; or poverty of speech, or of content of speech; odd beliefs or magical thinking; unusual perceptual experiences; and marked lack of initiative, interests, or energy. Prodromal features most commonly described in first-episode patients include: reduced concentration/attention; reduced drive and motivation, anergia; depressed mood; sleep disturbance; anxiety; social withdrawal; suspiciousness; deterioration in role functioning; irritability; thought-blocking phenomena; and disturbances in attention, perception, speech production, and motor function (6). Although prodromal signs and symptoms frequently present during the period immediately preceding the initial onset of psychosis, they are not specifically related to schizophrenia and are no longer included in the diagnostic criteria for schizophrenia.

Prognostic Implications

Despite the nonspecificity of signs and symptoms that occur during the premorbid phase, several of these characteristics are associated with the long-term clinical course of schizophrenia. Individuals with good premorbid psychosocial functioning tend to have a later age of onset, good response to antipsychotic medication, and a more benign course of illness characterized by fewer symptom exacerbations and higher interepisode functioning. Conversely, poor premorbid functioning tends to predict a more chronic, debilitating course. For example, individuals with limited social drive and emotional expression are more likely to have an earlier age of onset, worse social and occupational functioning, more prominent negative symptoms, and poorer response to antipsychotic medication.

Therapeutic Issues

Specific signs or symptoms that would warrant prophylactic treatment during the premorbid phase of the illness have not yet been identified. Due to the potentially serious adverse short- and long-term side effects associated with initiating prophylactic drug treatment in individuals who may not require such intervention to maintain adequate psychosocial functioning, a solid empirical basis must be established prior to the initiation of clinical interventions during this phase of illness. Clearly, the identification of signs and symptoms that precede illness onset and the development of early pharmacological and psychosocial intervention strategies is a critical area for continued research.

THE EARLY PHASE: ILLNESS ONSET AND DETERIORATION

Illness Onset: Clinical Characteristics

Identification of the initial episode of positive symptoms in schizophrenia is frequently difficult as the emergence of symptoms ranges from an acute to a gradual onset. In cases of relatively acute onset, dramatic and easily observed changes in cognitive and adaptive functioning may be observed over a period of several weeks to a few months. However, approximately 50% of patients demonstrate an insidious onset, with the earliest signs of the illness appearing years before the emergence of frank psychotic symptoms. In addition to variability in onset, there is also a wide range in duration between the onset of psychotic symptoms and initiation of treatment. Patients typically experience 12 to 24 months of psychotic symptoms before receiving treatment (7). However, there is often a considerable delay in obtaining psychiatric services in patients with a history of subtle deterioration and insidious onset, with studies reporting durations of untreated illness ranging up to 20 years (7).

Onset is often associated with a major life event, such as going off to college or military boot camp, which emphasizes the critical role that environmental factors play in determining the course of schizophrenia. During the early phase of the illness, positive symptoms tend to dominate the clinical presentation; negative symptoms appear much less frequently (2). The early phase of illness is characterized by considerable fluctuation and instability of both positive and negative symptoms, which are usually treatment responsive. Mood disturbances, including depression, anxiety, and agitation, are also common during the very early phase.

Therapeutic Issues

Effective and prompt intervention for the first psychotic episode is critical to optimal management of the early phase of schizophrenia, particularly in light of evidence that increased duration of untreated psychosis may predict worse outcome (8). A thorough and systematic effort at differential diagnosis is necessary when encountering a patient presenting with a first episode of psychosis, not only to identify potentially reversible neurological and medical causes of psychosis but also because treatment implications differ for various psychotic disorders. For example, patients with schizophrenia will need extended treatment with antipsychotic drugs, while those with psychotic symptoms secondary to a mood disorder will generally take such medications only for brief periods of time. Because the formulation of a diagnosis can be difficult in patients presenting with a first psychotic episode, it is important that data be collected from as many sources as possible (e.g., lab tests for illicit substances). Information from family members or others who are close to the patient is particularly helpful in this regard, since patients can be unreliable historians during an acute psychotic episode. Clinicians must also carefully assess the level of care and treatment setting that a given patient will require for optimal clinical management. Patients presenting with a first psychotic episode are often best served through inpatient hospitalization to ensure safety, to perform a careful diagnostic assessment, and to monitor symptomatology and treatment response.

Table 1 Summary of Treatment Strategies for First-Episode Schizophrenia Patients

1. Systematic and thorough formulation of diagnosis
2. Assessment of suicidality and appropriate level of care/treatment setting
3. Prompt initiation of antipsychotic medication to ameliorate psychotic symptoms
4. Establishment of treatment alliance
5. Provision of psychoeduction to patient and family
6. Work with patient and family to solve practical problems
7. Treatment of comorbid conditions

Selection of an effective antipsychotic medication to ameliorate the psychotic symptoms is the next critical task. The few relevant studies indicate that the rate of response to traditional antipsychotic drugs—e.g., haloperidol (Haldol)—among first-episode patients is as good as or better than the response rate in chronic patients (70%) (9). However, novel antipsychotics, such as risperidone (Risperdal), olanazapine (Zyprexa), quetiapine (Seroquel), and ziprasidone (Geodon) should be considered as a first-line therapy for first-episode patients when possible because of their improved efficacy and side-effect profile. Although the pivotal data for the efficacy of these medications come from studies of chronic patients, preliminary data on first-episode patients are promising (10). While antipsychotics are the first line in treatment, other medications should be considered for comorbid conditions, such as benzodiazepines—e.g., lorazepam (Ativan), clonazepan (Klonopin)—for anxiety, or antidepressants—e.g., fluoxetine (Prozac), sertraline (Zoloft)—if there is an accompanying depression. Fear of further mental deterioration, hopelessness, excessive dependence on treatment, or loss of faith in treatment may increase risk for suicide, which is particularly high for patients following illness onset (11). Thus, clinicians must vigilantly monitor suicidality during the very early phase of schizophrenia.

Psychosocial interventions involving the patient and, when possible, the family are also an important component of treatment in the early phase of schizophrenia. The critical task for the clinician is to develop an effective treatment alliance with the patient and his or her family to facilitate engagement in treatment, particularly compliance with medication. The formation of a trusting relationship is especially important when dealing with paranoid patients, which typically requires more time and greater patience on the part of the clinician. Although few controlled clinical trials of psychosocial treatments for patients with first-episode psychosis exist, supportive treatments for more chronic patients are applicable to this population.

An emotionally supportive, psychoeducational approach is the most effective means of engaging patients and their families in treatment. The basic elements of this approach include providing information about mental illness, facilitating the development of basic problem-solving skills, and crisis management. The stress-vulnerability model provides a useful, comprehensible framework for discussing the causes and prognosis of schizophrenia to patients and their families. These issues should be discussed in a manner that is frank and realistic while maintaining an empathic, hopeful attitude. Due to the fears, confusion, and cognitive disturbances that typically accompany a first-episode of psychosis, information should be presented gradually and expanded as the patient's symptoms remit.

Relapse and Deterioration: Clinical Characteristics

An accumulation of evidence suggests that clinical deterioration and instability characterize the first five years, approximately, following the onset of schizophrenia (1). These data are consistent with an active disease and deterioration process occurring during the early phase of schizophrenia, if not predating the emergence of psychotic symptoms. For example, structural brain abnormalities and global neurocognitive impairments are present in patients at the onset of illness (12,13). It is during the early phase that the majority of deterioration in symptomatology and adaptive functioning occurs, which may take only 6 months to 1 year to run its full course (14). Multiple episodes of symptom exacerbation alternating with periods of partial or complete remission of symptoms typically occur during this phase, as most patients suffering from schizophrenia will relapse. The risk of relapse and rehospitalization is highest within the first five years after illness onset (15).

Positive symptoms tend to dominate the clinical picture during symptom exacerbations but are usually treatment-responsive. Negative symptoms may increase in prevalence during this phase and can become increasingly persistent. Unfortunately, a return to the full premorbid level of functioning during remission is unusual in patients with schizophrenia. Cognitive impairments, once established, tend to remain stable and are associated with poor adaptive and occupational functioning (16). Mood disturbances and anxiety-related symptoms are also common as patients struggle to adjust to what is likely to be a chronic mental illness. Demoralization is particularly likely to occur in patients with good premorbid functioning and insight into their illness.

Considerable attention has focused on identifying symptoms and behaviors indicative of a "relapse prodrome" to facilitate intervention efforts prior to the re-emergence of psychotic symptoms. For most patients, relapse tends to be a gradual process that is preceded by a variety of noticeable changes lasting from a few days to several weeks or more. Putative indicators of a relapse prodrome include dysphoria, tension and nervousness, decreased appetite, difficulty concentrating and remembering, somatic concerns, and insomnia (17). Unfortunately, the specificity and sensitivity of these indicators are modest, making preventive interventions difficult. However, the emergence of such signs and symptoms, particularly in the context of relative clinical stability, is an indication for increased clinical monitoring and support. Relapse is often associated with exposure to stressors in patients' social environments, such as traumatic life events, daily hassles, or interpersonal stressors such as living in high–"expressed emotion" households characterized by critical attitudes, hostility, or overinvolvement toward the patient (18). Exposure to these sources of stress can result in relapse despite optimal maintenance drug therapy.

Therapeutic Issues

Therapeutic issues during this phase of schizophrenia center on 1) patients' choice to accept or reject treatment, 2) relapse prevention, 3) rapid intervention for symptom exacerbations, and 4) to the extent possible, assisting patients in their return to premorbid levels of functioning. Most treatment takes place in the community rather than in hospital or institutional settings. A multidisciplinary team approach to treatment is strongly recommended to ensure that patients receive comprehensive, coordinated, and continuous services. The level of care required by patients across the acute symptom exacerbations and remissions during the phase must be monitored and adjusted accordingly to provide the least restrictive setting that is safe and allows for effective treatment. Treatment of florid psychotic symptoms frequently requires inpatient hospitalization for patients who are incapable of caring for themselves, or at least increased clinical monitoring and support for patients with good social-support networks. As patients emerge from acute episodes, transition to a partial hospitalization program is frequently appropriate, with the eventual goal of transitioning patients to outpatient treatment settings after symptoms have stabilized.

Research strongly supports the efficacy of antipsychotic medications for treatment of acute psychotic symptoms and relapse prevention

Table 2 Summary of Treatment Strategies for the Early Phase of Schizophrenia

1. Determination of most beneficial antipsychotic medication, addressing problematic side effects
2. Work with patient and family to secure commitment to treatment
3. Monitoring of psychiatric status and suicidality
4. Assessment of most effective treatment setting
5. Treatment or referral for treatment of comorbid psychiatric disorders
6. Case management to facilitate access to services
7. Education of patients and families about prodromal symptoms to promote early recognition of episodes and initiation of treatment

during the first two years following the onset of the illness (9). Relapses occurring in patients who report consistently taking their prescribed antipsychotic medication should not necessarily be taken as evidence of treatment resistance, given the instability that characterizes this period. However, medication noncompliance, which occurs in approximately 50% of patients (19), remains the strongest predictor of relapse.

Many patients resist continued treatment because of side effects that accompany antipsychotic medications. The enhanced efficacy of novel antipsychotics for treatment of negative symptoms and their more favorable side-effect profile—particularly extrapyramidal side effects (EPS)—would be expected to improve compliance and permit longer periods of maintenance treatment. Careful monitoring of side effects and utilization of medication-management strategies, such as dosage adjustments, adjustments to the time of medication administration, and the use of adjunctive medications, are required to maximize the likelihood of treatment compliance. Indeed, clinicians must work hard to determine a medication that maximizes therapeutic benefit while minimizing troubling side effects. Another significant aspect of the clinician's work is to foster the patient's commitment to maximizing the benefits of his or her own treatment.

Clinicians must be acutely aware of the risk of suicide during this phase of illness, which is the leading cause of mortality in people suffering from schizophrenia (20). Risk of mortality is especially high in the young, during the early postdischarge period, and early in the course of the illness. Suicidality can be particularly difficult to assess and monitor in schizophrenia patients due in part to the similarities between depressive and negative symptoms. Many of the suicide risk factors are similar to those in the general population: being male, white, and socially isolated; having a depressive illness or history of suicide attempts; being unemployed; and experiencing recent rejection. Risk factors specific to schizophrenia include high IQ, high premorbid academic achievement, a deteriorating course with multiple exacerbations, awareness of loss of adaptive functioning, and having command hallucinations to kill oneself. In dealing with suicidality, rapid attention may curtail psychiatric and social morbidity, and the clinician should increase the level of observation and support (including hospitalization if necessary). For nonacute episodes of depression, clinicians may consider lowering medication dosage because neuroleptics may play a role in generating syndromes that mimic depression. Adjunctive antidepressant medications should also be considered for depression.

Patients in the early phase of schizophrenia are often ill prepared to find and maintain the multiple services they need to achieve adequate psychosocial functioning, which further increases risk of relapse. Among these basic needs, physical health, insurance, housing, financial, legal, and vocational issues are particularly common. Case management and social work services, particularly for patients lacking family resources, play a crucial role in treatment. Case managers can assist patients and their families in identifying needs, obtaining services (which patients are often unaware that they have access to), and, equally importantly, facilitating follow-through with receiving these services. Ideally, comprehensive integrated community services are applied in programs modeled on the Assertive Community Treatment (ACT) approach (21), in which patients are assigned to one multidisciplinary team (case manager, nurse, etc.) that has a fixed caseload and a high staff:patient ratio, and delivers all services when and where needed by the patient, 24 hours a day, 7 days a week. These programs have been shown to be effective in preventing rehospitalization, and facilitate continuity of care and communication among professionals.

Supportive therapy, which may be administered in individual or group formats, is useful in assisting patients to deal with problems in the "here and now." For example, clinicians may work with patients to identify and address precipitants of relapse or to improve communication, coping, and problem-solving skills. Psychotherapy is also useful in assisting patients to adjust to the many psychosocial effects of schizophrenia (see Chapter 1). Intensive, exploratory techniques (e.g., psychoanalytically based approaches) are not recommended for patients with schizophrenia as they may be overly stimulating and thereby prolong disorganization or precipitate relapse. As recovery proceeds, teaching patients to use relaxation exercises and cognitive reframing techniques can be beneficial. There is strong empirical support that family therapy interventions designed to educate families about schizophrenia, improve communication, and relieve family burden are effective in decreasing relapse rates (22). Teaching families to recognize prodromal symptoms can be particularly useful in minimizing risk of relapse.

Psychosocial interventions may also help to treat the many comorbid psychiatric conditions found in patients presenting for a first-episode of psychosis. For example, approximately one-third to one-half of psychotic patients present with comorbid substance use disorders (23). Substance use disorders are associated with more frequent and longer hospitalizations and other negative outcomes (e.g., homelessness, incarceration, HIV infection). Psychoeduation about substance abuse's adverse affects on the course and treatment of psychosis may be adequate for addressing relatively minor cases. However, if the substance use appears to be a more significant problem, referral should be made to a dual-diagnosis program that combines treatment of schizophrenia and substance use disorder after acute psychotic symptoms have been stabilized. Empirically supported psychosocial treatments for depression and anxiety have received empirical support and should also be considered as adjuncts to pharmacotherapy for patients who possess adequate insight and verbal abilities.

Prognostic Implications

Although some general predictors of course and outcome have been identified, overall predictive ability is quite limited. Several general characteristics of the early phase are prognostically significant for the long-term course of schizophrenia. Gradual symptom onset, which more commonly occurs in males, is often accompanied by negative symptoms during the early phase and is associated with poor long-term outcome, including more severe cognitive impairment and functional incapacity in social and work domains. A relatively sudden or acute onset is associated with wide variation of intermediate and long-term outcome, but is considered predictive of a more benign course of illness. Although the presence of mood disorder symptoms has historically been regarded as a good prognostic sign, more recent data raise uncertainty about this issue. Substance abuse is associated with poor long-term outcome. A number of studies suggest that a longer duration between illness onset and initiation of treatment with antipsychotic medication is associated with poor long-term outcome (8), including a recurrent pattern of poor treatment response and more severe and persistent positive and negative symptomatology. However, this should not preclude aggressive treatment in a patient with a long untreated

Table 3 Prognostic Implications of Clinical Presentation During Premorbid and Early Phases of Schizophrenia

Good prognosis
Late onset
Obvious precipitating factors
Acute onset
Good premorbid social, sexual, and work histories
Female
Married
Minimal comorbidity
Family history of mood disorders
Good support systems
Predominance of positive symptoms
Poor prognosis
Onset in youth
No precipitating factors
Insidious onset
Poor premorbid social, sexual, and work histories
Withdrawn, autistic behavior
Single, divorced, or widowed
Family history of schizophrenia
Poor support systems
Negative symptoms
Neurological signs and symptoms
History of perinatal trauma
No remissions in 3 years
Many relapses
History of assaultiveness

history because such individuals may still respond quite well to pharmacological intervention. Finally, responsiveness to biological treatments during the early phase of illness is predictive of better or worse long-term outcome.

THE MIDDLE PHASE: STABILIZATION

Clinical Characteristics

It is during the middle phase of the illness that patients tend to settle into a characteristic course of illness and adaptive functioning. An accumulation of research suggests that once a nadir in symptomatology and adaptive functioning has been reached (approximately five years following illness onset and treatment) a stabilization of symptoms tends to occur that persists into about the fifth decade of life (1). The clinical course displayed by patients after emerging from the early phase of the illness is often indicative of the longer-term course that will follow. Highly charged affects and positive symptoms tend to become less conspicuous as thought disorder and negative symptoms, such as reductions in ambition, initiative, emotional responsiveness, occupational level, and neglect of personal appearance, are slightly more stable during this phase of illness and, in some cases, may increasingly dominate the clinical picture. Negative symptoms may be associated with cognitive impairment and adaptive functioning deficits.

The illness course during the middle phase of schizophrenia typically follows the "rule of thirds." About one-third of patients have a relatively mild course characterized by few symptom relapses and good interepisode psychosocial functioning. Another third experience an intermediate course, with more frequent relapses and more persistent deficits in psychosocial functioning. The final third demonstrate a relatively severe and unremitting course, with an inability to maintain adequate self-care and a need for close supervision. Despite a plateau of symptoms during this phase, complications caused by the illness can lead to ever-increasing impediments for adaptive functioning. For example, competitive employment (regular jobs in the community as opposed to those provided directly by a rehabilitation agency) has been estimated at less than 20% for severely mentally ill persons and is probably lower for patients with chronic schizophrenia (24). Indeed, many patients lack competence in the domains of social and occupational functioning, which require skills that were either never developed or affected by the disruptive effects of the illness process.

Therapeutic Issues

Once the deterioration of the early phase of schizophrenia has stabilized and the clinical picture is clearer, it is critical to set realistic goals for outcome based on patients' cognitive abilities and available social-support network. For example, many patients cannot cope with time pressures and competition such that routine work in sheltered settings may be a more reasonable expectation than competitive employment. Relatedly, supportive housing may be a reasonable choice for patients who are incapable of independent living and self-care. Treatment interventions focus on maintenance of clinical stability and rehabilitative interventions to address long-term disabilities.

Table 4 Summary of Treatment Strategies for the Middle Phase of Schizophrenia

1. Determine optimal medication maintenance dosage
2. Consider depot preparation if compliance is inadequate
3. Place in optimal living conditions
4. Set realistic goals for outcome
5. Rehabilitate to restore social/occupational deficits associated with illness

Depending on patients' clinical status and available social supports, the optimal level of care and living conditions required must be assessed, which may range from independent living in the community with outpatient medication monitoring to supervised inpatient living settings. Pharmacological intervention focuses on maintenance treatment and relapse prevention. Medication management must balance both side effects and relapse risks in an effort to determine the minimum effective maintenance dosage. Clinicians should be ready to respond quickly to prodromal symptoms by adjusting medication and may prevent relapse risk by increasing clinical monitoring during periods of transition or impending stressors (e.g., changing living situations). For many patients, depot preparations are the best options during this phase of illness, particularly for patients who are consistently medication-noncompliant. Unfortunately, novel antipsychotics are not currently available in depot form.

Once acute symptoms have stabilized, many patients will ask to stop their medication (which also often occurs during symptom remission in the early phase). Dealing with this issue can be very difficult as there is currently no method for detecting which patients might achieve full recovery and not require long-term medication, although data suggest that the majority of patients (with or without medication) will relapse (e.g., Ref. 25). Educating patients and families about schizophrenia and the risks and potentially deleterious effects of relapse associated with not taking medication is critical. Following two to five years of successful treatment, it may be appropriate to determine whether some patients can tolerate a gradual dosage reduction and eventual discontinuation of medication in the context of close monitoring and psychosocial support. Only patients who are completely free of psychoses while on medication, and have not shown sign of previous relapse with dosage reduction, should be considered.

Psychosocial treatments during the middle phase of illness should focus on the development of skills to improve social and vocational functioning. A number of rehabilitation approaches have been shown to improve social-functioning abilities in stabilized schizophrenia patients, approaches that may also be used in the early phase of schizophrenia when appropriate. Social-skills training utilizes learning-theory principles to improve social functioning by helping patients to remediate problems in activities of daily living, employment, leisure, and relationships (26). These interventions typically break down complex social behaviors into simpler steps, which are subjected to corrective learning, practiced in role-plays, and applied in natural settings. In a variant of this approach, the cognitive-remediation model, the corrective learning process begins by targeting more fundamental cognitive impairments, such as attentional or planning deficits, with the theory that if the underlying cognitive impairment can be improved initially, this learning will be transferred to support more complex cognitive processes.

Vocational rehabilitation interventions have been shown to benefit patients who wish to work. In an effort to keep patients as functional and autonomous as possible in the community, various programs have been implemented to help them find and retain jobs (24). The formats of these programs include sheltered workshops, job support programs, and job clubs. Supported employment (SE), an intensive, multifaceted vocational rehabilitation program, has been shown to be an efficacious approach for helping patients to obtain and maintain competitive employment.

Psychotherapeutic interventions may be more complex and less structured and directive than those utilized in the early phase of schizophrenia for patients who are treatment-compliant and relatively free of positive or deficit symptoms. A large number of patients will continue to experience disturbing psychotic symptoms despite the best available medications. In recent years there has been a growing interest in developing and applying cognitive-behavioral interventions for patients with medication-resistant psychotic symptoms (27). These treatments focus on subjecting the content of delusions and hallucinations to reality testing. Interventions focus on rationally exploring the subjective nature of the psychotic symptoms, challenging the evidence for them, and utilizing cognitive techniques to help patients cope with their symptoms (e.g., cognitive reframing).

THE LATE PHASE

Clinical Characteristics

Kraepelin's classic description of schizophrenia as a degenerative disorder that invariably results in a grossly deteriorated end state has been revised in light of data indicating that many people with schizophrenia actually experience a gradual improvement in function and symptoms, or even a full remission during the late phase. This gradual improvement is typically not observed until after the age of 50. There is a tendency for the intensity of positive symptoms to diminish, and many patients with long-term impairments may regain some degree of social and occupational competence. However, the heterogeneity of schizophrenia in the late phase is similar to that in earlier phases in terms of the course of illness. Long-term follow-up studies (20 to 40 years) indicate that 21% to 57% of patients have a moderately good outcome (ranging from mild impairment to recovery), with the remainder achieving a more severe outcome (1). Positive symptoms clearly do not "burn out" in all geriatric patients and can remain highly prevalent even at this stage of the illness. Negative symptoms appear to be more severe in older patients than younger patients and are associated with cognitive impairment (28). In some patients with schizophrenia there is evidence of a very slow decline in cognitive functioning that is greater than the decline associated with normal aging but not nearly as precipitous as the decline in patients with neurodegenerative disorders (e.g., Alzheimer's disease).

Despite this more optimistic view, late-life schizophrenia patients present with many difficult management problems associated with both normal aging and factors unique to this phase of illness. Factors associated with aging in general that are particularly relevant to the treatment of patients with schizophrenia include physiological changes associated with the metabolism of medications, potential interactions with medications for emerging medical conditions, loss of mobility to obtain health-care services, and the loss of social support associated with the death of caretakers. With regard to unique factors, schizophrenia is associated with excess mortality and shorter lifespans compared with the general population (29), and the physical health of individuals with schizophrenia is often more typical of much older persons without the disorder (30). Depression is approximately 1.5 to 3 times more likely in patients with late life schizoophrenia as compared to the general elderly population (31). Additionally, a minority of late-life patients can have extremely severe cognitive impairments and meet criteria for an additional diagnosis of dementia (28), which profoundly affects self-care abilities. Despite the relatively optimistic long-term prognosis that has been demonstrated, the effects of years of dysfunction are rarely overcome and patients frequently continue to manifest signs of the illness throughout their lives. Although schizophrenia patients are overrepresented in nursing homes and state psychiatric institutions, the majority live in the community, where most receive little or no treatment beyond medication despite continued need. As the number of patients with late-life schizophrenia increases over the coming decades, the challenges of treating this population will also increase.

Treatment Issues

Given the complexities of managing patients in the late phase of schizophrenia, a coordinated, biopsychosocial approach to treatment is advisable (32). Patients in this phase require treatment for medical conditions that typically accompany aging. Symptoms and functional impairments may be associated with many causes in contrast to those found in earlier phases of the illness. Differential diagnosis of emerging physical problems or changes in mental status is critical. For example, elderly schizophrenia patients are at greater risk of developing delirium secondary to neuroleptics with anticholinergic properties than during earlier stages. These symptoms may mimic other conditions that accompany late life, and optimal, safe treatment requires accurate diagnosis.

Late-life schizophrenia patients demonstrate greater variability in tolerability and sensitivity to neuroleptics than patients in earlier phases. For example, akathesia, parkinsonian symptoms, and tardive dyskinesia tend to be more prevalent with increasing age (33). Side effects tend to occur more commonly in older schizophrenia patients, including sedation, orthostatic hypotension, anticholinergic reactions, and EPS. Additionally, absorption, metabolism, and excretion of antipsychotic medications differ considerably for late-life schizophrenia. While antipsychotics are the mainstay of treatment, dosages of neuroleptics for older patients are usually much lower (even one-third or less) than those used in younger adults (34).

The use of atypical medications has not yet been adequately evaluated in older adults. Clozapine may be especially problematic for older adults because of potential side effects (postural hypotension and sedation) and the frequent blood tests that are required. Given the gradual improvements that often accompany the late phase of schizophrenia, it may be appropriate to consider withdrawing antipsychotic medications under close clinical supervision. Unfortunately, there is little empirical information to guide this decision-making process.

The level of depression among community-residing older adults with schizophrenia is approximately 1.5 to 3 times the level in the general elderly population (31). Clinicians must pay attention to issues

Table 5 Summary of Clinical Strategies for the Late Phase of Schizophrenia

1. Assessment and coordination of medical health-care needs
2. Careful monitoring of medication dosages and side effects
3. Monitoring of potential adverse interactions with medications of medical conditions
4. Assessment of appropriate level of care based on cognitive, medical, and social-support factors
5. Careful differential diagnosis and treatment of emerging symptoms (e.g., depressive symptoms)
6. Facilitation of access to services (e.g., Meals on Wheels)

of possible medical etiology, and address whether such symptoms are caused or exacerbated by medication toxicity or medical conditions.

Clinicians must also deal with the issue of appropriate residential placement during this stage of the illness. In patients with severe cognitive deficits or debilitating medical problems, placement in a nursing home where constant care is available may be required. Many older persons with schizophrenia do not have family care providers available and are less socially connected than those without mental illness (35). For example, the death of parents, who are key caretakers for many persons with schizophrenia, frequently leaves middle-aged to elderly individuals with a dramatic reduction of social and financial support and at risk for decompensation and loss of residence in the community. The availability of social supports and the need to bolster this capacity are important considerations in treatment planning. Supported housing or residential treatment facilities may be appropriate for patients requiring supervision, and facilitating access to services such as transportation, home-care assistance, or Meals on Wheels may be indicated for aging patients living independently in the community.

Several individual psychological approaches with demonstrated efficacy in younger populations may be useful in treating older persons with schizophrenia (32). Capacity for communication, awareness of a problem, and capacity for retention and carryover should be considered when evaluating the appropriateness of psychotherapy. Psychological intervention should be matched to patients' level of need and ability, and should not create stress or cognitive overload.

CONCLUSIONS

Schizophrenia is a heterogeneous, multisymptom disorder, made more complex by its varied presentation cross-sectionally as well as prospectively. This requires a flexible perspective on the diagnosis and treatment of the illness. Inherent to this is an expectation that change will occur as the illness progresses despite the best-intended plans to create stability for the patient. In the early phase of schizophrenia most patients present with positive symptoms—less often, with negative symptoms—with both symptom types fluctuating but responsive to treatments. Cognitive dysfunction becomes apparent as the patient attempts to continue employment or school. In the middle phase, negative symptoms increase in prevalence, becoming at least as common as positive symptoms, and there is a greater degree of symptom stability. Cognitive symptoms can plateau, but also become a source of frustration for the patient and his family. In the late phase, there is gradual improvement of positive symptoms and social functioning, and negative symptoms may dominate the clinical picture. As we become more adept at medication and psychosocial interventions and apply them as early as possible it will become more evident whether these phases are immutable hallmarks of schizophrenia or potential areas of improvement and success.

REFERENCES

1. Davidson L, McGlashan TH. The varied outcomes of schizophrenia. Can J Psychiatry 1997; 42:34–43.
2. McGlashan TH, Fenton WS. The positive-negative distinction in schizophrenia: review of natural history validators. Arch Gen Psychiatry 1992; 49:63–72.
3. Davies N, Russell A, Jones P, Murray RM. Which characteristics of schizophrenia predate psychosis? J Psychiatric Res 1998; 32:121–131.
4. Fish B, Marcus J, Hans SL, Auerbach JG., Perdue S. Infants at risk for schizophrenia: sequelae of a genetic neurointegrative defect. Arch Gen Psychiatry 1992; 49:221–235.
5. American Psychiatric Association. Diagnostic and Statistical Manual of Mental Disorders. 3rd ed. Washington, DC: American Psychiatric Press, 1987.
6. Yung AR, McGorry PD. The prodromal phase of first-episode psychosis: past and current conceptualizations. Schizophr Bull 1996; 22:353–370.
7. Haas GL, Sweeney JA. Premorbid and onset features of first-episode schizophrenia. Schizophr Bull 1992; 18:373–386.
8. Wyatt RJ, Henter ID. The effects of early and sustained intervention on the long-term morbidity of schizophrenia. J Psychiatry Res 1998; 32(3–4):169–177.
9. Sheitman BB, Lee H, Strauss R, Lieberman JA. The evaluation and treatment of first-episode psychosis. Schizophr Bull 1997; 23:653–661.

10. DeQuardo JR. Pharmacologic treatment of first-episode schizophrenia: early intervention is key to outcome. J Clin Psychiatry 1998; 59(suppl 19):9–17.
11. Mortensen PB, Juel K. Mortality and causes of death in first admitted schizophrenic patients. Br J Psychiatry 1993; 163:183–189.
12. Mohamed S, Paulsen JS, O'Leary D, Arndt S, Andreasen N. Generalized cognitive deficits in schizophrenia: a study of first episode patients. Arch Gen Psychiatry 1999; 56:749–754.
13. Nopoulos P, Torres I, Flaum M, Andreasen NC, Ehrhardt JC, Yuh WT. Brain morphology in first episode schizophrenia. Am J Psychiatry 1995; 152:1721–1723.
14. McGlashan TH. A selective review of recent North American long-term followup studies of schizophrenia. Schizophr Bull 1988; 14:515–542.
15. Eaton WW, Mortensen PB, Herrman H, Freeman H, Biker W, Burgess P, Wooff K. Long-term course of hospitalization for schizophrenia. I. Risk for rehospitalization. Schizophr Bull 1992; 18:217–218.
16. Green MF. What are the functional consequences of neurocognitive deficits in schizophrenia? Am J Psychiatry 1996; 153:321–330.
17. Norman RMG, Malla AK. Prodromal symptoms of relapse in schizophrenia: a review. Schizophr Bull 1995; 21:527–539.
18. Butzlaff RL, Hooley JM. Expressed emotion and psychiatric relapse. Arch Gen Psychiatry 1998; 55:547–552
19. Fenton WS, Blyler CR, Heinssen RK. Determinants of medication compliance in schizophrenia: empirical and clinical findings. Schizophr Bull 1997; 23:637–651.
20. Fenton WS. Depression, suicide and suicide prevention in schizophrenia. Suicide Life Threat Behav 2000; 30:34–49.
21. Mueser KT, Bond GR, Drake RE, Resnick SG. Models of community care for severe mental illness: a review of research on case management. Schizophr Bull 1998; 24:37–74.
22. Bustillo J, Lauriello J, Horan WP, Keith S. The psychosocial treatment of schizophrenia: an update. Am J Psychiatry. In press.
23. Blanchard JJ, Brown SA, Horan WP, Sherwood AR. Substance use disorders in schizophrenia: review, integration, and a proposed model. Clin Psychol Rev 2000; 20:207–234.
24. Lehman AF. Vocational rehabilitation in schizophrenia. Schizophr Bull 1995; 21:645–656.
25. Wiersma D, Nienhius FJ, Sloof CJ, Giel R. Natural course of schizophrenic disorders: a 15-year followup of a Dutch incidence cohort. Schizophr Bull 1998; 23:653–661.
26. Bellack A, Mueser K. Psychosocial treatment of schizophrenia. Schizophr Bull 1993; 19:317–336.
27. Garety PA, Fowler D, Kuipers E. Cognitive-behavioral therapy for medication-resistant symptoms. Schizophr Bull 2000; 26:73–86.

28. Davidson M. Harvey PD, Powchik P, Parrella M, White L, Ynobler HY, Losonczy MF, Keefe RSE, Katz S, Frecska E. Severity of symptoms in chronically institutionalized geriatric schizophrenic patients. Am J Psychiatry 1995; 152:197–207.
29. Black DW, Fisher R. Mortality in DSM-IIIR schizophrenia. Schizophr Res 1992; 7:109–116.
30. Mulsant BH, Stergiou A, Keshavan MS, Sweet RA, Rifai AH, Pasternak R, Zubenko GS. Schizophrenia in late life: elderly patients admitted to an acute care psychiatric hospital. Schizophr Bull 1993; 19:709–721.
31. Cohen CI, Talavera N, Hartung R. Depression among aging persons with schizophrenia who live in the community. Psychiatr Serv 1996; 47:601–607.
32. Bartels SJ, Levine KJ, Mueser KT. A biopsychosocial approach to treatment of schizophrenia in late life. In: Duffy M, ed. Handbook of Counseling and Psychotherapy with Older Adults. New York: John Wiley & Sons, 1999.
33. Rosen J, Bohon S, Gershon S. Antipsychotics in the elderly. Acta Psychiatr Scand 1990; 358(suppl):170–175.
34. Jeste DV, Rockwell E, Harris MJ, Lohr JB, Lacro J. Conventional vs. newer antipsychotics in elderly patients. Am J Geriatr Psychiatry 1999; 7:70–76.
35. Semple SJ, Patterson TL, Shaw WS, Grant I, Moscona S, Koch W, Jeste D. The social networks of older schizophrenic patients. Int Psychogeriatr 1997; 9:81–94.

Index

Acamprosate, in alcoholism, 279
Acetylcholine, and tardive dyskinesia, 230
Activity scheduling, negative symptoms and, 200
ACT programs, 113
Acute dystonic reactions, risk factors, 226
Acute intermittent porphyria (AIP), 101
Acute laryngeal/pharyngeal dystonia, treatment of, 226
Acute psychosis, differential diagnosis of, 274
Acute psychotic episodes
- acute residential care, 115
- aggression, 128–129
- agitation, 128–129
- antipsychotic drug combinations, 123–124
- course, 108
- depot antipsychotic medications, 122–123, 133

[Acute psychotic episodes]
- electroconvulsive therapy, 127
- emergency room, 114–115
- guidelines, 127–134
- inpatient hospitalization, 115–116
- medical illness, 111
- medications, 118–127, 130–134
  - side effects, 133–134
- negative symptoms, 108, 110–111
- precipitating factors, 111, 130
- psychosocial issues, 134
- safety, 127–128
- symptoms, 109–113, 129
- treatment, 107–135
  - phases, 116–117
  - psychosocial, 132
  - setting, 113
  - voluntary vs. involuntary, 116

Acute residential care, in acute psychotic episodes, 115
Affective disorders, 57–58
Aggression, 110
- acute psychotic episodes, 128–129

Agitation, 109–110
  acute psychotic episodes, 128–129
Agranulocytosis, 149–150
  clozapine-induced, 236
AIP, 101
Akathisia, 110
  beta-blockers, 126
  treatment, 147, 226
Alcohol, toxicology screens, 93
Alcohol abuse, 63, 64, 91, 269
  biological markers, 94
  laboratory test, 93
  treatment, 279
Alcohol use
  self-reported reasons, 269
  and violence, 252
Alzheimer's disease, 63
Amphetamine abuse, 91
Amphetamines, toxicology screens, 93
Anticholinergic drugs, acute psychotic episodes, 125–126
Anticonvulsant drugs, treatment-refractory schizophrenia, 172–173
Antipsychotic drugs
  atypical
    extrapyramidal side effects, 112
    terminology, 214
  clinical setting, 217–225
  combinations, in acute psychotic episodes, 123–124
  depot, 133
  drug interactions, 222–225
  first-generation. *See* First-generation antipsychotic drugs
  pharmacological heterogeneity, 216
  with psychosocial interventions, maintenance treatment, 155–156
  psychotic relapse prevention, 142–143
[Antipsychotic drugs]
  second-generation. *See* Second-generation antipsychotics
  selection guidelines, 217–221
  side effects, 213–235. *See also* Extrapyrimidal side effects
    categorizing, 221–222
    identification, 220
    treatment, 225–238
  terminology, 214
  use, 217
Anxiety, 19–20
  benzodiazepines, 128
  clozapine, 216
  lorazepam, 128
Assault, potential, 13–14
Assertive Community Treatment (ACT) programs, 113
Assessment of Thought, Language, and Communication, 35–36
Attention, 187
  cognitive rehabilitation, 192
  neuropsychological tests, 75–76
  software programs, 192
Attentional focus, software programs for, 192
Attention/perceptual-motor-speed, neuropsychological tests for, 72
Atypical antipsychotic drugs
  extrapyramidal side effects, 112
  terminology, 214
Auditory cues, temporal vigilance and, 192
Auditory hallucinations, and risk of violence, 257–258
Auditory stimuli, reaction time, 192
Auxiliary ego, of interviewer, 23

Barbiturates, toxicology screens for, 93
Behavior, treatment goals for, 189
Benzodiazepines
  acute psychotic episodes, 125
  anxiety, 128

[Benzodiazepines]
  toxicology screens, 93
  treatment-refractory schizophrenia, 173
Beta-blockers
  acute psychotic episodes, 126
  akathisia, 126
Bipolar affective disorder, manic type, 56
Bisbee, Cynthia, 289
Bleuler, Eugen, 30
Blood-alcohol level, 93
Booklet Categories Test, 74
Botulinuum toxin injections and tardive dystonia, 229–230
BPRS, 39, 44
  factor-analytic work, 46–47
Brain tumor, signs and symptoms of, 97
Breath analysis, 93
Brief Psychiatric Rating Scale (BPRS), 39, 44
  factor-analytic work, 46–47
Brief reactive psychosis, 59–60

California Verbal Learning Test, 77
CAMI, 271
  characteristics, 272
Cancellation Test, 76
Cannabinoids, 92
Capgras delusions, risk of violence, 255
Carbamazepine, for treatment-refractory schizophrenia, 173
Carbohydrate-deficient transferrin, 93
Cardiac toxicity, 149
  guidelines, 237–238
Case management in comorbidity, 276–277
Catatonia, 111
Catatonic stupor, vignette, 4
Categories Tests, 74
Catharsis, moderating, 20–21
CBT, 184, 189–190, 195–197
  delusions, 197–198
  hallucinations, 199–200
Central nervous system, mass lesions, 96–97
Cerebrovascular events, 97–98
CET, 202
Chemical-abusing mentally ill (CAMI), 271–272
  characteristics, 272
Chemical dependence, etiology of, 269
Childhood factors, violence, 252
Chlorpromazine, trials, 165
Cholinomimetics, cognitive impairment, 83
Clinical scales for measuring EPS, 225
Clonazepam
  acute psychotic episodes, 125
  first-episode patients, 306
Clozapine
  acute psychotic episodes, 122, 127
  anxiety, 216
  cognitive impairment, 83
  drug trials, 165
  elderly, 317
  negative symptoms, maintenance treatment, 151–152
  psychotic relapse prevention, 144
  QTc prolongation, 237
  substance abuse, 278–279
  tardive dyskinesia, 229
  treatment-refractory schizophrenia, 166, 169–170
  weight gain, 235
Clozapine-induced agranulocytosis, guidelines, 236
Clozaril Support and Assistance Network (CSAN), 235
Clubhouse Model, 191
Cluster A personality disorders, 60–61
Cluster B personality disorders, 60–61

CMH, 115
Cocaine
  haloperidol, 269–270
  neuroleptics, 269
  toxicology screens, 93
Cognitive-behavioral interventions, 186
Cognitive-behavioral therapy (CBT), 184, 189–190, 195–197
  delusions, 197–198
  hallucinations, 199–200
Cognitive enhancement therapy (CET), 202
Cognitive impairments, 42
  maintenance treatment, 150–154
  rehabilitation, 82–83
  rehabilitation guidelines, 208
Cognitive/neuropsychological interventions, 186–189
Cognitive rehabilitation, 184
  attention, 192
  clinical description, 191–192
Command hallucinations, and risk of violence, 257–258
Communication, vignette, 4
Community mental health (CMH), 115
Comorbidity, treatment, 276–277
Comorbid neurobiology, 270–271
Complex partial seizures, 63–64
Computerized tomography (CT), 95–96
Computer programs, attention, 192
Concentration, in neuropsychological tests, 72, 75–76
Confrontation naming, neuropsychological tests, 73
Conjunctive feelings, 16
Continuous Performance Test, 75–76
Coping, 203–205
Crisis care, 115
CSAN, 235
CT, 95–96
Cytochrome P450, SGA metabolism of, 226
Deficit symptoms, 37, 43
  measurement, 37–39
Deficit syndrome, diagnostic criteria, 41
Delusional disorder, 59
Delusional projections, 8
Delusions, 32–33
  Capgras, 255
  CBT, 197–198
  collusion, 10
  evaluation, 129
  persecution, 253–254
  rehabilitation guidelines, 209
  threat/control-override, 255–256
  violence risk, 253–256
Dementia praecox, 69, 301
Demographics of violence, 251
Depot antipsychotic drugs, for acute psychotic episodes, 133
Depression, 40–41, 58–59, 113
  maintenance treatment, 150–154
Deterioration index, 73
Diabetes, 149
  weight gain, 234
Diagnostic and Statistical Manual of Mental Disorders (DSM-II), 31
Diagnostic and Statistical Manual of Mental Disorders (DSM-III), 31–32
  bipolar affective disorder, manic type, 56
Diagnostic and Statistical Manual of Mental Disorders (DSM-IV), 53
Digit Span and Arithmetic, 76
Disjunctive feelings, 16
Disorder of attention, 69
Disorganized schizophrenia, 16
Distribution method, CBT, 199
Dopamine
  psychosis, 215
  tardive dyskinesia, 230
Drug abuse, 63
Drug-induced disorders, laboratory tests for, 93
Drug-induced psychoses, 64–65

Drug screen, 93
Drug trials, adequacy of, 165–166
Drug use and violence, 252
DSM-II, 31
DSM-III, 31–32
  bipolar affective disorder, manic type, 56
DSM-IV, 53
Dual diagnosis, 271
  MICAA, treatment, 276
Dystonia, 226

ECA study, 250, 268
Ecstasy, 92
ECT
  acute psychotic episodes, 127
  treatment-refractory schizophrenia, 172–173
Educating Patients and Families about Mental Illness, 289
Education of family. *See* Family education program
EEG, 95
Elderly
  clozapine in, 317
  falls by, 149
Electroconvulsive therapy (ECT)
  acute psychotic episodes, 127
  treatment-refractory schizophrenia, 172–173
Electroencephalogram (EEG), 95
Emergency room, for acute psychotic episodes, 114–115
Empathy, vignette, 7
Epidemiological Catchment Area (ECA) study, 250, 268
Epilepsy, 94–95
  temporal-lobe, 63–64
Errorless learning principles, 82–83
Executive function
  components, 189
  deficits, 188
  neuropsychological tests, 72–75
  rehabilitation, 194–197

Extrapyramidal side effects (EPS)
  anticholinergic, 232
  cardiac, 237–238
  hematological, 235
  hepatic, 236
  measurement, 225
  ocular, 238
  tardive, 228–230
  treatment guidelines, 226–228

Factor-analytic work, 48–49
Falls by elderly, 149
Family Education in Mental Illness, 287–288
Family education program, 285–298
  attendance, 295–296
  beginning, 287–288
  content, 290
  evaluation, 295–296
  family member recruitment, 293
  literature search, 289
  maintenance treatment, 154–155
  materials, 291
  neglect, 286
  overhead presentations, 294–295
  population, 289–290
  presentations, 292–293
  recruitment, 293
  setting, 289–290
  staff training, 293–294
  survey, 288
  videos, 291, 294–295
Family studies of substance use disorder, 269
Fear
  of mental health professionals, 2
  of strangers, 8
Feighner criteria for bipolar affective disorder, manic type, 56
Finger Tapping Test, 78
First-generation antipsychotic drugs
  maintenance treatment
    cognitive deficits, 151
    depression, 151
    negative symptoms, 151

[First-generation antipsychotic drugs]
  psychotic relapse prevention, 142–143
Fluoxetine, for first-episode patients, 306
Fluphenazine
  acute psychotic episodes, 122–123, 133
  with psychosocial intervention, maintenance treatment, 155
  psychotic relapse prevention, 142–143
  treatment-refractory schizophrenia, 169
Flyers, use in family education program, 291
Focusing method, in CBT, 199
Fountain House model, 191
Furor diagnosticus, 21
Furor therapeuticus, 21

Galactorrhea, 149
Gamma-aminobutyric acid, tardive dyskinesia, 230
Gas chromatography-mass spectrometry (GC-MS), 93
Genetics of substance use disorder, 269
Grip Strength Test, 78–79

Hallucinations, 33
  auditory, 257–258
  CBT, 199–200
  command, 257–258
  evaluation, 129
  rehabilitation guidelines, 208
  violence risk, 257–258
Hallucinogens, 64–65
  abuse, 92
Haloperidol
  acute psychotic episodes, 122–123, 133–134
  cocaine, 269–270
  cognitive impairment, 83
  drug trials, 165
[Haloperidol]
  first-episode patients, 306
  negative symptoms, maintenance treatment, 152
  psychotic relapse prevention, 142–143
  treatment-refractory schizophrenia, 169
Hamilton Depression Scale, 40–41
Hatfield, Agnes, 287–288
Heart disease, 149
Hebephrenic schizophrenia, 16
Hepatic toxicity guidelines, 236
Homicide, potential for, 13–14
Hospitalization, for acute psychotic episodes, 115–116
Human immunoviruses, 98–99
Huntington's disease, 63
Hyperprolactinemia, 231–232
  treatment guidelines, 231–232
Hyperthyroidism, 101–102
Hypothyroidism, 101–102

Illicit drugs, 112
Immobility, 111
Independent living skills, 205–206
  rehabilitation guidelines, 209
Information-processing deficits, 76
Initial meeting
  patient ambivalence, 8–9
  rapport, 9–14
Inpatient treatment for acute psychotic episodes, 115–116
Integrated model, comorbidity, 276
Integrated psychological therapy (ITP), 202
Interictal psychosis, 94
Interviewing
  auxiliary ego, 23
  tips, 25–26
ITP, 202

Job skills, 204–205
  deficits, rehabilitation guidelines, 209

Kraepelin, Emil, 30

Language ability, neuropsychological tests, 72
Language function, neuropsychological tests, 73
Learning capacity, treatment goals, 188
Libido, loss of, 149
Life cycle
  early phase, 304–312
    clinical characteristics, 304–305
    differential diagnosis, 305–306
    prognostic implications, 311–312
    relapse, 307–308
    therapeutic issues, 305–311
  late phase, 315–318
    clinical characteristics, 315–317
    treatment issues, 317–318
  middle phase, 312–319
    clinical characteristics, 312–313
    therapeutic issues, 313–315
  premorbid/prodromal phase, 302–304
    clinical characteristics, 302–303
    predromal period, 303
    premorbid adjustment, 303
    prognostic implications, 304
    therapeutic issues, 304
Literature search, family education program, 289
Lithium, in treatment-refractory schizophrenia, 172
Living conditions, middle phase, 314
Long-term store, 75
Lorazepam
  acute psychotic episodes, 125
  anxiety, 128
  first-episode patients, 306
Lysergic acid diethylamide (LSD), 92

Magnetic resonance imaging (MRI), 95–96
Maintenance treatment, 141–156
  cognitive deficits, 150–154
[Maintenance treatment]
  combining antipsychotic drugs and psychosocial treatments, 154–156
  depression, 150–154
  drug side effects, 146–150
    neurological, 147–148
  negative symptoms, 150–154
  psychotic relapse prevention, 142–146
Major depressive episodes, 58
Major tranquilizers, terminology, 214
Marijuana, 92
MCT, 164
Medical illness, 113
Memory
  cognitive rehabilitation, 193–194
  neuropsychological tests, 75–76
Memory notebook, 193
Mentally ill chemical abusers and addicted (MICAA), 271
  characteristics, 272
  dual diagnosis, treatment, 276
Mental retardation, 62
Methamphetamine-induced psychoses, 65
Methylene dioxymethamphetamine, 92
Metropolitan St. Louis Psychiatric Center (MSLPC) family education program. *See* Family education program
MICAA, 271
  characteristics, 272
  dual diagnosis, treatment, 276
Misidentification syndrome and risk of violence, 254–255
Mnemonics, 193–194
Molindone, 234
Mood disorders, 57–58
Mood stabilizers, for acute psychotic episodes, 126–127
Motor speed, neuropsychological tests for, 78–79
MRI, 95–96

MSLPC, family education program. *See* Family education program
Multicenter Clozapine Trial (MCT), 164
Mushrooms, 92
Mutism, 111

Nalmefene, for alcoholism, 279
Naltrexone, for alcoholism, 279
Needs assessment, in family education program, 288
Negative symptoms, 36–37, 43
  maintenance treatment, 150–154
  measurement, 37–39
  primary vs. secondary, 37
  rehabilitation, 199–201, 208
  treatment-refractory schizophrenia, 168
Neophobia, 8
Neuroimaging studies, 95–96
Neuroleptic-induced movements, 227
Neuroleptic malignant syndrome (NMS), 233–234
  treatment guidelines, 233–234
Neuroleptics
  enhancing stimulants, 269
  extrapyramidal side effects, 111–112
  sensitivity, in late phase, 317
  terminology, 214
Neuropsychological tests, 72–79
  case examples, 79–82
Neurosyphilis, 99–100
NMS, 233–234
  treatment guidelines, 233–234
Nonpsychotic dysphoric states, 278
Nonsense syllable pronunciation, neuropsychological tests, 73
Norepinephrine, in tardive dyskinesia, 230
Novel antipsychotics, terminology, 214

Obsessive-compulsive disorder (OCD), 41–42
Obsessive-compulsive symptoms, 232–233
  treatment guidelines, 233
OCD, 41–42
Ocular toxicity guidelines, 238
Olanzapine
  acute psychotic episodes, 119–121, 127
  cognitive impairment, 83
  first-episode patients, 306
  maintenance treatment
    depression, 153
    negative symptoms, 152
  psychotic relapse prevention, 144–145
  tardive dyskinesia, 229
  treatment-refractory schizophrenia, 171–172
  weight gain, 235
Olfactory deficits, 75
Opiates, toxicology screens for, 93
Opioids, 92
  tardive dyskinesia, 230
Orientation Remediation Module, 192
Orthostatic hypotension, 148–149
Outpatient schizophrenics, alcohol use disorder in, 269
Outreach, comorbidity, 276–277

PANSS, 39, 43
  factor-analytic work, 46–47
Parallel model, comorbidity, 276
Paranoia, 8
Paranoid disorder, 59
Paranoid projections, 8
Paranoid psychosis, 92–93
Paranoid schizophrenia, vignette, 6
Patient ambivalence at initial meeting, 8–9
Patient compliance, evaluation of, 130
Patient interview, 1–26
  follow-up, 24–25

[Patient interview]
  initial meeting
    diagnosis, 12–13
    patient ambivalence, 8–9
    potential dangers, 13–14
    purpose, 10–12
    rapport, 9–14, 18
    therapeutic alliance, 12
    vignettes, 3–7
  length, 17–18
  physical setting, 17
  technique, 17–23
  theoretical considerations, 14–17
  timing, 17–18
  tips, 25–26
Patient resistance to continued treatment, 309
PCP, 64–65
  abuse, 91
  toxicology screens, 93
Peer groups and substance use disorder, 269
Perceptual-motor speed, neuropsychological tests, 78–79
Persecution delusions and risk of violence, 253–254
Personality disorders, 60–61
Personality traits, violence, 251–252
Phencyclidine (PCP), 64–65
  abuse, 91
  toxicology screens, 93
Positive and Negative Syndrome Scale (PANSS), 39, 43
  factor-analytical work, 16–17
Positive symptoms, 32–33, 43
  measurement, 33
Postictal psychosis, 95
Posturing, 111
Premorbid intellectual functioning
  neuropsychological tests, 73
Prescription drugs
  psychotic symptoms, 92
Privacy, vignette, 5, 7
Pseudoparkinsonism, management of, 147
Psilocybin, 92
Psychiatric diagnoses, operational criteria, 30
Psychological dialysis, vignette, 3
Psychosis, 109
  acute, differential diagnosis of, 274
  brief reactive, 59–60
  dopamine, 215
  as dream, 9–10
  interictal, 94
  not otherwise specified (NOS), 60
  paranoid, 92–93
  postictal, 95
Psychosocial interventions, 186, 190, 201
  with antipsychotic drug treatment
    maintenance treatment, 155–156
  early phase, 311
  maintenance treatment, 154–155
Psychosocial rehabilitation, 184
Psychosocial stressors, 112
Psychotherapeutic interventions, middle phase, 314–315
Psychotic relapse prevention
  antipsychotic drugs, 142–143
  guidelines, 146
  second-generation antipsychotic drugs, 143–146
Purdue Pegboard, 78

Quality of Life Scale, 39–40
Quetiapine
  acute psychotic episodes, 121
  cognitive impairment, 83
  first-episode patients, 306
  maintenance treatment
    depression, 153
    negative symptoms, 152
  ocular effects, 238
  psychotic relapse prevention, 145
  tardive dyskinesia, 229
  treatment-refractory schizophrenia, 172–173

Rapport, establishing, 9–14, 18

RDC, 31–32
  bipolar affective disorder, manic type, 56
Reaction time, to auditory stimuli, 192
Rehabilitation, 185–196
  cognitive, 184
    attention, 192
    clinical description, 191–192
  psychosocial, 184
  treatment goals, 188–189
  vocational, 314–315
Rehearsal, 194
Reitan-Klove Sensory-Perceptual Examination, 79
Relapse
  prevention, 142–146
  prodrome, 308
Research diagnostic criteria (RDC), 31–32
  bipolar affective disorder, manic type, 56
Reserpine, in treatment-refractory schizophrenia, 172
Residential care
  acute, 115
  late phase, 318
Respite care, 115
Risperidone
  acute psychotic episodes, 121–122
  first-episode patients, 306
  maintenance treatment
    depression, 153
    negative symptoms, 152
  psychotic relapse prevention, 144
  tardive dyskinesia, 229
  treatment-refractory schizophrenia, 170–171
  verbal memory, 153

Safety in acute psychotic episodes, 127–128
Scale for the Assessment of Negative Symptoms (SANS), 38–39
Scale for the Assessment of Positive Symptoms (SAPS), 33–34
Schizoaffectives, alcohol use disorder, 269
Schizophrenia
  clinical description, 73–79
  coping, 203–205
  diagnosis, 12–13
    frenzy to reach, 21
  differential diagnosis, 53–66
    excluding psychiatric illnesses, 56–62
    excluding psychotic disorders, 62–64
    excluding substance-induced psychotic disorders, 64–65
  disorganized, 16
  hebephrenic, 16
  laboratory diagnosis, 89–104
  life-cycle. *See* Life cycle
  paranoid, vignette, 6
  symptom clusters, 29–49
    cognitive impairments, 42
    defining, 44–46
    description, 32–42
    historical overview, 30–32
    importance, 47–49
    severity, 42–47
  symptoms
    differentiating negative and deficit, 48–49
    pragmatic assessment, 30–31
    severity measurement, 42–47
  treatment-refractory. *See* Treatment-refractory schizophrenia
Schizophreniform disorder, 57
Schneider, Kurt, 30
Scihzoaffective disorder, 57
SDMT, 79
Second-generation antipsychotics (SGAs)
  maintenance treatment
    cognitive deficits, 151–153
    depression, 151–153
    negative symptoms, 151–153

[Second-generation antipsychotics (SGAs)]
  psychotic relapse prevention, 143–146
  side effects, 223–224
  terminology, 214
  weight gain, 234
Sedatives, vs. disinhibiting compounds, 215–216
Seizure disorders, 94–96
  laboratory tests, 95–96
Seizures, complex partial, 63–64
Self-induced water intoxication, 229
Self-medication, for substance use disorder, 269
Sensitivity, vignette, 5
Sensory-perceptual function, neuropsychological tests, 72, 78–79
Sensory register, 75
Serial model, comorbidity, 276
Serotonin, in tardive dyskinesia, 230
Sertraline, in first-episode patients, 306
SGAs. *See* Second-generation antipsychotics
Shakow, David, 8
Short-term store, 75
Sialorrhea, anticholinergics, 126
Situational factors, and violence, 252
Skills training, negative symptoms, 200–201
Social isolation, 110
Social skills, 201–203
  impaired, 209
    rehabilitation guidelines, 209
  training, 155, 203
    guidelines, 203
Software programs
  attention, 192
Somatic etiology, 30
Spatial focusing, visual cues, 192
Speed, neuropsychological tests, 72
Speedballs, 92
Staff training for family education program, 293–294
Stimulant abuse, 91
Stroop Color and Word Test, 74–75
Substance abuse, 63, 112
  comorbidity, 268–270
  diagnostic issues, 271–275
  dual-diagnosis treatment, 112
  etiology, 269
  pharmacotherapy, 278–279
  prognostic implications, 311–312
  programmatic treatment, 275–278
  self-medication, 269
  self-reported reasons, 269
  treatment, 275–279
Substance-induced psychotic disorders, 64–65
  DMS-IV criteria, 273
  medications associated with, 274
Subtle cues, 22–23
Suicide
  potential, 13–14
  risk, 309–310
Sulpiride, in treatment-refractory schizophrenia, 173–175
Supportive therapy, early phase, 310–311
Surveys, in family education program, 288
Symbol-Digit Modalities Test (SDMT), 79
Systemic lupus erythematosus, 100

Tactile Finger Recognition Test, 79
Tarasoff rule, 248
Tardive dyskinesia, 148
  risk factors, 229
  SGAs, 229
  treatment, 229–230
Tardive effects, 228–230
  treatment guidelines, 228–230
Temporal-lobe epilepsy, 63–64
Temporal vigilance, 192

Terminology, antipsychotics, 214
Tests
  laboratory, 89–104
  neuropsychological, 72–82
Tetrahydrocannabinoids, 92
  toxicology screens, 93
Therapeutic alliance, 12
Thought disorder, 33–35, 43
  measurement, 35–36
Thought Disorder index, 35
Threat/control-override delusions, and risk of violence, 255–256
Thyroid disease, 101–102
Thyroid-stimulating hormone (TSH), 102
Toxicology screens, 93
Trail-making Test, 79
Tranquilizers, major, 214
Transference, 15–17
Treat, frenzy to, 21
Treatment noncompliance, 111–112
Treatment-refractory schizophrenia, 163–176
  alternative therapies, 172
  chronic hospitalization vs. poor symptom response, 167
  clinical description, 167–168
  conventional antipsychotic drugs, 169
  definition, 164–165
  drug treatment, 168–173
  guidelines, 174–175
  negative symptoms, 168
  neurobiology, 166
  new-generation drugs, 169–172
  prevalence, 166–167
  violence, 168
TSH, 102

University of Pennsylvania Smell Identification Test (UPSIT), 75
UPSIT, 75

Verbal ability, neuropsychological tests, 72–73
Verbal fluency, neuropsychological tests, 73
Verbal memory
  neuropsychological tests, 72
  risperidone, 153
Vigilance, software programs, 192
Violence, 110, 247–262
  anecdotes, 258–259
  assessment, 248–250
  case study, 261–262
  risk factors, 259–261
    general population, 251–252
    schizophrenia, 253–254
  schizophrenia, 250–251
  treatment-refractory schizophrenia, 168
Visual cues
  spatial focusing, 192
  temporal vigilance, 192
Visual processing, improving, 194
Visuospatial skills, 194
  impairment, 188
Vitamin B12 deficiency, 100–101
Vocational rehabilitation, middle phase, 314–315
Voices, and risk of violence, 257–258

Water intoxication, self-induced, 229
Waxy flexibility, 111
Wechsler Adult Intelligence Scales, 76
Wechsler Memory Scale-III (WMS-III), 78
Weight gain, 149
  diabetes, 234
  treatment guidelines, 235
White blood cell count, monitoring, 149–150
Wisconsin Card Sorting Test, 74
WMS-III, 78
Word fluency tests, 74–75
Working memory, 75, 187–188

Ziprasidone, 234
  acute psychotic episodes, 122
  adverse effects, 149
  psychotic relapse prevention, 145

About the Editor

John G. Csernansky is the Gregory B. Couch Professor of Psychiatry at the Washington University School of Medicine, St. Louis, Missouri, and Medical Director of the Metropolitan St. Louis Psychiatric Center, Missouri. The author or coauthor of numerous journal articles, book chapters, and books, he is a reviewer for the *American Journal of Psychiatry*, the *Archives of General Psychiatry*, and *Biological Psychiatry*, among others. A Fellow of the American Psychiatric Association and the American College of Neuropsychopharmacology, he is a member of the Society of Biological Psychiatry and the Society for Neuroscience. The recipient of the Donovan-Shear Award (2000) from the Mental Illness Coalition of St. Louis, Dr. Csernansky received the B.A. degree (1975) from Northwestern University, Evanston, Illinois, and the M.D. degree (1979) from the New York University School of Medicine, New York.

ISBN 0-8247-0642-0
90000
9 780824 706425